Healthcare Administration for Patient Safety and Engagement

Aleksandra Rosiek-Kryszewska
Nicolaus Copernicus University, Poland

Krzysztof Leksowski
Military Clinical Hospital, Poland & Nicolaus Copernicus University, Poland

A volume in the Advances in Healthcare Information Systems and Administration (AHISA) Book Series

IGI Global
DISSEMINATOR OF KNOWLEDGE

Published in the United States of America by
IGI Global
Medical Information Science Reference (an imprint of IGI Global)
701 E. Chocolate Avenue
Hershey PA, USA 17033
Tel: 717-533-8845
Fax: 717-533-8661
E-mail: cust@igi-global.com
Web site: http://www.igi-global.com

Library of Congress Cataloging-in-Publication Data

Names: Rosiek-Kryszewska, Aleksandra, 1981- editor. | Leksowski, Krzysztof, editor.
Title: Healthcare administration for patient safety and engagement / Aleksandra Rosiek-Kryszewska and Krzysztof Leksowski, editors.
Description: Hershey, PA : Medical Information Science Reference, [2018] | Includes bibliographical references.
Identifiers: LCCN 2017024070| ISBN 9781522539469 (hardcover) | ISBN 9781522539476 (ebook)
Subjects: | MESH: Patient Care Team | Patient Safety | Professional-Patient Relations | Patient Participation | Organizational Culture | Health Communication--ethics
Classification: LCC R859.7.S43 | NLM W 84.8 | DDC 610.289--dc23 LC record available at https://lccn.loc.gov/2017024070

This book is published in the IGI Global book series Advances in Healthcare Information Systems and Administration (AHISA) (ISSN: 2328-1243; eISSN: 2328-126X)

British Cataloguing in Publication Data
A Cataloguing in Publication record for this book is available from the British Library.

All work contributed to this book is new, previously-unpublished material. The views expressed in this book are those of the authors, but not necessarily of the publisher.

For electronic access to this publication, please contact: eresources@igi-global.com.

Advances in Healthcare Information Systems and Administration (AHISA) Book Series

Anastasius Moumtzoglou
Hellenic Society for Quality & Safety in Healthcare and P. & A. Kyriakou Children's Hospital, Greece

ISSN:2328-1243
EISSN:2328-126X

Mission

The **Advances in Healthcare Information Systems and Administration (AHISA) Book Series** aims to provide a channel for international researchers to progress the field of study on technology and its implications on healthcare and health information systems. With the growing focus on healthcare and the importance of enhancing this industry to tend to the expanding population, the book series seeks to accelerate the awareness of technological advancements of health information systems and expand awareness and implementation.

Driven by advancing technologies and their clinical applications, the emerging field of health information systems and informatics is still searching for coherent directing frameworks to advance health care and clinical practices and research. Conducting research in these areas is both promising and challenging due to a host of factors, including rapidly evolving technologies and their application complexity. At the same time, organizational issues, including technology adoption, diffusion and acceptance as well as cost benefits and cost effectiveness of advancing health information systems and informatics applications as innovative forms of investment in healthcare are gaining attention as well. **AHISA** addresses these concepts and critical issues.

Coverage

- Clinical Decision Support Design, Development and Implementation
- IT Applications in Physical Therapeutic Treatments
- Role of informatics specialists
- IS in Healthcare
- Rehabilitative Technologies
- IT Applications in Health Organizations and Practices
- Decision Support Systems
- Nursing Expert Systems
- Measurements and Impact of HISA on Public and Social Policy
- Medical informatics

IGI Global is currently accepting manuscripts for publication within this series. To submit a proposal for a volume in this series, please contact our Acquisition Editors at Acquisitions@igi-global.com or visit: http://www.igi-global.com/publish/.

The Advances in Healthcare Information Systems and Administration (AHISA) Book Series (ISSN 2328-1243) is published by IGI Global, 701 E. Chocolate Avenue, Hershey, PA 17033-1240, USA, www.igi-global.com. This series is composed of titles available for purchase individually; each title is edited to be contextually exclusive from any other title within the series. For pricing and ordering information please visit http://www.igi-global.com/book-series/advances-healthcare-information-systems-administration/37156. Postmaster: Send all address changes to above address.

Titles in this Series

For a list of additional titles in this series, please visit: www.igi-global.com/book-series

Novel Applications of Virtual Communities in Healthcare Settings
Christo El Morr (York University, Canada)
Medical Information Science Reference • copyright 2018 • 247pp • H/C (ISBN: 9781522529583) • US $235.00 (our price)

Handbook of Research on Data Science for Effective Healthcare Practice and Administration
Elham Akhond Zadeh Noughabi (University of Calgary, Canada) Bijan Raahemi (University of Ottawa, Canada) Amir Albadvi (Tarbiat Modares University, Iran) and Behrouz H. Far (University of Calgary, Canada)
Medical Information Science Reference • copyright 2017 • 545pp • H/C (ISBN: 9781522525158) • US $255.00 (our price)

Patent Law and Intellectual Property in the Medical Field
Rashmi Aggarwal (Institute of Management Technology Ghaziabad, India) and Rajinder Kaur (Panjab University, India)
Medical Information Science Reference • copyright 2017 • 257pp • H/C (ISBN: 9781522524144) • US $200.00 (our price)

Design, Development, and Integration of Reliable Electronic Healthcare Platforms
Anastasius Moumtzoglou (P&A Kyriakou Children's Hospital, Greece)
Medical Information Science Reference • copyright 2017 • 357pp • H/C (ISBN: 9781522517245) • US $205.00 (our price)

Cloud Computing Systems and Applications in Healthcare
Chintan M. Bhatt (Charotar University of Science & Technology, India) and S. K. Peddoju (Indian Institute of Technology Roorkee, India)
Medical Information Science Reference • copyright 2017 • 282pp • H/C (ISBN: 9781522510024) • US $205.00 (our price)

Handbook of Research on Healthcare Administration and Management
Nilmini Wickramasinghe (Epworth HealthCare, Australia & Deakin University, Australia)
Medical Information Science Reference • copyright 2017 • 825pp • H/C (ISBN: 9781522509202) • US $345.00 (our price)

IGI Global
DISSEMINATOR OF KNOWLEDGE

701 East Chocolate Avenue, Hershey, PA 17033, USA
Tel: 717-533-8845 x100 • Fax: 717-533-8661
E-Mail: cust@igi-global.com • www.igi-global.com

Table of Contents

Detailed Table of Contents

This chapter describes how managed healthcare is a systemic and institutional approach for cost management. It might be the remedy for increasing demand for limited human and material resources. In most of the developed countries the number of elderly patients with multimorbidity is increasing every year. This situation creates the necessity for implementing new policies based on cost-effective methods of diagnosis and treatment. Keeping quality high is crucial for patient safety, although cost reduction must occur to ensure the proper care for all. However, several ethical concerns are raised with these changes. The main is that although the physicians are focused on cost-effective procedures, they will take the patient's opinions into consideration. The outcome of an undermined relationship between doctors and their patients may be contrary to the reduction of the compliance and adherence may in fact increase the cost of services for specific patients. The proper communication patterns and post-discharge care is mandatory for limiting unwanted additional costs and benefits policy makers keeping patient satisfaction high.

This chapter discusses the leadership features that support the creation of an innovative culture of the organization, with particular emphasis on the attributes that are essential to building a competitive advantage in the medical services market. According to the concept of new management, managers are the initiators of change and development within the healthcare facility where they work. They require professionalism and a high level of competence which allows them to create and implement creative management solutions. Thus, the influence of management and the role of the leader in building competitive health care units is undisputed. Due to the specific nature of health care facilities, the ability to build trust, as well as the clear and precise communication of plans and visions, is gaining importance, in addition to knowledge and experience.

The purpose of this chapter is to point out that effective risk management, also in healthcare units, can contribute to the effective reduction of adverse events and, consequently, the compensation claims of the patients. Also defined is the concept of risk and outlines the necessary elements that should be included in effective risk management. As far as medical entities are concerned, risk management is primarily about dealing with adverse events. Conscious control and limiting the occurrence of these events affects patient safety in a medical facility.

This chapter describes how contemporary, dynamic development in all available human areas is unavoidable and necessary. However, along with the benefits and progress made by civilization, there is also a growing margin of vulnerability and unfavorable price developments. Professional burnout is becoming a global problem. It identifies the limits of current human capabilities to the serious phenomenon. In particular, nurses and medical rescuers, who are in direct contact with the patient, experience unpleasant symptoms of burnout.

Emergency medicine is a rapidly developing medical specialty which focuses on the diagnostic process, initial stabilization, and the treatment of patients suffering from acute illnesses or injuries. Emergency care can be provided in prehospital settings by emergency medical services, as well as in emergency departments. The primary providers of emergency care are: emergency medicine physicians, emergency nurses, and paramedics. Emergency medical personnel are required to be prepared to take decisive action at any time of day or night. It is essential for them to possess basic knowledge relating to psychology and an ability to utilize interpersonal communication skills. A critical role of medical workers in emergency settings is to provide a patient with emotional support coupled with medical assistance. Interpersonal communication skills depend on the personal abilities of an individual, however, these skills can be also enhanced through training and work experience.

This chapter describes how in recent decades, the concepts of social capital and quality of life have attracted the interest of both theoreticians and creators of social life. Both on the micro-, meso- and macrosocial levels, social capital has been viewed as one of the key elements of human well-being. Its positive influence on social well-being has been underlined by academics, practitioners of social life. In this chapter, the authors evaluate the relationship between social capital and the mental well-being of individuals. Through empirical analysis, the results of a representative research conducted among residents of one of the biggest Polish cities were examined. This concludes that social capital and social interaction are essential to the health of the individual.

This chapter describes how there are three major stakeholders in a patient's hospitalization: the patient, the healthcare providers, and the hospital. Satisfaction with the care and hospital experience is important to the patient because evidence suggests satisfied patients are more likely to adhere to self-care instructions and have better clinical outcomes. Hospitals have aimed to provide care and service that is highly satisfying to patients because it is the right thing to do and because reputation affects volume and revenues which in turn impacts the fiscal bottom line. Unfortunately, not all patients enjoy equal levels of satisfaction in the health care system. To succeed amongst today's competition; healthcare organizations must be patient-centered and win the loyalty of their patients by providing an outstanding patient experience, then retaining these patients, increasing the number of patients through positive word of mouth and continually delivering greater value.

When patients visit a doctor, they not only expect to be cured, but also to feel that they are taken care of. The patients like to be treated like guests, sit in a nice place during waiting for a doctor and feel that they are taken care of seriously at the reception desk. All these factors are important for the patients but the relationship with doctors seems to be the most valid. When the patients can choose a clinic where they want to make an appointment with a doctor, the owners and managers of the clinics try to persuade people to choose their clinic. Hence more and more often managers of the clinics try to find out the opinion of the patients, so scientists carried out the research on this phenomenon and called it Patient Satisfaction. This chapter presents the application of fuzzy sets and fuzzy relations to gather and analyze the information from patients and compute their contentment. Using classical logic is less appropriate because the patients can only choose two values: they are satisfied or dissatisfied. Fuzzy logic let the patients choose more phrases for their opinions.

Preface

Healthcare Administration for Patient Safety and Engagement looks at the complexity of healthcare in terms of management and patient safety. The topics discussed in the book are interdisciplinary, giving you a broad perspective on the health, safety and involvement of patients in the treatment process. Improving patient safety has led to a number of paradigms aimed at streamlining the management and operation of health care administration. Everyday practice shows that the issues contained in this book are taken up and widely discussed both in the medical and the managerial environment. Topics discussed in the book are relatively new. They change the perception of public hospitals and describe increased competition between private and public health care. Patients' expectations of medical care are also changing due to increased patient awareness and involvement in the treatment process. Varying patient expectations requires a change in the organization and building of leaders in the medical services market. These alterations also require teaching new skills in the medical services sector.

The ethical dilemmas presented in our book show how to communicate with patients in difficult situations and demonstrate the role of organizations in this process. The ethical issues of modern medicine and organizational culture described in this book may explain why an organization such as a hospital is focused on certain priorities, particularly in the context of patient safety and patient communication, ethical behavior, and quality medical procedures. The discussed role of patient communication and the ethical side of medicine is an important addition to the discussion of the controversial topic of treatment and patient safety.

The problems presented in the book focus on objectively assessing issues and drawing the reader's attention to the most important aspects.

The book was divided into two sections.

Section 1: Aspects of Management and Functioning of Administration in Healthcare
Section 2: Ethical Aspects Related to Patient Safety and Involvement in the Treatment Process

The issues described in Section 1 focus on effective management in health care to ensure the safety of patients in medical institutions. The issues discussed in this section are primarily addressed to managers, directors, and people who have an impact on the management and functioning of the administration in health care units. According to the concept of new management, managers are the initiators of change and development in the healthcare facility where they work. Professionalism and a high level of managerial competency allow you to create and implement creative solutions. An innovative approach plays an important role, which, through synergies with other factors, affects the competitiveness of healthcare institutions.

Section 2 describes the ethical aspects of patient safety and involvement in the treatment process. Attention to the ethical aspect of health care becomes extremely important at every stage of contact with the sick. Increasingly, universities are addressing this issue, in order to draw young students' attention to the humanistic approach to the patient. In this book, the authors also point out the role of clinical communication in health care settings. The chapters devoted to this topic represent the most important factors that significantly improve the safety and commitment to the patient at every stage of treatment.

Involving the patient in the treatment process is extremely important. In Part II of the book, the authors point out the patient and his role in assessing the quality of health care. Understanding the patient's point of view is the key to improving their satisfaction with treatment. Patients and their families focus their attention not only on the results of treatment, but they also comprehensively analyze factors affecting their safety during treatment. Additionally, in Part II the authors discuss the cooperation and involvement of all stakeholders in improving the safety and quality of the services offered. This is the essence of every system, including the health care system.

Cooperation and involvement of all stakeholders contributes to improving relationships, building a climate of security and respect. This cooperation, however, is prone to some risks that, in the face of competition in the medical services market, force the management to make informed decisions supported by substantive and constructive analysis. Due to the wide range of issues discussed, the book can also be used as a training tool for training new medical workers in terms of involvement and safety in health care settings.

Legal aspects have also been addressed, with the aim at providing a comprehensive look at these issues. They will be increasingly investigated and taught over the next ten years and that is why these issues are presented in our book.

The book contains 15 chapters devoted to the aforementioned aspects.

CHAPTER 1

This chapter covers issues related to health management and cost management. The authors also draw attention to the human factor and communication with the patient in order to achieve cost-effective benefits, quality and continuity of care.

CHAPTER 2

Authors pay attention to the innovative approach to managing healthcare. The departure from routine management aims to strengthen the position of the healthcare unit in the competitive market of medical services. Owing to the specific nature of health care facilities, confidence building is gaining in addition to knowledge and experience.

CHAPTER 3

In this chapter, the author defines the concept of risk and presents the necessary elements worth considering in effective risk management. As far as medical entities are concerned, risk management is primarily related to adverse events. Awareness of control and reduction of occurrence of these events affect the safety of patients in the medical institution.

CHAPTER 4

The topic of professional burnout is covered in this chapter. The burn syndrome is strongly associated with stress at work and chronic emotional stress experienced by an employee. The author points out that the effects of burnout symptoms are not only a personal problem of the individual, as it causes measurable organizational costs, and the phenomenon of burnout becomes a serious social problem. Therefore, the issue of burnout, in the context of organizational pressure, requires some extensive research and practical advice for contemporary work environments.

CHAPTER 5

This segment discusses the specific problems of emergency medicine. Strategic salvage goals are focused not only on the patient but also on the working conditions that medical staffs face.

CHAPTER 6

In this chapter the author discusses the activities of the medical community and its impact on improving public health. The actions taken are dealt with comprehensively in the health care system and analyzed in detail on many levels. This piece demonstrates that the actions undertaken relate not only to patient education, but also to the extent of the functioning of the healthcare organization, which should adapt to the needs of the changing environment (patient requirements, technology development, medical progress). The author analyzes the organizational, technological, and psychological aspects as well as factors influencing human behavior. The approach to assessing the performance of the medical environment in a comprehensive way is consistent with the latest world health trend.

CHAPTER 7

This chapter discusses the issues of patient safety and involvement in the treatment process. Authors emphasize the role of patient engagement in quality assessment of health care. Understanding the patient's point of view, the authors say, is the key to improving the quality, effectiveness, satisfaction and safety of patients.

CHAPTER 8

In this selection, the author points out that the sense and need for security are the most basic needs of man. The basic concepts of patient safety and well-being are discussed. The importance of both factors for the hospital treatment process as well as the consequences of patient insecurity and its impact on the patient's biopsychosocial status are presented.

CHAPTER 9

Here, the author draws attention to the quality of life. She is looking for relationships between social capital and subjective quality of life. The data obtained was examined to test the hypothesis that social capital is related to the psychological well-being of individuals.

CHAPTER 10

This chapter presents the satisfaction of the patient. The author gives guidance to managers and explains why patients' satisfaction, quality of care are important for success in health care.

CHAPTER 11

In this article, the authors present the use of fuzzy sets to collect and analyze information from patients and to calculate their satisfaction. The use of fuzzy logic allowed patients to choose more phrases for their opinions. At the beginning of the study, researchers should employ experts who are familiar with the health care system.

CHAPTER 12

In this chapter the author presents the issues of clinical communication in the therapeutic team. Success in this area depends solely on the understanding of the rules governing the communication process and the implementation of these principles by all team members. The author emphasizes that the positive relationship in the therapeutic team is also determined by the motivational system: it must be homogeneous, fair and transparent.

CHAPTER 13

In this chapter, the authors analyzed the relationship between the overall satisfaction of the physician and his / her ability to communicate with the patient. It has been noted that both general satisfaction with life and satisfaction with such an important element as professional activity can be an important psychosocial resource, which greatly improves the quality of professional duties. Because work is an important part of our lives, it must be rewarding and give us a chance to grow.

CHAPTER 14

This chapter is devoted to aspects of a physiotherapist's work; those who must be able to recognize many limitations and contraindications. According to the authors, it is worthwhile to direct attention to a professional approach to the patient and the role of physiotherapists in building these relationships.

CHAPTER 15

The chapter deals with issues of interpersonal communication, taking into account many perspectives. The authors point out the interconnection of people by a common system of message encoding and decoding. The opening of the European gateway makes intercultural communication ubiquitous and this includes health care. International assignments require new, culturally-minded doctors. This chapter outlines the challenges, barriers and solutions in the aforementioned area, based on the personal experiences of the authors.

The book focuses on both the theoretical and practical aspects of management, commitment and patient safety, which are backed up by the experiences of the authors. The publication addresses consumers interested in health care management, health care professionals responsible for improving patient safety, as well as medical students and patients who are interested in the topics discussed above.

Aleksandra Rosiek-Kryszewska
Nicolaus Copernicus University, Poland

Krzysztof Leksowski
Nicolaus Copernicus University, Poland

Acknowledgment

The editors of this book would like to thank all those who took part in the process of preparing of this book, and all those who contributed the material for the book. The editors would also like to thank peer-reviewers, especially PhD Anna Rosiek and Professor Aleksander Goch, for they commitment and the effort in the process of review.

Section 1

Aspects of Management and Functioning of Administration in Healthcare

Chapter 1
Managed Healthcare: A Temporary Trend or a New Standard for Providing Health Services?

Karolina H. Czarnecka
Medical University of Lodz, Poland

Filip Pawliczak
Medical University of Lodz, Poland

ABSTRACT

This chapter describes how managed healthcare is a systemic and institutional approach for cost management. It might be the remedy for increasing demand for limited human and material resources. In most of the developed countries the number of elderly patients with multimorbidity is increasing every year. This situation creates the necessity for implementing new policies based on cost-effective methods of diagnosis and treatment. Keeping quality high is crucial for patient safety, although cost reduction must occur to ensure the proper care for all. However, several ethical concerns are raised with these changes. The main is that although the physicians are focused on cost-effective procedures, they will take the patient's opinions into consideration. The outcome of an undermined relationship between doctors and their patients may be contrary to the reduction of the compliance and adherence may in fact increase the cost of services for specific patients. The proper communication patterns and post-discharge care is mandatory for limiting unwanted additional costs and benefits policy makers keeping patient satisfaction high.

DEFINITION OF THE MANAGED HEALTHCARE

General description of the managed health care term usually contains two elements of equally high importance - cost reduction and quality improvement. (Kongstvedt, 2012; Sekhri 2000) By far it is the simplest and most objective definition describing its nature in every case. However, managed care is not homogenous across the globe. Primary solutions were modified to satisfy political and financial needs of different countries. The development of managed care system and its variations was forced by rising

DOI: 10.4018/978-1-5225-3946-9.ch001

health demands and costs. Preserving the high quality of care caused the reduction of availability of the health services due to relative shortness of funds. The idea of managed health care is to implement optimal diagnostic, therapeutic and organizational procedures for cost reduction and quality maintenance or improvement. (Tobin, 1997) Due to such solutions greater number of patients may receive proper care in adequate moment.

The idea of managed care is thought to be an American invention. However, system is adapted in several countries worldwide. It is well known in Great Britain, Australia, Russia, New Zealand, Croatia, Hungary. Some parts are also introduced in the Netherlands, Germany and Israel. (Stein, 2016) Managed health care is being also implemented in Poland as a part of national health care system reorganization. The project is called Coordinated Health Care (orig. Koordynowana Opieka Zdrowotna – KOZ). The most precise Polish definition was created by Polish Association of Managed Care (orig. Polskie Towarzystwo Koordynowanej Ochrony Zdrowia - PTKOZ). It states that managed health care means organized activities of system participants for achieving cost-effective benefits, quality and continuity of patient care (Fedorowski, 2017). According to PTKOZ managed care should also fulfill several requirements. It has to be:

- Complex and integrated
- Controlled organizationally
- Dynamically reactive towards stakeholders demands
- Modern and of high quality
- Valuable and effective
- Referring to solutions proven as correct in different parts of the world

Polish government and main stakeholders interpreted, coordinated, or managed health care as unified actions of several types of providers such as hospitals, ambulatory care units, basic health care providers, rehabilitation facilities, administration and prophylaxis for better health and financial outcome. (Banaś, 2016) The payment is done after whole process of diagnosis and treatment is finished according to standards & procedures. Every detail of this multistage plan has to be reported. Patient is being coordinated by one qualified person and there is no need for him to find proper provider for specific procedure to be done. All of his effort is to enter the process and agree or not to proposed methods of diagnosis and treatment. As the providers are connected into public network their ability to fulfill these requirements is probable. The most important factor of Polish interpretation is that the managed care system will be public and the only funding will be national. The aim of policy makers is to provide health care for every citizen of Poland regardless if they have insurance coverage or not (NFZ materials, 2017).

Types of Managed Health Care Organizations

The main managed care organizations (MCOs) existing at US market are not described in existing literature as specified individual health care plans. They are rather presented as continuum of solutions of the same issue. The main purpose they are designed for is to reduce the total health care cost. Some of them are more efficient, others are more consumer- or provider-friendly but unfortunately, more expensive. The evolvement of all presented MCOs is the answer for imperfection and insufficiency of insurance and health benefits models present in US in the first half of 20th century. (Kongstvedt, 2001)

Most popular types are listed below. Short characterization is added for better understanding.

- **HMO Model:** Health plans combining traditional insurance model with organized health service providing system. The responsibility of quality is on the side of payer. The HMOs contracts with individual physicians, health care facilities, hospitals and ambulatory care units to achieve full access to health care.
- **PPOs (Preferred Provider Organization):** Health benefits plans are contracted with a specified network of providers in which all covered health services can be obtained without additional payments. It allows negotiated and rapid payment rates. Utilization management is introduced and the consumer choice of other providers (non contracted) is preserved.
- **EPOs:** Same as PPOs without possibility to choose providers being out of the contract.
- **IPA Model:** Benefits plans are contracted with physicians associated in organizations offering medical services to usually non-HMO patients.
- **POS Plans:** Based on Primary Care Physicians (PCP) paid through capitation payment. Typically, the PCP are „gatekeepers" referring patients to more specialized health care facilities when necessary. The more sophisticated care is needed, more of payments are done through reimbursement.

BRIEF HISTORY OF MANAGED HEALTH CARE

The official beginning of the managed care era in the USA dates back to 1970s. Before that moment, health benefits, employers' insurance plans and recently developed Medicare and Medicaid were the main parts of American health care system. The overall cost of health services increased dangerously in previous years resulting in public debate over the possible ways of fending off the crisis as situation became one of the most important challenges for national policy makers. It is the moment in time, when one of the most popular managed care organizations were developed – the health maintenance organizations (HMOs). They were proposed by their strongest protagonist - Dr. Paul M. Ellwood and advised to Richard Nixon, who was the first American President to transform non-for-profit health care system into for-profit model. The first form of managed health care was implemented as US Congress passed „The Health Maintenance Organization Act" in 1973. This document was successful as it resulted in growing number of HMOs and slowly eliminated traditional health insurance plans. In 1982 the Tax Equity and Fiscal Responsibility Act passed which allowed Medicare system to pay HMOs on a capitated basis. The aim was to provide more benefits for the same amount of money. The goal was achieved as it covered also the prescribed drugs, which were not reimbursed earlier. Public acceptance for the idea of HMOs grew as it offered additional benefits such as child & women's preventive visits, several preventive services. The consumers satisfaction increased and it settled ground under the HMOs development in next years. In 1982 Medicare introduced different form of payment resulting shorter hospitalizations due paying for class or group of diagnoses instead of reimbursing the total cost of patients care during the time of hospitalization.

Preferred Provider Organizations (PPOs) appeared in Denver in 1970s. System was based on negotiations that provided discounts in hospitals for employers of interested companies creating the extra benefit plans for their employees. The idea of these discounts was beneficial for the hospitals as the competition was high and preferred hospital was more likely to survive. Discounts were satisfying for the employers as the cost-sharing was more acceptable.

The golden age for managed health care started in 1990s. Its rapid growth observed in that time referred mostly to appearance of many new specialized HMOs and sector consolidation.

In 15 years – between 1984 to 1999 – the commercial enrollment of private HMOs grew from 15.1 million to 104.6 million. PPOs development also occurred in that time resulting equal share of market among them and HMOs. After initial phase, the market of managed care organizations started to consolidate, as bigger, national structures became powerful enough to absorb smaller, local plans. The situation allowed to transform some of non-for-profit plans into for-profit businesses. Physicians also started to gather in and moved away from private practices toward group practices. Hospitals eventually consolidated as well as their network provided better clinical care. Several connected health facilities had also stronger negotiating position and were preferred as more stable as providers for big commercial plans.

Speed of managed health care growth and ways of its development created movement against it. In literature it is called as managed care backlash. The rage of the consumers raised due to new situation when the system of managed care was the only one to limit unnecessary medical decisions as not cost effective. Patients felt left without the proper care. The commercialization of the structures of the system only exacerbated this trend as plan makers put more effort into saving and creating profits than spending on proper treatment. Many more problems arose in that dynamic moment, but the main challenges concerning public opinion were delayed or denied payments. Struggling with those issues resulted in new policies and legal acts implementing standardized procedures protecting the patients and resolving the problems of underpaid or discriminated providers as every facility willing to accept the general terms could join HMOs plans thus they should be paid equally. The industry also responded to overwhelming negation of the managed health care as they slightly changed the form of the system by opening access by eliminating the „gatekeepers". The results were easy to predict as the perception of the system and public opinion correlated with the general health care cost. Becoming more consumer-friendly, the HMOs affected the overall budget negatively.

The managed health care became mature in previous decade revealing more consistent approach. Some of the health plans were expanded, more standardized procedures were implemented. Unfortunately, the increase of health care cost resulted in higher prices of insurance coverage, thus number of people deciding to live without health insurance increased up to 17% in 2009 (Boland, 1991; Kongstvedt, 2012).

History of Managed Health Care in Poland

In Poland, the historical beginning of health care system is dated back to first years after regaining independence (1920s and 30s) (Ćwiąkała-Małys, 2013). The system was only for around 7% of population and it was typical Bismarck health and social insurance model. After II World War the system was transformed into Semashko health care model, which was created especially for physical workers of public factories and farmers. Private business owners were left without access to national health care till 1970s. The demand of this group was supplied by group practices of doctors which supplemented national health care system. In mid 70s, the ambulatory care units, primary health care sector and hospitals were unified. In the beginning of the 90s the communism was over. Since then most of the Polish health care experts suggest that Poland has no health care strategy. Most of further changes were implemented as emergency interventions. During the time of economic transformation of Polish polity, health care system moved away from communistic centrally planned economy into free market reality. The health care cost became a major issue for providers which split into individual facilities. The central budget funding was transformed into multiple health insurance model. 16 individual public health insurance plans were created for each voivodeship and 1 central for whole country. The main issue with such organization was that patients could not be treated in different voivodeship as prices and payments differed between the plans. This situation raised concern whether constitutional privilege of equity in access to health care was preserved. Government presented plan for creating one central national health care funding organization (orig. Narodowy Fundusz Zdrowia – NFZ) in the first half of 2000s. (Atłachowicz, 2013) The idea was to appoint independent organization with its own budget as the nationwide payer. The system connected all health insurance plans and based on obligatory contribution. The providers had to sign agreements with NFZ and fulfill the contract. Patients' diseases were classified into homogenous groups of patients. It provided ability to control the cost as payment was done after the diagnosis and proper treatment was reported with the list of procedures. The private providers could also start in the contests to obtain vital contracts. It was the moment when industry of health care providers grew rapidly, especially in overestimated procedures which allowed to build up enormous profit. Unfortunately, such situation left the public hospitals with the most expensive and underpaid cases resulting in growing number of units in debt. Irregular funding and fee-for-service system as well as demographic situation of Poland resulted in increase of total health care cost. The limited contracts extended the time of awaital to publicly unacceptable level. Even though the NFZ is very efficient organization (only 1% of its budget is for operational purposes), the public dissatisfaction arose. (Puchta, 2014)

The idea of managed health care appeared in public discussion in the middle of 2010s. First managed health care companies were private businesses offering health services for corporations' employees. The biggest existing up to now are LuxMed, Medicover and Enel-Med. They possess their own providers as well as subcontractors for contracting procedures not possible to be obtained inside the company. Public sector had to create the foundation for future health care reforms implementing managed health care into existing insurance model. The national and local health needs map were created showing what parts of the country are left without proper medical access. Next step is to connect all public and key health facilities in the network of providers allowing proper coordination. (Mądrala, 2013).

Figure 1. Scheme presents process of diagnosis and treatment of a single patient in a managed healthcare model proposed in Poland. All of the providers are connected with each other. The payment is done after finishing of the treatment in the end of the process when patient comes back to PCP.

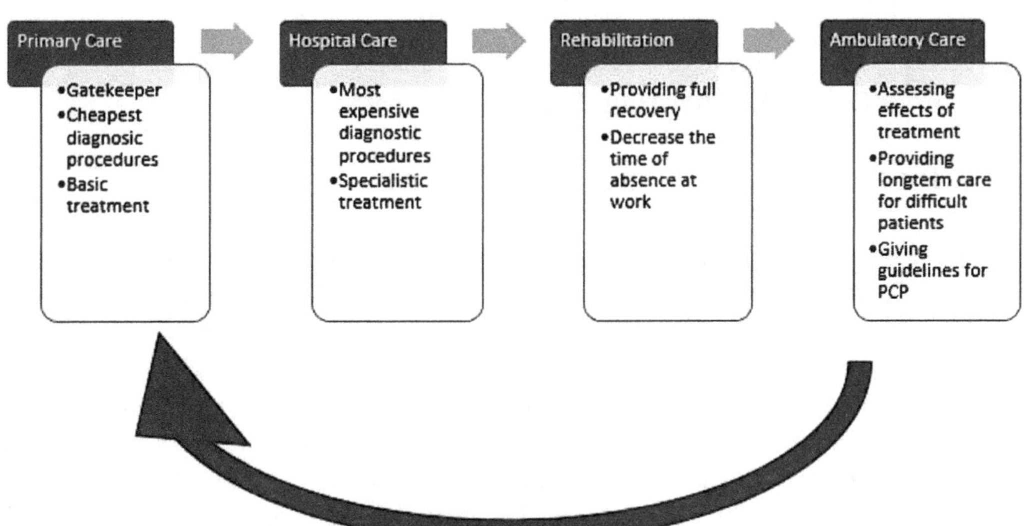

Managed Health Care as New Standard for Providing Health Services

According to WHO the overarching objectives of the health system for which this system is designed are: 1) the continued improvement of the health status of the population (which should be measured with the use of clear, comparable, objective and transparent meters); 2) satisfying consumer needs of patients in the use of services entities health system; 3) ensuring solidarity in financing health care. The health system should be built on a set of principles, in particular subsidiarity, universality, pluralism, decent legislation, equality of patients and stakeholders involved in health care, Principle of innovation and plasticity, and evidence based health policy. (Mądrala, 2013). In the context of coordinated care becomes very important that the condition of equality of patients and those involved in the processes of health care and the universality of the system is difficult to reach because of the expenditure that has to be incurred. It should be emphasized that the list of participants in the health care system includes not only patients, medical service providers (clinics, hospitals, medical staff) and main payer - market regulator, but also educational entities, companies (manufacturers of medicines, medical and rehabilitation devices,), employers (employing patients with chronic diseases), Private Payers (companies, private insurance), central and local Authorities and Non-governmental Organizations. (Kongstvedt, 2001; Boland, 2001; Mądrala, 2013)

As managed health care spreads across the world since 1970s its position in the global health approach becomes stronger. World Bank agreed to help introducing managed health care in Poland & other countries as it's more stable financial system than previous one. Its role in implementing new financial plans in health care rises. On the other hand, WHO experts debate if US example of backlash may be the reason to be more cautious in implementing managed care worldwide. However, even if managed health care model is not fully accepted, the basic elements may be used to provide savings. Every country has to organize its health care system on its own to fulfill expectations of its citizens. Health budgets in every country, developing or developed, are too short to provide satisfying results. Managed care is a tool & prescription for more precise spending of the funds on particular procedures. It is not ideal resolution for every case and it creates some challenges, but in the end, it might still be the only way to cure the financial problems of health providers. The global forecast for managed health care based on tendencies predicts that it will become the most common approach and it will become standard model for future generations of health care policy makers.

CHALLENGES FOR THE MANAGED HEALTH CARE

Challenges for the Managed Health Care: Complexity Approach

One of main issue in coordinated care is to plan in advance the actions, programs and financing for the basic care, hospitalization and interventions on the regional, national and in case of Europe – European level. Creating the plan for the coordinated care of patients in certain age, with one chronic disease and without the coexisting diseases is already complex. The basic care approach uses the linear model – diagnosis of the disease, introduction of the treatment or rehabilitation, patient monitoring and evaluation of treatment effectiveness. When we consider wide range of patients, with different secondary diseases, with diverse access to the healthcare, the linear model is insufficient. The managed healthcare system has to response for more health challenges i.e. health inequalities among one population and in different countries, differences in already established healthcare model, ageing of the populations, easy access to the Over the Counter (OTC) drugs and dietary supplements instead of professional diagnosis and treatment, problem of drug interactions in coexisting chronic diseases. Planning the activities and action in managed health care require thorough analysis of these challenges, but also involvement of all stakeholders in those actions. And what is very important it also require change in the approach to the patient – enabling the co-management of treatment and diagnosis process.

Creating new, more efficient, prevention and treatment programs for public healthcare (dedicated for the potential users of the managed healthcare system) should be based on complexity approach. (Rutter, 2017) This approach may help in reduction of the proportion of unsuccessful health care actions compensate for health inequalities that are interfering in the prevention or treatment actions. In planning coordinated care one of the most complicated action is to link numerous elements, that are affecting each other, in order to plan activities and healthcare procedures. (Rutter, 2017; Diez, 2011). Equally important it is to create a health system considered as an ongoing process, subject to evaluation and implementing multiple changes quickly. And dependent on all participants in the system, where changes can be proposed either by patients, physicians, other health professionals, insurance companies, companies producing medical devices, aids etc. This means that the effectiveness of the system should be monitored from below by its users a greater degree than it is in the systems used so far. The system Health care systems have multiple, independently managed, interrelated subsystems that affect each other (Ruter, 2017). Changes in these systems are dynamic, therefore the management of the health care system should not be carried out solely by the main payer (ie the National Health Fund). Due to the principle of subsidiarity (social institutions can not interfere in matters with which Individual entities are able to manage themselves) and the principle of equality of entities management actions should be implemented on the basis of extensive consultations with system participants including: patients, medical service providers, companies, employers, educational entities, central and local Authorities, NGOs and all payers in the systems.

Challenges for the Managed Health Care: Global Innovation on Local Scale

Many successfully driven interventions in one region or country may not be applicable in other countries. The effect of the intervention is dependent on many factors, which may be referred to as socio-economic but not directly from the prosperity of society. Without deep analysis of the needs of all users of the health care system the creation a well-functioning coordinated care system is unattainable. Failure to take account of some user needs may result in system inconsistency or increase the cost of running curative, preventive or informational programs. The historical, political, sociological, cultural and technical context should be take into consideration in order to plan the principles of a dynamic system that meets the needs of all users of the care system (Greenhalgh 2017).

Challenges for the Managed Health Care: Effective Communication

One of main issue of current medicine is effective communication among healthcare specialists and between physicist and patients. In both types of communication misunderstandings, interpretation problems or gaps in communication may result in an incorrect diagnosis, delays in taking the right therapeutic routes, or lack of proper continuation of the treatment.

One of the reasons for the problems in communication between doctors, nurses and other healthcare practitioners is the lack of direct communication (Shannon, 2012). In hospitals, day-care centers or outpatient clinics the information about the patient health condition, disease course, performed examinations and results of diagnostic analysis must be present in written form: in paper documentation, or in database. This cause the situation where exchanging information about patient health is often processed only by reading and interpretation of the files or analysis reports added to the documentation. On the other hand, lack of personnel and the reimbursement system based on the number of patients examined rather than the quality of the medical visit are causing shortening of the time dedicated for each patient. Other observed communication problem is no compensation of direct communication effort by healthcare management system (Shannon, 2012). That is why many physicists, instead of contacting other specialist in order to discuss the patient results, are focused only on interpretation of the written reports (Ventola, 2014). “According to communication experts and physician leaders, the dearth of direct communication between physicians is caused by several overlapping factors. Primary among these are disincentives for communication that exist in the current health care system…” (Shannon, 2012). In time-pressure atmosphere and work overload misspelling and errors in the written reports can occur, even when using error-reporting systems. Based on the reports, the cause of the made mistakes should be analyzed and actions taken to tackle communication problems. Such actions are possible if all participants in the health care process report errors or problems with understanding the message. It depends on profession or function f. ex. reporting errors is more likely by the nurses, than physicists or pharmacists (Wolf, 2008). Patients also can report errors, however most of them probably would not notice this kind of errors, until the visit in the pharmacy or next visit in the clinic. It depends to a great extent on the knowledge of patients or their families about health, treatment or drug interactions. So the more aware is the patient, the greater he will be able to successfully use the facilities of coordinated care. (Shannon, 2012) In coordinated care all participant should be focused on passing clear messages, avoidance of misapprehension and reporting of detected errors. Especially, if in the adopted care model, where for convenience, the number of patient visits at the clinic, and the number of meetings with specialists is limited, and the direct contact is substituted by phone or internet contact, or through the application. Also in model of coordinated care with the important role of coordination centers the communication is very important, as the patient is not necessarily meeting a physician.

Once the position of the patient in the Healthcare system will be redefined, and the level and manner of communication will be improved, the patient may gain the ability to take active part in decision making process. The complete Healthcare system improvements are very difficult to introduce because of the need for comprehensive change on different levels of the healthcare system. In opposite simple improvements in communication between patients and healthcare specialists and among them can lead to significant changes in the management of the treatment process and the reception of health care performance.

Absence of proper communication between the healthcare specialists and patients may also lead to very dangerous consequences i.e. failure: to follow recommendations for follow-up visits, to take the recommended screening tests, to keep the recommended diet, to take medications, or follow the order of rehabilitation activities. All mentioned above can lead to lack of proper continuation of treatment, lengthen the time of taking medicines (painkillers), prolongation of the recovery time, or even significant deterioration of health until re-hospitalization.

In coordinated care one of the main issues is the patient ability to take part in decision making process for his/her healthcare procedures. In order to co-decide on the course of treatment processes 3 general changes in the relation between the patient and the healthcare represent must be reached. First of all, change in the care system regarding the health procedures and documentation that is required by the hospitals or outpatient clinics -simplifying and clarifying the procedures f. ex. presenting algorithms of actions to be taken in diagnostic or rehabilitation process understandable for patients; preparing lists pd demanded documentation prior to the visit; creating atmosphere of professionalism. Secondly change the way patient is regarded by the Healthcare provider/ Healthcare system from Unconscious user, patent to Conscious user, service recipient and finally, payer. Tertiary there is a strong need of communication process improvement. From patient's point of view the information on the health status or proposed procedures that he/she is obtaining from healthcare specialist is too complex because of using specialist clinical language and detailed documentation attached. Improper communication may also result from too short information being conveyed or the use of many, incomprehensible for patients, abbreviations.

Challenges for the Managed Health Care: Communication via Social Media

Patients often seek information about their health through internet, especially when they feel uninformed or when the information in their medical records is difficult to understand (medical jargon). Under the influence of information found on the internet, especially on blogs and discussion forums often created by non-professionals, patients sometimes decide to change the physician's recommendations on medication, diet or rehabilitation. (Wald 2007). To dispel doubts about the prescribed medicines and their side effects patient need to make an appointment for another visit. Often instead of waiting for a visit, relying on information from the internet, patient modifies treatment itself. In many cases those actions can strongly interfere the treatment plan and doctors will not know about this change in real time. Even reading the news from official scientific journal can lead to the misunderstood and ally proven. To prevent such situations, physicians or healthcare professionals should be available to patients in real time. It should be acknowledging to patients that the information they can retrieved from many internet sources is uncensored, impersonal, and biased, full of advertisement and product placement. (Segal 2012) On the other hand the information obtained from professional sources as medical journal web pages or medical services of the Health institutes may cause that patients under the influence of information on adverse effects of medicines they use, decide to stop taking these medicines. While it may be that the potential threat does not affect their condition, patients will take action without consulting their doctors, which may result in their health deteriorating. (Segal 2012).

Using the internet based media can help patients in many ways – in recognizing the symptoms of disease, helping patients make informed health care choices, choosing the appropriate medical specialty. (Wald 2007) For chronic ill patients using the internet media can have additional advantage – creating the online support community. The positive impact of using social media in patient awareness has been already proven in musculoskeletal medicine, cardiology, vascular and orthopaedic surgery. (Indees, 2013; Curry, 2014; Herron, 2015) The most important among them: popularisation of new therapeutic approaches, increasing patient awareness, information about the goals of the various medical specialties or dissemination of knowledge about preventive actions. (Indees, 2013) The possibility of spreading the information to many users in more direct way, in short time (much shorter than publication of results of clinical investigations in medical journals), also with use of informal language, it all together shortens the distance between healthcare professionals and society. (Indees, 2013; Herron, 2015) However there is a potential danger of losing the authority of physicians by shifting of conventional notions due to the change in the doctor to patient relationship. (Wald 2007).

There are many web pages where patients can obtain information about the competence of physicians f. ex. portals presenting physicians ranking and patients views on their attitudes, professional behaviour, ability to communicate medical information in an understandable way for "ordinary customers". On the other hand, doctors, health centres and hospitals use other resources than official websites to improve contact with patients f. ex. professional networking sites – LinkedIn or MedTube (on YouTube), social networking sites and blogs Facebook, Twitter, Instagram. However, contact with patients through social media like Facebook or Tumbrl poses many risks. (Herron, 2015). Those risks of using social media in communication with patients should not be underestimated. The use of social networks or microblogs brings the threat of easy spreading of the inadequate information (f. ex. campaigns against vaccination, the promotion of dietary supplements described as drugs), promotion of not-medicinal practices, that can postpone the diagnosis of treatment. (Herron, 2015). Professional approach can also be seen as ability to divide the presented official info versus private opinions (Denencke, 2015).

In case of social networks and applications, one of the most important issue is the safety of the private data stored and/or shared by users. Data exchanged between physicians and patients and between healthcare professionals should be protected to the greatest extent possible (Denencke, 2015). In case of the patient-physician contact via social media the confidence of interchanged information depends on site licensing agreement or consent to access the data that any user must express to use the application. Lack of safety can lead to the situation of unauthorized access information on the health or planned treatment (Denencke, 2015). In case of Coordinated care where part of the interchanged information can be send directly from the medical devices used by patients the safety of data is guaranteed by the device application. Often data are analysed on the service site, so unauthorized access information can be secured (Herron, 2015; Denencke, 2015).

In conclusion the use of new means of communication between a health care specialist and patients, especially websites, dedicated services, blogs and social media, combined with the use of telemedicine solutions will hopefully create new healthcare systems providing patients with selected information. (Herron, 2015) Such systems will also help to reach specialists in the appropriate field and will allow for the adaptation of therapeutic or preventive activities in response to the needs of the local community. (Greenhalgh, 2017) Dedicated services will provide the opportunity for a better exchange of knowledge between the specialists, and will give better platform for developing ideas, creating new strategies for health interventions creative work. However all the mentioned above challenges should be taken in consideration in order to create smart health system.

In our opinion the essential features of such a system should be to devoid of unnecessary activities, adapting global programs to the local scale (i.e. to the needs of the local community), focusing on the credibility of the presented information, using of social media with caution, taking into consideration the security of stored and transmitted data and placing the patient in the position of the legitimate user of the system.

REFERENCES

Atłachowicz, J. (2013). Historia ubezpieczeń zdrowotnych w Polsce [History of health insurance in Poland]. Retrieved from http://wartowiedziec.org/index.php/zdrowie/aktualnosci-i-ekonomia/14708-historia-ubezpiecze-w-polsce

Banaś, I., & Zając, M. (2016). Koordynowana opieka zdrowotna –cele i zasady organizacji [Coordinated healthcare - goals and principles of organization]. Retrieved from http://akademia.nfz.gov.pl/wp-content/uploads/2016/06/Koordynowana-opieka-zdrowotna-cele-i-zasady-organizacji.-Izabela-Bana%C5%9B-Magdalena-Zaj%C4%85c.pdf

Boland, P. (2001). *Making Managed Healthcare Work: A Practical Guide to Strategies and Solutions.* Jones & Bartlett Learning.

Curry, E., Li, X., Nguyen, J., & Matzkin, E. (2014). Prevalence of Internet and social media usage in orthopedic surgery. *Orthopaedic Review*, *6*(3). PMID:25317312

Ćwiąkała-Małys, A., & Łagowski, P. (2013). Ewolucyjny obraz przekształceń systemu ochrony zdrowia w Polsce [The evolutionary picture of the transformation of the healthcare system in Poland]. *Przegląd Prawa i Administracji*, *93*, 90–101.

Denecke, K., Bamidis, P., Bond, C., Gabarron, E., Househ, M., Lau, A. Y., & Hansen, M. (2015). Ethical Issues of Social Media Usage in Healthcare. *Yearbook of Medical Informatics*, *10*(1), 137–147. doi:10.15265/IY-2015-001 PMID:26293861

Diez Roux, A. (2011). Complex systems thinking and current impasses in health disparities research. *American Journal of Public Health*, *101*(9), 1627–1634. doi:10.2105/AJPH.2011.300149 PMID:21778505

Fedorowski, J. J. (2017). Definition of KOZ. Retrieved from http://ptkoz.org/definicja-koz

Herron, P. D. (2015). Opportunities and ethical challenges for the practice of medicine in the digital era. *Current Reviews in Musculoskeletal Medicine*, *8*(2), 113–117. doi:10.1007/s12178-015-9264-0 PMID:25786848

Indes, J., Gates, L., Mitchell, E., & Muhs, B. (2013). Social media in vascular surgery. *Journal of Vascular Surgery*, *57*(4), 1159–1162. doi:10.1016/j.jvs.2012.09.065 PMID:23321344

Kongstvedt, P. R. (2001). *The Managed Health Care Handbook*. Jones & Bartlett Learning.

Kongstvedt, P. R. (2012). *Essentials of Managed Health Care*. Jones & Bartlett Publishers.

Kripalani, S., LeFevre, F., Phillips, C. O., Williams, M. V., Basaviah, P., & Baker, D. W. (2007). Deficits in communication and information transfer between hospital-based and primary care physicians: Implications for patient safety and continuity of care. *Journal of the American Medical Association*, *297*(8), 831–841. doi:10.1001/jama.297.8.831 PMID:17327525

Lee Ventola, C. (2014). Social Media and Health Care Professionals: Benefits, Risks, and Best Practices. *P&T*, *39*(7), 491–499, 520. PMID:25083128

Mądrala, A. (Ed.). (2013). System ochrony zdrowia w Polsce - Diagnoza i kierunki reformy, AKADEMIA ZDROWIA 2030 [Health System in Poland - Diagnosis and directions of reform, HEALTH ACADEMY 2030].

Official materials of the National health Fund in Poland. (2017). Koordynowana opieka zdrowotna w Polsce [Coordinated healthcare in Poland]. Retrieved from http://akademia.nfz.gov.pl/ook/

Puchta, P. (2014). *Polish Healthcare System in Transition - Perceptions of the OLD and NEW Systems.* Dayton, Ohio: Wright State University.

Rutter, H. R., Savona, N., Glonti, K., Cummins, S., Finegood, D., & Greaves, F. (2017). The need for a complex systems model of evidence for public health. *Lancet.* doi:10.1016/S0140-6736(17)31267-9 PMID:28622953

Segal, S. (2012). Saving patients from Internet health information. Retrieved from: http://www.kevinmd.com/blog/2012/02/saving-patients-internet-health-information.html

Sekhri, N. K. (2000). Managed care: The US experience. *Bulletin of the World Health Organization,* 830–844. PMID:10916920

Stein, K. V. (2016). *Integrated Care around the world. Examples to help improve (primary) health care in Poland.* Warszawa: Narodowy Fundusz Zdrowia – Centrala Departament Analiz i Strategii.

Stille, C. J., Mazor, K. M., Meterko, V., & Wasserman, R. C. (2011). Development and validation of a tool to improve paediatric referral/consultation communication. *BMJ Quality & Safety, 20*(8), 692–697. doi:10.1136/bmjqs.2010.045781 PMID:21339312

Stille, C. J., McLaughlin, T. J., Primack, W. A., Mazor, K. M., & Wasserman, R. C. (2006). Determinants and impact of generalist specialist communication about pediatric outpatient referrals. *Pediatrics, 118*(4), 1341–1349. doi:10.1542/peds.2005-3010 PMID:17015522

Tobin, C. (1997) What is managed health care? Retrieved from https://nfb.org/images/nfb/publications/vodold/mngdcare.htm

Wald, H. S., Dube, C. E., & Anthony, D. C. (2007). Untangling the Web – The Impact of Internet Use on Health Care and the Physician-Patient Relationship. *Patient Education and Counseling, 68*(3), 218–224. doi:10.1016/j.pec.2007.05.016 PMID:17920226

Wolf, Z. R., & Hughes, R. G. (2008). Error Reporting and Disclosure. In R.G. Hughes (Eds.), *Patient Safety and Quality: An Evidence-Based Handbook for Nurses* (Ch. 35). Retrieved from: https://www.ncbi.nlm.nih.gov/books/NBK2652/

Chapter 2
The Impact of Management and Leadership Roles in Building Competitive Healthcare Units

Aleksandra Rosiek-Kryszewska
Nicolaus Copernicus University, Poland

Anna Rosiek
Ross-Medica, Poland

ABSTRACT

This chapter discusses the leadership features that support the creation of an innovative culture of the organization, with particular emphasis on the attributes that are essential to building a competitive advantage in the medical services market. According to the concept of new management, managers are the initiators of change and development within the healthcare facility where they work. They require professionalism and a high level of competence which allows them to create and implement creative management solutions. Thus, the influence of management and the role of the leader in building competitive health care units is undisputed. Due to the specific nature of health care facilities, the ability to build trust, as well as the clear and precise communication of plans and visions, is gaining importance, in addition to knowledge and experience.

INTRODUCTION

The key challenge facing health care leaders is to implement policies and procedures to improve the functioning of the unit and to ensure competitiveness in the healthcare market. The responsibility that managers take to plan, direct and coordinate medical services requires knowledge, experience and commitment. This is not an easy task as emerging health care and growing competition in the medical services market pose new challenges. Healthcare management is an exciting and rapidly growing area of health care. There is a continuing need for professionally trained health care managers. It is important that the manager is competent and able to achieve the target goal, such as safe and high quality patient care. The

DOI: 10.4018/978-1-5225-3946-9.ch002

quality and safety of a healthcare facility depends on many factors (Brasaite, Kaunonen, Martinkenas, Mockiene, Suominen, 2016). The most important are:

- A culture that promotes security excellence
- Planning and providing services that meet the needs of patients
- Availability of human, financial, physical and information resources – to provide care
- Sufficient staff and other service providers
- Current rating among healthcare facilities and improvement of results

The healthcare management area is open and increasingly diverse. The manager's role is to coordinate all aspects of the healthcare facility to ensure smooth functioning. The medical field includes not only patient contact, but also co-operation with insurance companies, accounting procedures, information systems management for the introduction and monitoring of patient records and expensive medical equipment, and the management and motivation of staff. Since a healthcare facility is a company, all of this must be achieved in a cost-effective and safe way for the patient. This requires the ability to coordinate, motivate and organize work to make the right decisions. The medical team must be in sync and well-coordinated, so that the medical care will provide high standards of medical services. No doubt, management is needed to support and coordinate services provided within a healthcare unit. Understanding the role of leaders and their impact on organizational effectiveness requires knowledge of the strategy and organizational culture of the work environment in which the members of the organization can make the right decisions (Ferlie & Shortell, 2001). A number of researchers have identified strategies and factors that work well for organizations, including health care. These include:

- Consistent leadership with common goals;
- Supporting a culture of organization;
- Employee involvement;
- Team development in the work environment;
- Patient- response strategy - high quality care and patient safety;
- Strategies to improve patient involvement in the treatment process.

The role of a leader in building and sustaining high quality care and competing health care units requires careful analysis. Applying strategies, compromises and making key decisions leads to success. Shared goals and coordinated action in health care settings are key to improving quality, safety, and the building of competitive health care facilities (Huczyński & Buchanan, 2007).

Significance of Management Competencies in the Health Services Sector

The necessity of having highly competent health care staff is due to the variability of the sector, where, with decreasing financial expenditures, management is required to increase the efficiency of healthcare facilities management while minimizing costs. Under such conditions, making rational decisions that result in efficient and effective management is a must in building competitive health care units. Managers of health care have the right and moral responsibility to ensure the safety and quality of health services provided. Forming and effectively executing missions, building visions and organizational strategies, shaping the positive image of organizations in the external environment (Oleksyn 2006) and psychosocially enabling efficient human resource management are required. Also, as distinctly noted in the model of F. Delamare Le Deist and J. Winterton, - the ability to deal with one's ability to learn and reflect, and the ability to deal with uncertainty, play a significant role in the structure of managerial competences. However, managing an organization and acting in a successful way is required by the manager and supervised in a systematic and transparent manner. Mintzberg made a division of manager roles taking into account the knowledge, commitment and decision-making logic. As seen in Figure 1, three main groups of managers are presented: interpersonal, informational and decision-making.

Interpersonal Roles

- **Figurehead:** Occupies a high position, but does not allow this to affect decision;
- **Leader:** Builds positive relationships with employees, motivates them and encourages them to develop further, communicates goals, supports and gives feedback, but also oversees progress;
- **Connector:** Maintains a contact network outside the work unit for information.

Information Role

Information roles include the reception, collection and dissemination of information.

- **Monitor:** Collects and analyzes information that may affect the operation of the organization, conducts careful observation of the environment, ensures all collected information is stored to streamline activities
- **Distributing Information:** Disseminates information to other people and parts of the organization, conveys information internally obtained from various sources; Reliably fulfilling this role requires both the ability to filter information and delegate.
- **Ombudsman:** Provides official information inside and outside the organization. Utilizes tools such as the press, the Internet, Twitter and social media updates to provide critical information about current activities.

Figure 1. Own study based on Dr. Henry Mintzberg

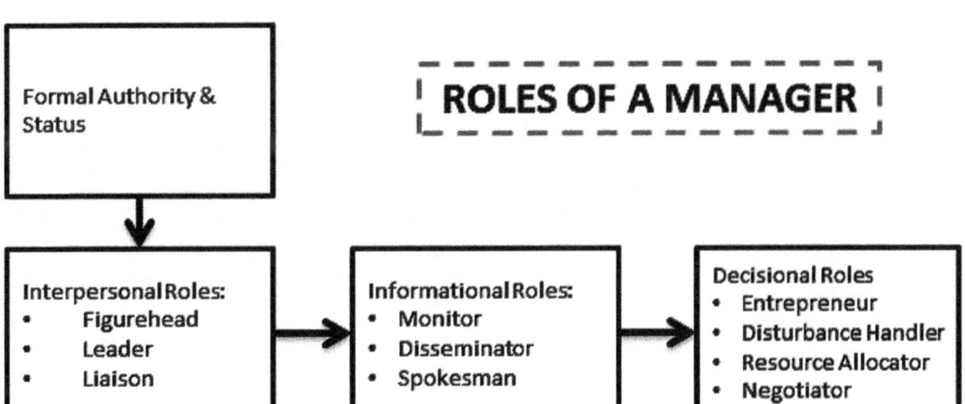

Role as a Decision Maker

- **Entrepreneur:** His task is to initiate, design and implement change, encourage innovative solutions and take risks associated with it;
- **Managing Disturbances:** A leader takes corrective action when the organization encounters important and unexpected difficulties, reduces conflicts, solves problems, and provides support;
- **Distributing Resources:** Your role is to distribute resources within your organization such as time, equipment, human resources and finances. He is responsible for allocating and supervising financial, material and human resources;
- **Negotiator:** He represents the organization in major negotiations affecting the areas of responsibility of the manager, the interests of the group, and compromises.

The Role of Manager in Health Care

The management of a medical institution, especially a hospital, requires specialized management skills and cannot be performed alongside of the medical profession. In the case of the private medical sector, the key is not only the construction of modern hospital infrastructure but also the planning and organization of hospital functions. Health sector managers must also remember that sustainability is a cornerstone of effective functioning, the objectives of which are to meet the needs and expectations of the different stakeholders. In the medical field, dialogue and mutual respect are needed at every step. The construction of a patient-friendly hospital is not just an investment in modern equipment that enables non-invasive procedures. It must also enables faster recovery. Without trust between the hospital management and its medical and administrative staff, it is impossible to build open relationships between doctors and patients, which are critical both in the treatment process and in the patient's trust in the medical institution. Private medical companies are increasingly understanding the principles of social responsibility and the benefits that this strategy brings. Under conditions of increasing market competition, it benefits not only companies but equally benefits their patients and partners. In order to achieve certain managerial intentions in the future, it is necessary to allocate resources appropriately in the planning, organizing and personnel management stages. Table 1 describes the management stages that significantly affect management in medical care.

Table 1. Stages and functions of management

Planning	Requires direction, priorities and purposes
Organization	The key element of this function is the fusion of competence and responsibility
Personnel Management	Refers to the acquisition and maintenance of human resources through the application of different strategies (Personal development, financial grants, etc.)
Controlling	Monitor activities and, in the event of failures, take corrective measures to increase efficiency
Managing	Actions within this function involve initiating efforts through effective leadership, motivation, and communication with subordinate employees

Own study.

LEADERSHIP

Vision, understanding and self-confidence are definitely the foundation of effective leadership. In the literature, many scholars agree with the definition that leadership is the process of influencing, without using coercion, the shaping of organizational goals, motivating behaviors, attaining goals, and supporting organizational culture (Hatane, Siagian, Octavia, Cummins, Wang, Demerouti, & Le Blance; 2017). The best leaders communicate their vision clearly and often enough, they are open to new ideas, new approaches, but they are constantly aware of the direction both the team and the organization are leading. They create a vision, announce it and lead their team to the goal (de la Billiere; 2007). The large number of diversified players in the healthcare market means that, in each particular case, the leader will perform his or her own tasks in a particular way, managing a particular institution and its staff, and offering patients a specific portfolio of services (Frączkiewicz-Wronka, & Austen-Tynda A, 2009). . The leader's role is to lead the team, pointing the way to the goal. It is the main link between the functioning of the whole healthcare facility. The main tasks of the managing person include:

- Setting goals and defining the factors that will guide them;
- Ensuring efficiency and communicating information to coworkers;
- Organizing work and structures;
- Analyzing necessary actions, decisions and relationships;
- Motivating and informing employees;
- Creating a responsible and effective team of people.

In regards to the issues of leadership, it should be noted that it can be considered in many aspects. Table 2 shows the dimensions of leadership according to J. Kouzes and B. Posner.

Leadership Models

There are many theories of leadership models. For decades, leadership theories have been the source of numerous studies. In reality and in practice, many people have tried to define what allows authentic leaders to distinguish themselves from the mass! Some theories are based on behavioral research and claim that leadership can be learned, while others believe these are innate traits (Nichols, Cottrell, 2014).

Table 2. Own study based on James M. Kouzes, Barry Z.Posner "The Leadership Challenge"

Taking on Challenges	Inspire a Common Vision	Enable Others to Act	Determining the Road	Motivating
Look for opportunities to make changes	Creating a vision	Collaborate by promoting common goals	Consistency within the declared value system	Appreciating the contribution of others to the success of each project
Risk taking	Encourage co-workers to achieve common goals	Building trust	Planning small successes that strengthen engagement	Celebrating achievements
Learning from mistakes		Increasing the freedom of co-workers	Giving example to others	

This means that certain qualities such as intelligence, sense of responsibility, creativity and other values are attributes of a good leader. Gordon Allport, an American psychologist, identified about 18,000 personality traits (Matthews, Deary & Whiteman, 2003, p. 3). Leadership Theory focused on analyzing the distinctive mental, physical and social characteristics in order to gain a better understanding of what is a hallmark or a combination of common features among leaders. Gordon Allport's studies are among the first to bring to the study behavioral leadership. When considering leadership in the health care market, one can look at the behavior of a person who is a leader. What qualities should a leader have in order to successfully manage a subordinate organization? At present, most of the researchers are analyzing five leadership models that practitioners believe are essential to building leadership.The first one is the leader who builds his leadership on expert knowledge and continuing education. Its strength is determined by an open mind and the ability to quickly identify niches that allow the company to maintain its place in the market. Weaknesses include being too detached from reality and attached to new theories instead of focusing on the details of action. The second is a leader based primarily on the strength and constancy of his character. Usually these positive character traits bring unexpectedly good results - especially in a distributed environment that loses its priority without a strong "leader". Unfortunately, when other perspectives come into play, the stubbornness of their reasoning can be fatal and can lead to the breakup of the sector. This is especially true if the team embodies more of a strong personality.

The third type of leadership is a "situational leader", who uses his own emotional maturity and experience to manage the project effectively. Usually it is a person who neatly moves in both macro- and microscale, both at the level of strategic decisions taken at the board level and at the level of individual teams. This type of manager can be eclipsed by the most dynamic members of his team. The disadvantage may be that in companies that develop very dynamically, they are easily marginalized by other managers with more expansive personalities. The ability to juggle a wide and narrow perspective sometimes leads to confusion and too easy justification for failures, all of which are not understood by the manager alone. The fourth type of manager is a person based primarily on hard methodological knowledge and management experience. It is a person who does not shirk even in the face of the greatest problems and delays, because usually she has seen worse things. Unfortunately, as often happens with experts, they occasionally disregard the real problems that arise out of the training examples presented in training. They are also reluctant to admit defeat, which in the long run can mean stagnation and the ceasing of development. Lastly, the fifth type of leader rated by the specialists is the "reactive" manager, i.e. the one who maintains the focus of the project in the proper response to problems. This is the kind of conciliator that is useful for all the projects that are in conflict. Its weakness is often the tendency to "shortcut" walking and activities that have ad hoc goals, without the due attention to the realization of far-reaching plans.

According to John Kotter (2005), the leader should:

- **Set the Direction of Development:** Defining the vision of the organization for the future and formulating its implementation strategy. It requires the leader to formulate conclusions based on the observation of reality, multi-faceted thinking and strategic thinking. He should be able to synthesize data and information. One of the most important leadership skills in this area is the ability to communicate your vision to others and encouraging them to take risks. Envisioning is not the same as planning and distinguishing a leader from a manager;

- **Unite People:** At the same time, leaders should understand their goal and vision and work to implement a strategy to achieve it. It requires impact on everyone who is successful in implementing the strategy (both units and teams). Communication skills such as credibility, empathy, the ability to convey a part of competence, and control are needed to effectively bring people around vision and strategy. This area also provides opportunities to develop and solve problems in the team;
- **Motivate and Inspire Action:** The leader should motivate and inspire employees so as to encourage their ability to make changes and overcome obstacles within the workplace. He should be able to see talents in people with whom he works, allow them to pursue their ambitions, and recognize and praise them to strengthen their self-esteem. Motivation and inspiration require the ability to involve people in decision-making, feedback, coaching, rewarding success, and allowing others to take leadership roles. (Kotter, 2005).

Leadership is difficult to grasp and cannot be unequivocally described. There is no universal recipe for success in management. Every man is an individual collection of qualities and needs. Each organization is unique and has a specific system of authority. In every system of power there are persons who have the power of possessing and who are subject to surrender. The leader, however, is not the authority based on the formal role, but rather based on the informal role, as the source of knowledge and leadership skills, character traits, behavioral style, norms and values. One of the many desirable features of a leader in the work place is the ability to work with subordinates. This skill gains momentum when we realize that the organization's most important resource is its employees. Their work directly affects client satisfaction - the patient and his expectations. The Figure 2 illustrates Blanchard's leadership models that help guide the direction of development.

Figure 2. Ken Blanchard's servant leadership model: SERVE
Own study based on K. Blanchard, P. Hodges, The Servant Leader. Transforming Your Heart, Head, Hands & Habits, Countryman, Nashville, Tennessee 2003.)

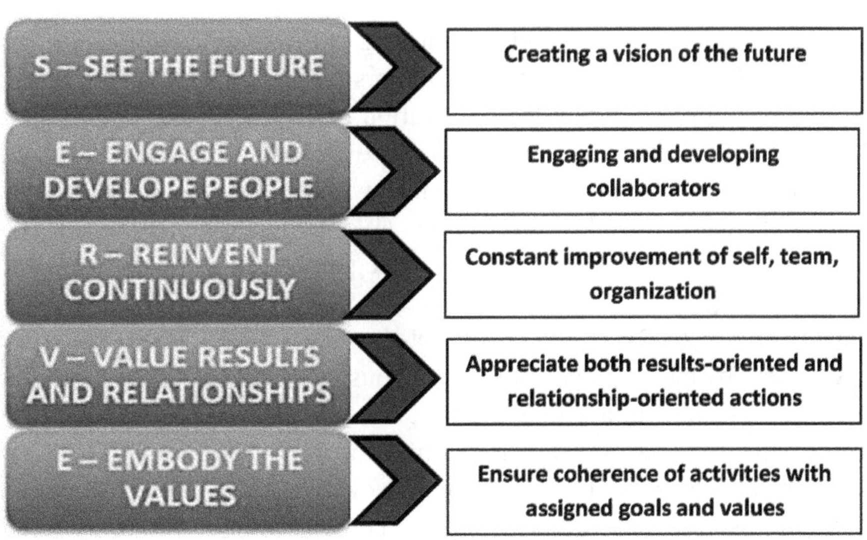

HUMAN RESOURCES IN HEALTH CARE

The relationship between human resources and healthcare is very complex. The effective management of the health system depends to a large extent on the proper management of its human resources. This problem becomes particularly important in a situation of their limitation. Human resources are understood in the literature of the subject as a source of qualification and ability of all persons operating in a given system. The concept of using human resources is based on the belief that a person should be "placed" in a facility where his individual abilities meet with a particular opportunity to do something unique. It represents an optimistic vision, resulting from the conviction that "work is the place where the success of man meets the success of the world" (M.Adamiec, 2000). A healthcare provider needs the knowledge of qualified and reliable medical staff to ensure the proper provision of healthcare services and reduce patient complaints. In a perfectly managed company, people engage in goals, using their capabilities for the good of the organization. In practice, however, what seems obvious and transparent can be a bit more difficult. How do you induce people to act? How do you encourage them to achieve their goals? Moreover, do the inherent characteristics of the leader affect the smooth operation of the organization?

Employees constantly watch their superiors. They expect support, examples, appreciation, and respect from them. They come to the organization primarily because of its reputation. They want it to develop and encourage growth in a professional manner. Leaving the workplace, however, is most often caused by improper co-operation with the supervisor. The leader works for his subordinates, and subordinates want to work for his supervisor. Employees come to work to offer superior skills and time. Whether the clients-patients will be satisfied and what the organization gains depends very much on the attitude of their leader. Every employee has unused decks of ideas, inventions, abilities. The leader's role is to see these qualities and motivate the subordinates. Motivated employees are able to put more effort into their work and achieve better results than those who lack motivation. Efficient management should combine both the company's goals and the goals of the individual employees, as this motivates them.

Motivating

Human resources are essential for the smooth functioning of the health care system. From the point of view of the economics of remuneration, medical workers play a significant role in health budgets in most countries (Vujicic, Marko, Zurn; 2006). Motivation is closely linked to job satisfaction. In turn, this keeps workers in the workplace (Luoma, 2006). The retention of health workers reduces the costs of the health care system by seeking and employing new workers (Deussom, 2014). As many countries experience shortages of qualified health care workers (World Health Organization, 2005), the loss of doctors and nurses, in particular, can have serious consequences for the health and safety of patients (Eastwood, 2005). In keeping with the satisfaction of health care workers, a well-functioning motivational system helps (Franco, Miller, 2002). An important factor for motivation, effectiveness and satisfaction is the individual assessment by the employee of the righteousness or the rightness of the reward received. Justice can be defined as the ratio of a worker's work to his or her rewards compared to awards received by others for similar expenses. Classical division of motivation methods distinguishes two main groups of stimuli - material and non-material. In management theory, it is noted that non-economic motivational methods can be more effective than reward or punishment. Excessive weighting to control financial incentives leads to ineffectiveness in employee management. It also turns out that financial incentives have a long-lasting effect, unlike others, whose effects disappear quickly. People's actions are a string of choices. Employees can establish the relationship between performance and desired outcomes. Theories of motivation try to answer the questions:

- What motivates people to act?
- Why do people choose specific behavior?

Motivation is influenced by a complex set of social, professional and economic factors (Deussom, 2012). There are many reasons why health care workers remain motivated and decide to stay at work. Often, a more important role in maintaining motivated health care workers is played by intangible incentives. Feeling satisfied with work and well performed duties and patient satisfaction is one reason for strong motivation. Factors affecting employee motivation and satisfaction are also career development, adequate compensation and satisfactory working and living conditions (Deussom, Jaskiewicz, 2012). However, many authors also point out that the same factors may be the cause of the reduced activity of health care workers. Each of these problems - or their combination - can lead to dissatisfaction. Doctors and rural workers often point to limited career development as a demotivating factor (Kotzee, Couper, 2006). The lack of opportunities to pursue a career and the lack of opportunities to improve the qualifications of medical workers are important reasons for dissatisfaction. In clinics and hospitals in Tanzania, medical workers are often asked to perform tasks that go beyond their practice but without proper training. This can lead to frustration and demotivation (Manongi & Marchan, 2006). This also raises concerns about the quality of health services and patient safety. Another issue is maintaining positive relationships with management and co-workers (Zakariasen, 2006). Proper communication with colleagues can improve employee satisfaction and motivate employees.

Motivational strategies should address these complex issues in a holistic way: provide opportunities for career advancement, make efforts to ensure appropriate working conditions, and promote positive workplace relationships, including the Joint Learning Initiative (2004). Ensuring safe and pleasant working conditions improves productivity and also affects the quality and safety of services provided at health care facilities. It is also important to support employees through management. Compliance with employee motivational principles is key to maintaining a qualified medical staff. This can be achieved by employing appropriately trained managers who deliberately set clear and understandable goals while meeting the expectations of employees (Henderson, 2008; Bonenberger, 2012; Rowe, 2005). Employee time and constructive feedback are powerful incentives to motivate and motivate employees to work and professionally develop (World Health Organization, 2006).

COMPETITIVENESS IN THE MARKET OF MEDICAL SERVICES

Considering the possibility of building competitive health care units, consideration should be given to the conditions of operation - current and future, positive and negative effects of the external environment as well as the various interdependencies arising from competition between rivals. Management literature presents and analyzes the sources of competitive advantage from different perspectives without defining this concept (Doligalski, 2013). It is understood that competitive advantage is the achievement and maintenance of an overriding position by the company towards more competitors. An entity that has achieved such a position within the market is able to offer customers - services or goods better than the ones offered by competitors. This means better service, lower price, higher standard of service or more comprehensive satisfaction of customer needs (Wait, 2012). According to P. Kotler, only "a company that gains more knowledge about customer needs, perceptions, preferences and behaviors will gain a competitive advantage." The same author states that "companies can gain competitive advantage on a variety of factors, such as higher quality, speed, security, customer service, design and reliability, lower costs and lower prices" (Kotler, 2004).

Hospitals compete with each other by offering services desirable in the medical services market that provide professional medical care and high quality of service. Specialist hospital services, which use state-of-the-art technology, are an incentive for patients to take treatment in a particular healthcare unit. However, the health care peculiarities are high and constantly rising costs in spite of efforts to reduce them. Unfortunately, cost increases do not go hand in hand with improved quality. Medical services are limited to currently accepted procedures or standards that are not always at the highest level. Competition in the medical services market is desirable and should be transformed (Hardin, Kilian, Spykerman, 2017). In healthy competition, continuous improvement and the introduction of innovative solutions is a stimulus to progress and change. To begin this process, however, the approach of both payers and providers of healthcare services must change - from a purely material outlook of "how much does a service cost" to "what benefits will the patient receive for the innovation used?". According to M.E. Porter, this is an extremely important aspect of building the competition. That is, to measure and report the effects of treatment and the activities of medical institutions in terms of the universal availability of information for all stakeholders in the health care system. He also points out that effective competition and efficiency in health care in every country can be said when they have, among others, the following properties (Porter, 2007):

- Healthcare centers focused on creating value for patients, not just on cost reduction
- A universal method of measuring the effects and costs of treatment for each patient
- Health care providers who take into account the entire patient care cycle (long-term care)
- Not only local but also regional and national competition
- Measuring and reporting the effects of treatment and the activities of medical facilities; At the same time, having the universal availability to share information with all health care system stakeholders
- Innovative activities that are rewarded, which tend to increase the value for patients;
- A process of integrating medical care

The role of adequate measures and methods of measuring competitiveness in health care is still a topic of open discussion and an important field for research exploration. Research conducted in the health care sector reviews competition in several aspects. The relationship between competition and the quality of health care was examined (Zwanziger and Melnick, 1996; Enthoven, 1993; Kassirer, 1995; Chassin, 1997) as well as between competition and the cost of the health care system (Robinson & Luft, 1985, Robinson & Luft, 1987, Robinson & Luft, 1988, Zwanziger & Melnick, 1996; Zwanziger & Melnick, 1988; Robinson, 1991). In addition, the relationship between competition and patient satisfaction was examined (Miller, 1996, Brook and Kosecoff, 1988). These studies show that competition can benefit patients over time. Improving quality and processes leads to lower costs, which in turn results in increased patient satisfaction. Particular attention should be paid to the impact of competition, in the context of the unstable external environment, the mission and strategic goals of the healthcare organization and its internal environment in terms of the quality of health care and the costs of the health care system, and how they relate to patient satisfaction. Traditional health care competition includes one or more components (i.e. prices, top-quality products or services). Competition can also be based on new technology and innovation. The key role of competition in healthcare is the ability to create a mechanism to reduce healthcare costs. Competition in a positive aspect eliminates inefficiencies that would otherwise result in high production costs that will ultimately be passed on to patients through high health care and delivery costs. Porter and Teisberg point out the positive health care competition characterized by the following features:

- Preventing stagnation
- Improving the quality of care
- A shift towards innovative treatments
- Better diagnosis and treatment of diseases
- Correct supplier information, treatment and alternatives for specific conditions

Competition remains important in the healthcare sector and covers all stakeholders, such as suppliers, payers, and patients.

PERSONS PROVIDING CARE (DOCTORS, MEDICAL STAFF)

Competition between doctors has always existed. However, it was mainly based on professionalism and quality of work. The patient was more likely to go to a doctor who was able to make a more accurate diagnosis and successfully cure the patient. Until recently, such competition had an effect on income, but only in those few cases where the doctor had a private practice, if not he still received a fixed salary from the payroll. At present, competition has become a widespread phenomenon, directly affecting the incomes of most physicians. With the existence of competition and its growing role we have to reconcile that this is simply a fact. It should, however, be based on strict rules. Anxiety raises the fact that its nature and ways of practicing by some doctors dangerously approach those practiced in trade and service industries.

In the medical services market, strong competition among medical staff is fueling modern technologies and research that attract the best medical professionals. It encourages doctors and medical workers to migrate and change jobs.

Medical Supply Units (Hospitals, Clinics, Nursing Homes)

Healthcare units, like other organizations, need to develop a long-term concept of efficient action that will best harness their potential and capabilities. Hospitals and health care units compete with each other both for the patient, the medical staff and the payer (Harris and McDaniel, 1993). The most important challenge facing the health care system is the improvement of the quality and effectiveness of the operation, including the appropriate allocation of resources to the individual healthcare segments, to meet patients' needs at an optimum level. In the battle for trust of payers and patients, the key strengths will be the security and quality of the services and the efficiency of the facility. These conditions are definitely conducive to the further development of the private medical sector. This is a significant signal as the private market is already an important part of the health care system and often provides access to both outpatient and hospital care. Providing comprehensive medical care at various stages of treatment - from primary care, through specialist care, to hospital treatment, ensures the right level of patient safety and comfort. Therefore, the complexity of medical care is an important criterion for the competitiveness of health care units.

Medical Service Payers

Medical service payers provide health care financing through contracting, defining the mechanisms and methods of financing and monitoring the performance of contracted benefits. Payers must make an informed choice when deciding on plans to purchase medical services.

To better understand the nature of competition in health care, Zwanziger and Melnick (1996) proposed a model for the analysis of two types of healthcare markets:

- **Quality (Non-Material) Competition:** Related to the quality of the services provided; In this case, the patient's choice of health care provider is related to the choice of doctor and the quality of services provided to the individual. Hospitals generally compete for patients through efforts made to employ the best professionals and care for safety, high quality of service and patient satisfaction with care (Aaron, 1991).
- **Price Competition:** Price is an important factor in the acquisition and retention of patients, especially in the private medical sector.

When considering price competition from an economic point of view, the importance of prices in shaping the relationship between demand for medical supplies and their supply is distorted by many factors. As a result, the rise in prices of medical services in specific cases may cause a reduction in the supply of services, as a decrease in purchasing power will result in a decrease in demand (Jaworzyńska, 2014).

McGuire draws attention to the fact that healthcare maximization is not the primary and only criterion for action; doctors (medical professionals) are not always constrained by market demand (because they largely shape the demand); they usually do not affect the price (McGuire 2000).

In health care, competition can take place in the following spheres:

- Between public and private service providers in relation to patients (competition K1)
- Between public and private service providers in relation to the third-party payer (K2)
- Between third party payers in relation to patients (K3)
- Between service providers in relation to the central authority, i.e. The Ministry of Health (K4)

There is no competitive relationship between the payer and the public funder in countries such as Poland, where there is a centralized system of health fund raising, due to the regulation of cash flow directly by the state. Sometimes a so-called. "Competitiveness of regions" is spoken about in regard to the process of allocating public funds to healthcare. However, it is rather a matter of transparent rules for the distribution of funds between regions. In the object sense, competition can be played on:

- Access to a specified number of patients (KB),
- Access to public funds through contracts (KC);

- Access to the patient's financial resources, transferred in the form of insurance premium or tax (KD);
- Access to budget funds financing eg highly specialized procedures (KA).

These types of competitive interactions are found in the practice of European states in different configurations and different intensities, depending primarily on the means of financing the system and the number of third party providers and payers available to the patient in free choice. This situation does not apply to the classical planned market, where there is only one entity, usually the local health administration (monopson), on the buyer's side. The development of a rival mechanism between health care providers for access to funds from a third party payer (K2) is aimed at achieving greater economic efficiency. With this type of competition, sometimes referred to as "public competition" or "directed competition", is the use of the payment system incentives (payment method agreed in the contract) that determines whether the payer pays for benefits actually rendered or services only planning. Sometimes, these two solutions are described as - in the first case - the mechanism of "money flowing behind the patient", and in the second one - "money flowing in front of the patient".

Competition in the Formula "Money Flowing Before the Patient"

The requirement for service contracts through negotiation with the payer creates, on the one hand, the risk of losing the source of funding for services and, on the other, offers the prospect of coverage for a larger volume of services. This decision of the payer determines available services and what extent will be paid from the general health insurance (Bismarck model: Germany, the Netherlands), general taxes (Beveridge model: UK, Finland, Sweden) or mixed funds (involving both sources: Greece, Italy, Portugal, Spain).

Figure 3. Competitive relationships ($K_1 – K_4$) and possible areas of competition ($K_A – K_D$)
Study: Iga Rudawska "Health Care, Market Aspects and Marketing", issued by PWN.

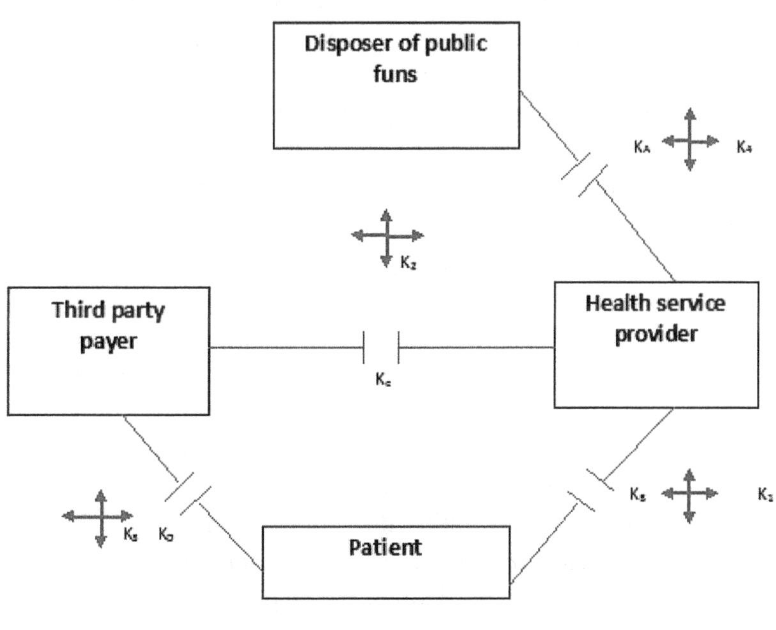

The Polish system is more similar to the Beveridge model, as the contribution of universal health insurance is a "parapodat" (part of personal income tax - PIT). This access to public funds held by the public payer determines to a large extent the competitive position of healthcare institutions. Having adequate financial resources determines the ability of an establishment to stay on the market. Separating the function of the supplier from the functions of the health care buyer, which exists in the competitive mechanism for the payer funds, has the following advantages:

- Third party payers may limit the asymmetry of information between the patient and the provider by setting up a patient counseling service;
- Third party payers can monitor the performance of service providers and perform comparative analysis, thereby stimulating qualitative changes;
- Third party payers, concluding contracts with multiple level providers (primary care and specialists), have the ability to coordinate these levels of care.

These favorable phenomena can occur within the assumption that:

- There is no monopoly position of the payer (the position currently occupied by the payer in Poland, Sweden and the UK);
- The payer has full information;
- There is no informal connection between payers and service providers.

Monopson is a situation where one payer purchases services on behalf of patients. However, it does not play the role of their attorney, nor does it feel the need to go beyond the function of the service buyer. Expansive knowledge of prices and costs does not allow the payer to make reliable comparative analyzes. When the third condition is not fulfilled, the non-economic factors that determine the conclusion of a contract distort the regulatory and allocation function of competition. The allocation of funds at the payer's disposal does not take place according to the criterion of efficiency and effectiveness. This also does not achieve the desired distribution of resources, guaranteeing their intended use.

Solving problems arising from the monopolistic position of the third party may be used to introduce a multiplicity of entities on the payer's side. However, there are still threats such as the rejection by insurance companies of the so called Negative risk group (avoiding joining an insured group of people whose health is worse than average and for which the likely cost of treatment will be higher than average), and "cream market" (allowing only healthy and affluent patients to be covered by insurance contracts). Violates the principle of solidarity because of both the uneven distribution of risk and the escalation of inequalities in the health status of citizens. The phenomenon of "cream sprays" from the insurance market is a concern for states with a core health insurance system. Previously practiced solutions are: the state guarantee of access to a defined range of benefits paid by public payers and introduction of a mechanism of financial compensation between payers. Financial equalization, though rooted in access, restricts competition to the obvious detriment of the quality of services offered. The proposed mechanisms to address incentives to motivate payers to act as advocates for the interests of patients are widely discussed in the European forum. The final choice of a route is dependent on past experience, in particular on market transparency. In turn, limiting the problem of informal systems that determine the contracting system is conducive to the management of managerial positions, unencumbered or political bias, or false professional solidarity with a particular service provider.

Competition in the Formula of "Cash Flow Following the Patient"

Stimulation of the market mechanism in health services can also take place within the "money-for-the-patient" formula. In this case, the amount of cash flow to the provider is determined by the final beneficiaries of the services - the patients choosing a particular service provider. The scope of their choices may vary and cover different levels of care. Characteristic here is the phenomenon of patient preference mobility for service providers, giving rise to the functioning of the K1 competition mechanism. Paying a service provider proportionally to the number and type of services actually provided is more beneficial from a microeconomic perspective. It stimulates positive quality competition and competition for market share. Furthermore, admission of private sector participation favors the pursuit of innovative competitive functions. However, the qualitative competition is related to the lack of excellent information. Without it, patients may be inclined towards attractive but not necessarily needed services, which increases the total cost of health care. Benefiting from the patient's perspective, the open-source financing system, which leads to unrestricted access to all medical services, promotes a "moral hazard" and thus leads to increased costs and expenses.

SUMMARY

The complexity of the health care system requires efficient management to ensure patients' safety and high quality of services. The conflicting needs of patients, families, suppliers, payers and regulators make health care institutions the most complex organizations in modern society. Each unit must operate independently; however, coherence and coordination are needed at each stage to ensure patient safety. At this stage, the role of the health care manager becomes essential. Its task is to make sure that organizational tasks are performed in the best way to achieve the goals set. Striving to maintain a competitive advantage in the medical services market is increasingly demanded by healthcare providers. This involves attracting customer-clients with a steady cash flow, which in turn affects the complex fulfillment of their needs. Ultimately, management decisions affect the overall performance of the healthcare facility, which translates into ensuring patients receive the highest level of medical care and access to modern treatment. Competition and ever-increasing patient demands make medical practitioners and their managers extremely flexible. The heterogeneity of medical services allows caregivers to standardize services. Thanks to such solutions, stagnation is prevented, the quality of services is improved and there is a return to innovative treatment methods. Building a competitive healthcare facility is the primary responsibility of a healthcare manager, since the benefits of such management are important to all stakeholders.

REFERENCES

Adamiec, M., & Kożusznik, B. (2000). *Zarządzanie zasobami ludzkimi: aktor-kreator-inspirator*. Katowice.

Blanchard, K., & Hodges, P. (2003). *Transforming Your Heart, Head, Hands & Habits*. Nashville, TN: Countryman.

Bonenberger, M., Aikins, M., Akweongo, P., & Wyss, K. (2014). The effects of health worker motivation and job satisfaction on turnover intention in Ghana: A cross-sectional study. *Human Resources for Health*, *12*(43), 10–1186. PMID:25106497

Brasaite, I., Kaunonen, M., Martinkenas, A., Mockiene, V., & Suominen, T. (2016). Health care professionals' skills regarding patient safety. *Medicina*, *52*(4), 250–256. doi:10.1016/j.medici.2016.05.004 PMID:27697239

Cummins Fred, A. (2017). *Agile Enterprise Leadership. In Building the Agile Enterprise* (2nd ed., pp. 333–368). doi:10.1016/B978-0-12-805160-3.00011-9

Czekaj, J. (2012). *Podstawy zarządzania informacją*. Kraków: Wydawnictwo Uniwersytetu Ekonomicznego w Krakowie.

de la Billiere, S. P. (2007). Przywodztwo, [w:] Biznes – Zarządzanie firmą cz. 2, praca zbior. Wyd. PWN, Warszawa.

Deussom, R., Jaskiewicz, W., Dwyer, S., & Tulenko, K. (2012). Holding Health Workers Accountable: Governance Approaches to Reducing Absenteeism (Technical Brief 3).

Doligalski, T. (2013). *Internet w zarządzaniu wartością klienta* (p. 222). Warszawa: Oficyna Wydawnicza SGH.

Eastwood, J. B., Conroy, R. E., Naicker, S., West, P. A., Tutt, R. C., & Plange-Rhule, J. (2005). Loss of health professionals from sub-Saharan Africa: The pivotal role of the UK. *Lancet*, *365*(9474), 1893–1900. doi:10.1016/S0140-6736(05)66623-8 PMID:15924988

Ferlie, S. (2001). *Improving the Quality of Health Care in the United Kingdom and the United States: A Framework for Change. University of London*. Berkeley: University of California.

Frączkiewicz-Wronka, A., & Austen-Tynda, A. (Eds.) (2009). Przywództwo w ochronie zdrowia.

Gierszewska, G. (2016). Male i średnie przedsiębiorstwa, innowacyjność, konkurencyjność- głos w dyskusji [w:] Grzeszczyk T.A.: Wybrane problemy wzrostu innowacyjności i konkurencyjności przedsiębiorstw. Oficyna Wydawnicza Politechniki Warszawskiej, Warszawa.

Hardin, L., Kilian, A., & Spykerman, K. (2017). Competing health care systems and complex patients: An inter-professional collaboration to improve outcomes and reduce health care costs. *Journal of Interprofessional Education & Practice*, *7*(June), 5–10. doi:10.1016/j.xjep.2017.01.002

Henderson, L. N., & Tulloch, J. (2008). Incentives for retaining and motivating health workers in Pacific and Asian countries. *Human Resources for Health*, *6*(1), 18. doi:10.1186/1478-4491-6-18 PMID:18793436

Rowe, A. K., de Savigny, D., Lanata, C. F., & Victora, C. G. (2005). How can we achieve and maintain high-quality performance of health workers in low-resource settings? *Lancet*, *366*(9490), 1026–1035. doi:10.1016/S0140-6736(05)67028-6 PMID:16168785

Huczynski, A., & Buchanan, D. A. (2007). *Organisational Behaviour* (6th ed.). Harlow, England: FT Prentice Hall.

Jaworzyńska, M. (2014). Market equilibrium in the health market- the theoretical background. Annales Universitatis Mariae Curie-Skłodowska, XLVIII(2).

Joint Learning Initiative. (2004). *Human Resources for Health: Overcoming the Crisis*. Cambridge, MA: Harvard University Press.

Kotler, P. (2004). *Marketing od A do Z*. Warszawa: PWE.

Kotter. J. (2005). Co właściwie robią przywódcy? [What Do Leaders Do?]. *Harvard Business Review*.

Kouzes, J.M., & Posner, B.Z. (2012). The Leadership Challenge: How to Make Extraordinary Things Happen in Organizations.

Luoma, M. (2006). Increasing the Motivation of Health-care Workers. Capacity Project Technical Brief 7.

Manongi, R. N., Marchant, T. C., & Bygbjerg, I. C. (2006). Improving motivation among primary health care workers in Tanzania: A health worker perspective. *Human Resources for Health*, *4*(1), 6. doi:10.1186/1478-4491-4-6 PMID:16522213

Matthews, G., Deary, I., & Whiteman, M. (2003). *Personality traits*. Cambridge: Cambridge University Press. doi:10.1017/CBO9780511812736

McGuire [2000] – T. McGuire, Physician agency, w: Handbook of Health Economics, red. A. J. Culyer, J. P. Newhouse, vol. 1A. (2000). Amsterdam: Elsevier.

Miller, F. L., Bennett, S., & Kanfer, R. (2002). Health sector reform and public sector health worker motivation: A conceptual framework. *Social Science & Medicine*, *54*(8), 1255–1266. doi:10.1016/S0277-9536(01)00094-6 PMID:11989961

Mintzberg H.; Managing on three planes. Journal: Leader To Leader, vol. 2010, no. 57, pp. 29-33.

Nichols, A. L., & Cottrell, C. A. (2014, August). Cottrell Catherine A. What do people desire in their leaders? The role of leadership level on trait desirability. *The Leadership Quarterly*, *25*(4), 711–729. doi:10.1016/j.leaqua.2014.04.001

Oleksyn, T. (2006). *Zarządzanie kompetencjami. In Teoria i praktyka* (p. 30). Kraków: Oficyna Ekonomiczna.

Penc, J. (2006). *Sztuka skutecznego zarządzania*. Kraków: Oficyna Ekonomiczna.

Porter M.E. (2007). Competitive Strategy.

Semuel, H., Siagian, H., & Octavia, S. (2017, February). The Effect of Leadership and Innovation on Differentiation Strategy and Company Performance. *Procedia: Social and Behavioral Sciences*, *237*(21), 1152–1159. doi:10.1016/j.sbspro.2017.02.171

Vujicic, M., & Zurn, P. (2006). The dynamics of the health labour market. *The International Journal of Health Planning and Management*, *21*(2), 101–115. doi:10.1002/hpm.834 PMID:16846103

Wang, H.-J., Demerouti, E., & Le Blanc, P. (2017). Transformational leadership, adaptability and job crafting: The moderating role of organizational identification. *Journal of Vocational Behavior*, *100*(June), 185–195. doi:10.1016/j.jvb.2017.03.009

World Health Organization. (2006). The world health report: 2006: working together for health. *World Health Organization.* Retrieved from http://www.who.int/whr/2006/en/

Zakariasen Kenneth, L. (2006, Summer). The importance of process in building an executive leadership team: A case study. *Healthcare Management Forum*, *19*(2), 6–10. doi:10.1016/S0840-4704(10)60816-2 PMID:17017759

Chapter 3
Management of Risk and Adverse Events in Medical Entities

Bożena Pieczka
Higher School of Economy in Bydgoszcz, Poland

ABSTRACT

The purpose of this chapter is to point out that effective risk management, also in healthcare units, can contribute to the effective reduction of adverse events and, consequently, the compensation claims of the patients. Also defined is the concept of risk and outlines the necessary elements that should be included in effective risk management. As far as medical entities are concerned, risk management is primarily about dealing with adverse events. Conscious control and limiting the occurrence of these events affects patient safety in a medical facility.

INTRODUCTION

Each company to take a risk to achieve the planned results. A free market creates both opportunities for extra profits and the risk of loss as a result of unfavorable changes in the business environment and mistakes within the organization. Therefore, more and more companies are choosing to implement a risk management system. The same situation applies to healthcare units. The primary goal of every healthcare provider is to provide health care services in the highest possible quality.

Quality of services affects the safety of the patient in the context of achieving the goal of treatment – full recovery, as well as avoiding the risk of complications as a side effect of treatment. It is important to be aware that the complications, that accompanies the healing process, can be a part of the process itself. The point is to avoid or minimize the potential risk of culpable complications. The essence of each system, including healthcare, is the cooperation of its participants and their cooperation.

Such cooperation, however, is prone to certain types of risk, which, in the age of competition on the medical services market, have to force management authorities to take conscious decisions supported by very substantive and constructive quantitative analyzes. All institutions that act as stakeholders in

DOI: 10.4018/978-1-5225-3946-9.ch003

the healthcare system – i.e. public payers such as the National Health Fund, the government, local governments, healthcare providers, and finally a single patient - coexist and work together within a single health system and at the same time are functioning as independent units. Each of the parties is exposed to their own risks, but also determines the emergence of such risks in other exchange groups on the market. Risk management, therefore, must be systemic, integrating all the processes taking place in a given unit.

Risk Management: The Essence and Legal Conditions

Risk management is a relatively new branch of management science, focused on the reasonable minimization of risks that the organization is exposed to.

In Poland, the genesis of risk management is reflected in the Legal Act On Public Finances from 27 August 2009.

Starting in 2010, management audits have been introduced in Poland as a way of directing and overseeing the public finance sector, with the aim of managing the effectiveness, efficiency and adequacy of all processes.

According to art. 68 of the Legal Act On Public Finances, management control is all activities undertaken to ensure that objectives and tasks are implemented in a lawful, effective, economical and timely manner.

A relevant part of management control is risk management. These are the procedures, policies and coordinated actions taken by both the management of the entity and its employees, which, by identifying and analyzing risks and identifying adequate risk responses, increase the probability of meeting and accomplishing the objectives.

The head of this unit plays a key role in the shaping and subsequent functioning of the risk management system at the public-sector unit level. His attitude and commitment influence how the risk management is perceived by the other employees. The cited law puts on him the responsibility for ensuring adequate, efficient and effective management control. The unit manager must therefore seek to create an effective risk management system.

In the Statement No. 6 of the Minister of Finance (6th December 2012) on detailed guidelines for the public finance sector in the area of risk planning and management, there are detailed instructions on how to conduct this process to be effective

For this reason, the state-owned medical institutions are obliged by law to carry out management control and, consequently, conduct risk management (Statement No. 23 of the Minister of Finance). This requirement is respected in particular by the founding bodies of the medical entity, which are: local authorities, universities and the Ministry of Health.

The Definition of Risk

The term risk comes from the ancient Greek word *riza*, which meant the reef, the basic danger in ancient shipping, and from the beginning was being seen as a symbol of serious threat in uncertainty.

Tadeusz Kaczmarek (2010) points out that: "the first work in the field of risk referred to research into the probability of occurrence of particular events and were published in the 17th century by B. Pascal, Ch. Huygens, E. Halley and n. - creators of probability theory and precursors of statistics" (p. 11).

Risk management in economy appeared at the break of the 1940s and 1950s, mainly as an insurance linked risk. Thereafter, the procedure was raised to financial risk (in the context of abuse in this area), then to other areas of business such as health safety, information security, etc.

The first and second World War overthrew the myth of perfect society and the noble human race. What is more, we have doubts as to whether the world can grow safely. At the same time, different areas of risk were being discovered and explored. As a result of these circumstances, a new discipline, called Risk Management, was started, which in a logical, orderly and consistent manner dealt with a diversified risk. Its dynamic development started mainly in the United States.

Among other things, risk management has been extended to capital markets where efforts have been made to manage assets rationally and thus avoid losses or minimize them. This was an attempt to go beyond accidental and random events.

Kaczmarek (2010) points out that:

... history of risk management includes important economic, political, military, scientific and technological events in the past 20th century. What kind of events? First of all, these were wars, and among them the Russian-Japan War, First and Second World War, Korean War, dozens of conflicts located on different continents, producing the first car, invention of television, computer. Other groundbreaking events: this is the Great Crisis of the Thirties, the rise and fall of totalitarian systems (fascism and communism), the invention and production of the atomic bomb, the construction of nuclear power plants, ecological hazard and global warming. This list can be supplemented by other incidents, such as the sinking of the passenger ship "Titanic", the environmental disaster of the chemical factory in Seveso (Italy), nuclear reactor explosion in Chernobyl (Ukraine), Challenger disaster (USA), abduction of the Exxon Valdes ship, the WTC terrorist attack in New York City (9/11/2001). Finally, we should mention frequent earthquakes in different regions of the world, hurricanes, typhoons and cyclones. All these events stimulated the development of a new interdisciplinary field from the border of management and economic sciences, called diversified risk management... (p. 29-30).

At the moment there are many standards in risk management in Poland. Many of them are included in legislation, many in international and national standards, others are recommendations from individual international organizations and associations. Each of them defines basic ways of behaving in a given field or area of activity.

Szomanski (2012) points out that the only standard that is covering the entire risk management system in an organization is ISO 31000: 2009 (ISO 31000: 2012 for Poland, published on March 5, 2012). This standard specifies the principles and general guidelines for risk management. The doctrine did not work out a final meaning for the term "risk". This standard definition of risk is associated with uncertainty: the risk is the result of uncertainty with regard to established objectives.

Taking into account all aspects of understanding this concept, the risk can be defined as an uncertainty of occurrence of undesired event. Given the fact that risk is a permanent feature of any organization, it should be identified in each area of any business.

Benefits of the Risk Management Process

Risk management is all the procedures, policies and coordinated action taken by both the management of the entity and its employees, which, by identifying and analyzing risk and identifying adequate response to risk, increase the likelihood of achieving the objectives and accomplishing the task (Communication No. 6, Ministry of Finance, 2012, p. 2).

The primary goal of the health care risk management process, is to ensure patient safety by integrating the various processes from medical, management and supportive areas. In this area, the risk can be measured and monitored by financial losses and health damage.

The benefits of running this process are as follows (Szomański, 2012):

- **Risk Management Creates and Protects Value:** It contributes to a possible demonstration of increased confidence in achieving goals and improving the service quality.
- **Risk Management Should Be an Integral Part of All Processes in the Organization:** Properly integrated into all processes, risk management is part of management responsibility and an integral part of all organizational processes, including strategic planning, which contributes to reducing uncertainty and optimizing risk and is bringing measurable benefits.
- **Risk Management Is a Part of Decision-Making:** Helping decision-makers to make wise choices, prioritize actions, and identify alternative directions.
- **Risk Management Clearly Addresses Uncertainty:** Taking into account uncertainty, its nature, and how it can be identified, analyzed and evaluated helps to deal with uncertainty.
- **Risk Management Should Be Systematic, Formalized, and Timely:** Only doing so contributes to continuous improvement in efficiency and to achieving consistent, comparable and credible results.
- **Risk Management Should Be Based on the Best Available Information:** Risk management should be customized to the external and internal determinants of the organization and the risk profiles existing in the organization. Only then will it produce the expected results. Risk management should take into account human and cultural factors, recognize opportunities, perceptions and intentions of people inside and outside the organization that can facilitate or hinder achieving goals, thus reducing uncertainty in decision-making and pointing to countermeasures. Risk management should be transparent, holistic and ensure, that appropriate and timely involvement of particular decision-makers remains relevant and up-to-date.
- **Risk Management Is Dynamic, Repetitive, and It Responds to Changes:** When internal and external events take place, knowledge levels and conditions change, new risks emerge, some risks change and some of them disappear. Monitoring and risk review will be used to ensure that the organization is still well informed about the uncertainty of its activities and can take preventive actions.
- **Risk Management Simplify Constant Improvement:** Risk management can indicate the direction of change in the environment, priorities of actions and possible losses, if these events occur. All this makes it possible to take reasonable countermeasures. It is also worth to mention that proper usage of countermeasures takes place only when they are involved in risk management.

STAGES OF RISK MANAGEMENT

The risk management process consists of four basic stages (Choma, 2011):

- Risk identification
- Risk analysis
- Risk assessment
- Risk monitoring and control

The basic condition for the effectiveness of any risk management system is to adapt it to the unit.

Risk Identification

According to detailed guidance for public finances sector entities in the area of risk planning and management, annexed to Communication No. 6 of the Minister of Finances dated 6 December 2012, the introduction to risk management is to have the correct definitions of the objectives and tasks of the entity. Then a systematic assessment of their implementation is carried out. Goals need to be set so that it is not only possible to identify and analyze risks, but primarily to effectively manage the institution. The obligation to set objectives and prepare the work plans for the individual, and to report on the implementation of these plans, is a necessary condition for the proper management of the unit.

While planning, you two basic groups of objectives can be distinguished:

1. Strategic
2. Operational

Strategic goals should be the result of the established mission and vision. The goals are rather fixed and apply to a longer period of time. Operational objectives should result from strategic objectives, be more dynamic, include a shorter period (e.g. year) and relate to specific activities that will be implemented. Strategic goals can also be seen as the most important goals of the whole entity, while the operational objectives can be seen as the goals of the individual units, that are needed to achieve the strategic objectives.

If an entity defines objectives in both perspectives, risk management should also address both. Types of risk come from different sources and can be classified according to different criteria. One way to analyze health care risk is to assign it and refer to each of the parties in the process of exchanging medical services, including: the patient, the payer and the healthcare provider.

Nieszporska (2012) suggests that in order to identify key risks in a medical facility, it is first necessary to recognize the external and internal conditions in which the facility operates.

According to Okoniewska (2015), the most important risks of a medical entity concern the proper management of contracts with the National Health Fund (or the Ministry of Health). There are also financial risks, adequate debt management policies (if it exists), and a cost control policy. Substantial risk in medical entities is the risk associated with the medical activity, i.e. the risk of occurrence of undesirable events. The occurrence of undesirable events can be a source of danger resulting in patients' claims.

In general, the risks in a medical entity can be divided into:

- **Strategic (External) Risks:** i.e. risk of mission, purpose, risks related to the code of ethics, changing regulations, perception of the external and internal context
- **Operational Risk (Internal):** Organizational, technical, technological and legal risk associated with human resources management (Okoniewska, 2015)

In any case, the risk should be related to goals/tasks. The identification of the risks by the medical entity should be individualized. For this purpose, negative events that occurred in the past can be used. Knowledge of these events allows us to create a catalog of events that we want to counter in the future. We know from experience what events have occurred and, above all, how these adverse events influenced the medical entity. This helps to create internal procedures that, based on past experience, will minimize or prevent the occurrence of these adverse events. The risk should be identified at such a level so that specific actions can be taken to prevent its occurrence. It is essential that all risks are individually assigned to risk owners, who are responsible for managing and monitoring each risk and its consequences. First and foremost, the risk owner should have the appropriate decision-making skills and qualifications sufficient to ensure the effective management of his risk (Giebel, 2012).

For the survival and development of a healthcare provider, three interrelated elements are crucial:

1. Obtaining and maintaining appropriate certificates and accreditation, confirming the high quality of the provided services
2. Contracts with institutional payers, in particular including the national health fund
3. Accounting liquidity

Risk Analysis

When the medical entity identifies the risks (which should be analyzed to determine the likelihood and potential effects), then the acceptable risk level can be established.

Doing a risk analysis will allow to draw up a risk map, that graphically presents how each risk is assessed and draws attention to those critical risks, that require further action. It indicates areas requiring especially careful monitoring and those that do not require special attention. Such risk hierarchy is essential for the risk management process.

The medical entity should make the choice of how to analyze the risk by adapting it to its needs (Communication No. 6 of the Ministry of Finance, p.15).

Risk Assessment

Risk assessment is made based on identified and measured risks. When evaluating, it is important to keep in mind both the probability of occurrence and the impact of a risk.

Some risks are subjected to numerical analysis, such as financial risk. For other types, like reputational risk, it is only possible to use subjective judgment. Nevertheless, it seems necessary to create a framework for risk assessment adapted to the business profile. This assessment should to be strictly based on objective and independent evidence.

Spot risk assessment allows to sort the types of risk according to their weight or criteria. Based on this, a hierarchy of actions taken to reduce risk can be made.

Documentation and Risk Monitoring

In risk management it is important to document assessment of the identified risk sources, which should be done in a way that facilitates the monitoring and identification of risk priorities. Once the risks have been ranked, the entity should consider taking action to monitor it. The nature of control activities depends on the extent to which the company can accept the risk, and the extent to which it can control it.

The monitoring and risk management process involves observing the identified risks, implementing response plans and assessing their effectiveness, checking if the preventive actions taken in response to the risks produced expected results, or do they require modifications. In addition, the purpose of risk monitoring is to determine whether any unidentified events have occurred.

Risk monitoring includes:

- Reviewing, to determine whether the risk has changed,
- Checking whether spot risk analysis is still relevant,
- Ensuring the effectiveness of the existing control mechanisms,
- Monitoring the development of agreed risk management activities.

Choma (2011) states, that "the risk management process should be based on the writing regular reports by the responsible people. The frequency of their reports should be regulated by the internal policy of the entity"(p.19).

RISK MANAGEMENT IN MEDICINE

The risk that comes with performing medical activity, and the legal responsibility of the provider before the patient and the public, were already known in ancient times. Hammurabi Code of 1750 BC imposed severe penalties (such as a loss of hands) to healers who treated patients ineffectively or contributed to their death. The medics, realizing that they can do harm to their patients while bearing responsibility for it, started to set themselves ethical principles. The most famous is the Hippocratic Oath "First of all, do not harm" (from Lat. *Primum non nocere*), which until today is taken by young doctors - a medical oath. It contains the code of ethics.

In the 20th century, expectations and demands considering physicians have increased significantly, although it remains clear to all that it is impossible to completely prevent injury and harm resulting from the provided services.

In all countries medical risk management systems have evolved in response to the growing number of high costs claims caused by medical errors. The United States was undoubtedly a pioneer in this area.

Among the causes of the development of risk management in medicine can be mentioned ("*Rozwój zarządzania ryzykiem w medycynie,*" pp. 2-3,4):

1. **Changes in Medicine:** The introduction of new technologies and medicines, that can cause side effects and undesirable effects. These two factors were the cause of the difficulties and put the patients at risk. In addition, the progressive professionalization of medicine makes the process of treating patients possible for many healthcare providers, increasing the risk of treatment discontinuation.

At the same time more and more, sick patients are being admitted for treatment, and the length of hospitalization is systematically decreasing, increasing the number of ambulatory services.

2. **Commercialization of Medical Services and the Competition Between Healthcare Providers:** Medicine is slowly losing its uniqueness and is becoming another sector of economy. The current patients are increasingly becoming consumers of medical services. This increases the requirements for healthcare providers and expects a positive outcome without side effects.
3. **Social and Legal Reasons:** Growing public awareness and widespread access to medical information, increasing patient involvement in treatment decisions, increasing criticism towards doctors and hospitals and increasing value of compensations and redresses - all of this result in a growing number law suits.
4. **Increasing Complexity of Healthcare Systems:** The process of treatment increasingly leans towards the diversification of medical services, and patients are admitted to different specialists, often taking place in different facilities. In such circumstances the risk of errors and adverse events increases. The deployment of teamwork and the rapid exchange of information between professionals can inhibit the growth of adverse events in healthcare facilities in Poland.

Another change, that accelerated the development of risk management, was putting the responsibility on the medical institutions. In the past they were often treated as a kind of hospice - the responsibility for their patients was solely on the physician. The process of evolution in this area began with the changes in the justice system in USA. As a consequence, regulations and procedures were introduced that required the hospitals to supervise doctors' work.

The importance of risk management in medicine has grown, its goals and scope have gone beyond its original framework covering a number of different areas, including: supporting legislative efforts in medical issues and providing an continuous guidance in this area. This way the risk management affects the whole health policy.

Initially, clinical risk management was based on a retrospective analysis of adverse events, but over the years significant prevention and quality control aspects of also became more important.

Proactive medical risk management (prophylactic or proactive clinical risk management) is based on an assessment of the current functioning of the treatment system. This approach is intended to support the prevention and mitigation of adverse events, including those, that have not taken place in the past.

Health services are activities with a specific ethos, related to significant social expectations. It is both a business and a public mission. Regardless of the form of ownership, the healthcare provider must be focused on creating and maintaining a stable relationship with the surroundings.

The social mission of the healthcare service operator and his economic interest require building of the most stable relations with the social environment.

So it can be said, that quality management and risk management are the fundamental pillars of strategy and organization (Opolski & Waśniewski, 2011).

ADVERSE EVENTS: KEY RISK IN THE MEDICAL FIELD

As already mentioned in this material, the primary goal of the medical entities is to ensure the quality of health services, which directly increase patient safety for optimal treatment conditions.

In medical entities the risk takes a specific form of adverse events. Recommendations from the Commission of the European Communities on patient safety, including the prevention and control of healthcare associated infections - COM (2008) 837 final version - point out that 8-12% of patients admitted to hospitals in EU suffer from adverse events. According to the Commission, the members of the EU should develop a system to record and analyze the scale and causes of adverse events, and develop effective solutions and responses.

The cited message shows that the most common adverse events include, among others: healthcare-associated infections, medicine-related events and complications after a surgery procedure. Some adverse events are related to the specific risks associated with the necessary treatments or medications. However, other medical errors are caused for example by: diagnostic errors, failure to take a correct action according to test results, prescription, delivery or administration of the wrong medicine, or at the wrong dose, or harmful combination with another medicine, or a failure of a medical product.

Based on research conducted in the EU it is assumed, that 8-12% of hospitalization causes negative health consequences, pensions and rehabilitation benefits, of which 70% are avoidable (based on the Recommendation of the European Union Council on patient safety and prevention from health-related infections, 9 June, 2009 / C 151/01 and other arrangements considering the quality in protection of patients health and safety).

According to the recommendations of the National Consultant in Nursing (Kruk-Kupiec, 2011), in the medical sector - in the medical field - risk management is reduced to management of adverse events. Its primary purpose is to eliminate the dangers that may occur while a patient is in the hospital.

In this place it is necessary to define the concept of an adverse event. According to the definition adopted by the Health Quality Monitoring Center (Accreditation Standard Series, 2009), adverse events are harm and damage caused during treatment or as a result of it, not related to the natural course of the disease or the patient's condition.

Carrying out an informed hospital policy for medical risk management - Adverse events - increases the safety of patients treated in this entity and reduces the potential risk of financial claims. More and more hospitals get the certificate of accreditation, which means compliance with the standards of the Health Monitoring Center and the ISO quality management standards.

The accreditation certificate is of paramount importance in healthcare, because it confirms that the hospital that holds it is a safe one. It means, that a hospital in the strategy of its operation performs an ongoing analysis of the occurring adverse events. It identifies, collects and analyzes data on adverse events related to the patient, i.e., the management of risk. It is, however, essential to use the conclusions from the analysis in order to prevent adverse events from arising in the future.

A consequence of the occurrence of risks associated with adverse events are the claims of patients. Patients can pursue their claims in proceedings:

- Judicial
- In front of the regional medical events committee, which does not rule out court proceedings (according to the patient rights act of 6 November 2008 and the patient rights ombudsman)

The form of protecting the medical entity from patients' claims is to have insurance policies with a broad range of protection (compulsory OC, insurance policies, etc.).

Claims for Compensation

An effective risk management process, including in particular the management of adverse events, should minimize the scale of potential claims for compensation.

Analysis and Statistics

The functioning risk management system defines the so-called weak points of the medical entity, by identifying individual risks and take actions against their occurrence.

In recent years, by increasing the awareness of the rights of patients, the number of court cases is growing rapidly. The medical documentation is therefore of great importance in court proceedings.

In Poland, the number of claims considering professional responsibilities increases annually by an average of 14% and is higher than the European average. According to a CBOS study from 2014, every third Pole in the study said, that he or she was a victim of a medical error or, at least, an oversight, omission, incompetence of the doctor, e.g. by the usage of specific "nomenclature", like calling the patient a "petitioner" or an "individual".

According to the data of the Patient Rights Office from the Ministry of Health, it is clear that non-compliance with the rights of the sick person is mainly due to hindering them from accessing medical services, not communicating (in an accessible and understandable manner) all information about their health status to the patients, and - what should be emphasized - difficulties in obtaining medical records. Also in these cases medical documentation concerning the events that are the subject of the complaint is of crucial importance (Marcinkowski, Kaczmarek, Herfort, Szozda & Żaba, 2011).

Year after year, the number of patients referring to various types of hospital complaints is increasing. The most common is infection, poorly performed surgery or improper treatment in emergency ward.

More and more patients are suing medical institutions. Not only because of the obvious damage caused by medical malpractice or neglect, but also more often in case of a formal failure to provide medical services - such as refusing or giving access to medical information, abnormalities in the information procedure about patient health status and their consent to certain benefits.

The Patient Rights Ombudsman in Poland is legally obliged to report annually how well the patient's rights are respected (art.58 of the Patient Rights Act and the Patient Rights Ombudsman). According to a report published for the year 2015 (accepted by the Council of Ministers in July 2016), over 71,000 various types of reports, complaints and signals from patients have been send to the Office of the Patients' Rights Ombudsman. This is the highest number since the Ombudsman's election in 2009. In his opinion it means, that the public awareness of patients' rights is ever-growing and the level of respect for patient rights is unsatisfactory.

There are many factors influencing the situation. The main problem has always been the same – the underfunding of the healthcare system. However, in addition to financial factors, the influence of management, the organization of providing healthcare services in medical entities, the attitude of medical practitioners to the patient and the non-compliance by entities to the law also became relevant.

Particular attention is placed on the most frequently reported cases and complaints from patients, including not respecting patients' rights to health services and the right to medical records.

It is becoming increasingly common that the abuse of patients' rights ends in a courtroom, as is described later in this article.

To conclude, patients are aware of the rights they have in the healthcare system. As a consequence of such a state of affairs, the medical entities are more at risk of patients claiming compensation for situations that have occurred in the treatment process, even if these situations do not lead to harm. They may be a consequence of not respecting the patients' rights, which is guaranteed by the Patient Rights Act and the Patient Rights Commissioner.

The BFP law team, led by lawyer Jolanta Budzowska, developed a report on the investigation of acts related to the so-called medical errors in polish hospitals and the analysis of cases taken to the voivodship committees. It was made as a part of the "Safe Hospital - Safe Patient" project, commissioned by the Center for Quality Monitoring in Healthcare from cases of medical events completed in 2012-2013. 183 cases were investigated, which ended with the final settlement of district courts in 2011-2013. According to the report, the injured patients are often newborns (10,38% of cases), which in most cases refers to adverse events directly related to childbirth and neonatal perinatal care.

Biggest group of victims were patients with bad or very bad financial situation. 81,97% of all the suits demanded amounts up to 300,000 PLN. A little over 1% of patients demanded over 1 million PLN.

Only in 40% of cases the court admitted to the patient and report the occurrence of a culpable incident. The basis for the decision was most often the recognition, that there was a lack of due diligence in the treatment. Surgical human error has been identified as the cause of almost one in ten identified adverse events (9.66%) - a surgical error should be understood as a error in the technique of performing the particular surgery. There was also a high level of medical emergencies (the cause of 8.28% of adverse medical events identified), identically to a diagnostic error in the absence of diagnostic tests (the cause of 8.28% of reported adverse medical events). Diagnostic error in the form of incorrect diagnosis occurred in 4.14% of cases of adverse medical events. Abnormalities in patient autonomy as well as medical documentation accounted for a total of 13.79% of the hospital's financial claims. Failure to choose a course of treatment, i.e. a medical error in the form of an outdated or abnormal treatment or lack of proper treatment, makes 5.52% of reported adverse medical events. Organizational errors caused by inadequate hospital management have been identified as 3.45% of the causes of reported adverse events.

The most important component of the compensation for patients is financial redress. The average amount of compensation awarded was 101,950.00 PLN. In 0.55% of all cases redress was awarded in the amount of over 500 000 PLN. While in about 10% of all cases the amount of compensation was over 100 000 PLN (9.84%). The amount of compensation was usually in the range of up to 75 000 PLN (25.68%) - Budzowska (2015).

Jurisdiction

Medical Error

Article number 4 of the statement on the professions of doctor and dentist (from 5th December 1996) about errors in medical art states, that a physician is required to practice his profession in accordance with the indications of current medical knowledge, the methods and means of prevention, diagnosis and treatment available to him in accordance with the principles of professional ethics and with due diligence. Failure to perform according to newest medical knowledge will be referred to as medical error or medical malpractice.

The harm suffered by a patient as a result of medical activities is defined as any injury to a legally protected property, with two types of damage: material damage (personal or property damage) and non-material damage (physical suffering or moral harm).

Determining the extend of the harm means comparing the state, in which the patient would have been if not for the incorrect treatment - and the condition resulting from this procedure. In the Supreme Court opinion, that the cause and effect link between the doctor's conduct and the resulting injury doesn't have to be reliably established, since it is usually not possible in "medical cases" - and in most cases, it can only be named high level probability or predominant probability and very rarely as certainty or exclusive fault. An important element in assessing the correctness of treatment is to determine what kind of activities the physician has done in due time, if he had performed the necessary additional tests, or if there was a consultation with a doctor of the appropriate specialty. A patient, who claims compensation for harm in medical entity, must prove the correctness of his or her claims, including the guilty verdict. The doctor is not presumed guilty, because he or she is only obliged to provide with due diligence in the treatment of a patient, absence of which has to be proven to the doctor.

In court proceedings, however, the physician should prove that he performed his duties correctly and acted in accordance with the principles of medical knowledge - and the patient claiming compensation must provide evidence of the contrary. The patient isn't usually an expert in the medical field, so it is very important to have a investigation of the evidence. The most important is the medical documentation - very often scant and illegible (Marcinkowski et al., 2011).

The law in numerous judgments states, that the causal link between the error of the physician and the deterioration of the patient's health, or the reduction of the chance for his improvement do not need to be established with certainty, only the high probability of the existence of such a compound is enough. The likelihood of causal linkage to one of these causes (SC judgments: July 5, 1967, I PR 74/67, OSN 1968, No. 2, item 26 and June 7, 1969, II CR 165/69, OSPiKA of 1969, No. 7-8, item 155, dated 13 June 2000, V CKN 34/00, Lex No. 52689, 17 May 2007, III CSK 429/06, Lex No. 274129).

Often the courts grant patients high compensation not just for medical errors committed by doctors, but for infringement of patient rights.

Violation of Patient Rights

The Supreme Court in its verdict of April 27, 2012 (file No. V CSK 142/11) pointed out, that pursuant to Art. 19a of the first act on healthcare facilities (this event took place under the previous version on the law on healthcare institutions; in the current legal status this regulation corresponds to Article 4 of the Patients' Rights Act), in the event of a culpable infringement of the patient's rights referred to In art. 18, paragraph 2 and 3 and art. 19, paragraph 1-4, the court may award the injured person compensation for the material harm suffered under Art. 448 of the Civil Code included in art. 19, paragraph 1, point 1 the right to healthcare services claimed by the claimant justifies the expectation of the patient that the therapeutic and diagnostic methods that meet his / her needs will be based on proven and up-to-date methods and will therefore be of adequate quality. Adoption of the culpable infringement of the patients' rights will be justified in the case of medical staff failing to perform a diagnostic test for the patient, who is not physically diagnosed at the same time, because there was no diagnosis at all (Nesterowicz, M. (2013). Gloss to the above sentence. OSP 6 (61), LEX No. 1222168).

As well pointed out in the literature and the judiciary (Highest Court judgment of 29 May 2007, V CSK 76/2007, OSNC (2008) no 7-8, item 91), financial claims are resulting from the infringement of the patients' rights and arising from art. 445 § 1 of the Civil Code. They have a distinct character and define the liability of perpetrators for separate unlawful acts. Art. 445 in related with art. 444 § 1 of the Civil Code. Treats for the compensation of harm resulting from body injury or health disorders, deprivation of liberty, etc., while Article 19a of the healthcare facilities act protects the dignity, privacy and autonomy of the patient regardless of the outcome of the chosen treatment and the effectiveness of the procedure. Their functions are also different: compensating in the first one and disciplining and compensating the other.

Legal protection includes, in addition to the violation of personal rights covered by the above calculation, also a violation of the right to appropriate medical care, that may result in a person suffering a negative mental experience, discomfort or loss of confidence in the healer, even if he has not caused medical harm. There is no need to meet the condition of injury to a person for him/her to get financial compensation, it may be granted for the very fact of the infringement and does not dependent on the simultaneous occurrence of such injury. If, however, patients' rights are not respected (e.g. any delays in the treatment or diagnostic examination) and it results in personal injury, health discomfort or only a deterioration of his or her health, he or she may claim redress - 445 of the Civil Code to compensate the damage, for the costs of treatment and other costs and expenses.

SUMMARY

Every economy exists in a risky environment and every sector of the economy is exposed to risk or uncertainty. Depending on the type of human activity, risk is understood differently and its multiple factors determine the use of various methods of its measurement, control and management.

Of particular importance is the risk associated with the health system, and, therefore, to the complex system not only by its structure but also by the multidimensional nature of services. Risk management in healthcare facilities requires not only medical, but also social, ethical and legal considerations (Lisowska, 24.11.2016).

Despite the fact that the number of adverse events in this sector is practically unlimited, a modern medical entity who seeks to stay competitive on the market with the right level of service needs to conduct a risk management process, in this case medical risk management (risk of adverse events). Identifying risks and then applying them in an economic assessment of a facility commonly used in the world are a guarantee for effective risk management.

In the opinion of Rafał Holanowski, CEO of Supra Brokers SA, presented at one of the sessions of the XII Health Market Forum (Warsaw, 26-27 October 2016), appropriate standardization of procedures for the reporting of adverse events is a very important element of avoiding risks in hospitals. Healthcare is recognized worldwide as one of the areas, that are most at risk for human error. Therefore, a key element in the implementation of the risk management process and a committed and co-responsible staff, that will understand the purpose of the process that is being implemented.

There is a pool of unforeseen and unavoidable adverse events, such as age or the physiological state of the patient. But there are also events that can be prevented. No doctor is able to guarantee complete therapeutic success and every benefit, even if performed exemplarily there is still a risk.

In the light of such necessities, but also of the real possibilities and situations in which healthcare institutions are currently located in Poland, special attention is paid to the skillful identification of these risks, the exclusion of them, and, in the case of complications, the minimization of risk.

Running an effective risk management process can give measurable financial gains through increasing the institution's competitiveness in the medical services market, but also by reducing potential claims for patients' compensation.

REFERENCES

Act of 27 August 2009 on Public Finance (Journal of Laws of 2016.1870 with later amendments).

Act of December 5, 1996 on the profession of doctor and dentist (Journal of Laws of 2015.464 amended).

Banaszak-Holl, J., Levitsky, S., & Zald, M. (2010). *Social movements and the transformation of American health care*. Oxford, CA: Oxford University Press. doi:10.1093/acprof:oso/9780195388299.001.0001

Borkowski, G. (2012). *Zarządzanie ryzykiem*. Katowice, CA: Uniwersytet Ekonomiczny.

Bukowska-Piestrzyńska, A. (2007). Marketing usług zdrowotnych. Warszawa, CA: CeDeWu.

Buła, P. (2015). *System zarządzania ryzykiem w przedsiębiorstwie, jako element nadzoru korporacyjnego*. Kraków, CA: Uniwersytet Jagielloński.

Centrum Monitorowania Jakości w Ochronie Zdrowia. (2009). *Zestaw standardów akredytacyjnych*. Kraków: CMJ.

Choma, A. (2011). Zarządzanie ryzykiem. *Think*, *4*(8), 12.

Ministry of Finance. (n.d.). Communication No. 23 of the Minister of Finance of 16 December 2009 on standards Management control for the public finance sector (Official Journal 2009.15.84).

Ministry of Finance. (n.d.). Communication No. 6 of the Minister of Finance dated 6 December, 2012 on detailed issues Guidelines for the public finance sector in planning and management of risk (Official Journal 2012.56).

Cutler, D. M. (2004). *Your money or your life: strong medicine for America's health care system*. Oxford, CA: Oxford University Press.

EC. (2009) Retrieved 20.02.2017 from: http://ec.europa.eu/health//sites/health/files/patient_safety/docs/council_2009_pl

European Union. (n.d.). Recommendation of the Council of the European Union of 9 June 2009 on security The patient and the prevention and combating of infections related to health, 2009 / C 151/01. Technical Report (2008) Improving Patient Safety in the EU developed for Commissioned by the European Commission, the RAND Corporation. Retrieved 09.03.2017 from https://pl.wikipedia.org/wiki/Kodeks_Hammurabiego

Frączkiewicz-Wronka, A. (2012). *Wykorzystanie analizy interesariuszy w zarządzaniu organizacją zdrowotną*. Katowice, CA: Śląsk.

Gabryś, E. (2009). Zarządzanie ryzykiem w szpitalach publicznych w Polsce. In R. Holly & J. Suchecka (Eds.), *Szpital Publiczny w polskim systemie ochrony zdrowia. Zarządzanie i gospodarka finansowa* (pp. 93-115). Łódź-Warszawa, CA: Agencja Wydawnicza Sowa.

Glossmann, J.P., Schliebusch, O., Diehl, V., Walshe, R. *Lean management in hospitals: potentials and limitations*. Munich, CA: Med Klin.

Graban, M. (2011). *Lean Hospitals. Improving Quality, Patient Safety, and Employee Satisfaction*. Wrocław, CA: ProdPublishing.

Hamrol, A., & Mantura, W. (2011). *Zarządzanie jakością Teoria i praktyka*. Warszawa, CA: PWN.

Holanowski, R. (2016, 27 października).Ryzyko kliniczne, czyli uczmy się na błędach, aby było ich coraz mniej [wypowiedź zarejestrowana podczas XII Forum Rynku Zdrowia, Warszawa 26-27 października 2016 roku]. Obtained from http://rynekzdrowia.pl

ISO. (2012, March). ISO 31000: 2009 Risk Management. Rules and Guidelines - Polish edition PN ISO 31000.

Jajuga, K. (2014). *Zarządzanie ryzykiem*. Warszawa, CA: PWN.

Jędralska, K. (2010). *Niepewność jako źródło paradoksów strategicznych. W: J. Lichtarski, H. Jagoda (red.) Kierunki i dylematy rozwoju nauki i praktyki zarządzania przedsiębiorstwem*. Wrocław, CA: Uniwersytet Ekonomiczny.

Judgment of the Supreme Court: July 5, 1967, I PR 74/67, OSN of 1968 No. 2, item. 26 and of 7 June 1969, II CR 165/69, OSPiKA of 1969, no. 7-8, pos. 155, dated June 13, 2000, V CKN 34/00, Lex No. 52689, 17 May 2007, III CSK 429/06, Lex no. 274129); Gloss to the judgment of M. Nesterowicz, Lex No. 1222168, OSP 2013/6/61.

Kaczmarek, T. T. (2010). Filozofia ryzyka – nowe tendencje w gospodarce globalnej. W: T. Kaczmarek (red.), Zarządzanie ryzykiem-ujęcie interdyscyplinarne (s.:11-14,29-30). Warszawa, CA: Difin S.A.

Kasiewicz, S. (2011). *Zintegrowane zarządzanie ryzykiem przedsiębiorstwa w Polsce*. Warszawa, CA: Wolter Kluwer.

Kodeks Etyki Lekarskiej. (n.d.). Retrieved 09.03.2017 from http://www.nil.org.pl

Kruk-Kupiec, G. (2011) National Consultant in Nursing, Consultant's recommendations National nursing field for good nursing practice, Safe Hospital - Safe Patient, Risk Management of Adverse Events, Project Safe medical practice. Retrieved 21.08.2012 from http: // www.mz.gov.pl

Krzakiewicz, K. (2008). *Kognitywne podejście do zarządzania strategicznego. W: J. Rokita (red.), Ku nowym paradygmatom nauk o zarządzaniu*. Katowice, CA: GWSH.

Kutryba, B., Kutaj-Wąsikowska, H., & Tombarkiwewicz, M. (2015). *Zdarzenia niepożądane. Analiza przyczyn źródłowych zdarzeń niepożądanych*. Kraków, CA: Centrum Monitorowania Jakości w Ochronie Zdrowia.

Lichtarski, H. Jagoda (red.), *Kierunki i dylematy rozwoju nauki i praktyki zarządzania przedsiębiorstwem*. Wrocław, CA: Uniwersytet Ekonomiczny.

Lisiecka, K. (2003). Zarządzanie jakością usług zdrowotnych. Warszawa, CA: Instytut Przedsiębiorczości i samorządności.

Monkiewicz, J., & Gąsiorkiewicz, L. (2010). *Zarządzanie ryzykiem w działalności organizacji*. Warszawa, CA: C.H. Beck.

Nieszporska, S. (2008). Jakość usług szpitalnych w ocenie pacjenta. In K. Ryć, & Z. Skrzypczak (Ed.), Ochrona zdrowia i gospodarka. Mechanizmy rynkowe a regulacje publiczne (pp. 197-205). Warszawa, CA: Zarządzania Uniwersytetu Warszawskiego.

Opolski, K., Dykowska, G., & Możdżonek, M. (2005). Zarządzanie przez jakość w usługach zdrowotnych. Teoria i praktyka., Warszawa, CA: CeDeWu.

Opolski, K., & Waśniewski, K. (2011). Zarządzanie jakością i ryzykiem w usługach zdrowotnych. Warszawa, CA: CeDeWu.

Pasowicz, M. (2012). Zarządzanie podmiotami leczniczymi – bezpieczeństwo pacjentów i sposoby ograniczania ryzyka szpitali. Kraków, CA: Krakowskie Towarzystwo Edukacyjne sp. z o.o. – Oficyna Wydawnicza AFM.

Patient Rights Patent and Patient Rights Act of 6 November 2008 (Journal of Laws, no. 2016.186t.j. With later meme).

Perechuda, K., & Kowalewski, M. (2008). *Zarządzanie komercyjną firmą medyczną*. Warszawa, CA: Wolters Kluwer.

Rozwój zarządzania ryzykiem w medycynie (2017). Retrieved 01.03.2017 from http://www.madanes.pl

Simon, H., & Dietl, M. (2007). *Tajemniczy mistrzowie XXI wieku. Strategie sukcesu nieznanych liderów na światowych rynkach*. Warszawa, CA: Difin.

Staniec, K. Klimczak, M. (2008). Panorama ryzyka. W: I.Staniec& J. Zawiła-Niedźwiecki (red.), *Zarządzanie ryzykiem operacyjnym*. Warszawa, CA: C.H. Beck.

Tarczyński, W., & Mojsiewicz, M. (2001). *Zarządzanie ryzykiem*. Warszawa, CA: PWE.

The Act of 6 November 2008 on Accreditation in Health Care (Journal of Laws No. 2016.2135).

Trela, A. (2016). Zarządzanie jakością w działalności leczniczej. Warszawa, CA: Wiedza i Praktyka.

Założenia do projektu ustawy o jakości w ochronie zdrowia i bezpieczeństwie pacjentów. (n.d.). Project of 20 January 2017. Retrieved 21.01.2017 from http://www.legislacja.rcl.gov.pl

Chapter 4
The Impact of the Attitude of Medical Staff From Burnout on the Level of Ongoing Medical Services

Anita Wójcik
10 Military Hospital, Poland

ABSTRACT

This chapter describes how contemporary, dynamic development in all available human areas is unavoidable and necessary. However, along with the benefits and progress made by civilization, there is also a growing margin of vulnerability and unfavorable price developments. Professional burnout is becoming a global problem. It identifies the limits of current human capabilities to the serious phenomenon. In particular, nurses and medical rescuers, who are in direct contact with the patient, experience unpleasant symptoms of burnout.

INTRODUCTION

The concept of burnout is a very trendy, popular and widely used term. Basically, the term can be seen as the mark of the modern times. Although originally, we have been in contact with this phenomenon (not yet a concept) in the story of Graham Greene, *A Burn-Out Case*. That is where the author presents the main character who openly demonstrates his "overall fatigue". Despite his professional fame, financial and, you would think, social comfort he is definitely forced to declare that he has had enough. His psychosocial fatigue has brought him to a situation where he reevaluates his life and views. The decision of social alienation and living deep in a bush, away from the civilization echoes is not as much an escape as a way of saving his being, the wreckage of his suffocated *ego*. Later, as a result of the carried out analysis and research, psychology would call that way of dealing with stress a reset, which restores an emotional balance. In the literature that was the first case of such an immeasurable revealing of a burnout symptom (Schaufeli, Enzman, 1998).

DOI: 10.4018/978-1-5225-3946-9.ch004

The emergence of the sole concept of burnout is not an artificial stimulation. That term rather constitutes the outcome of a spontaneous, but evolving problem of specific occupational groups. In principle, it should be assumed that used for years ordinary term or a metaphor has been an anchor to bring attention to the existing internal problem of escalation of the professional life on a human being as the biopsychosocial entity. Something what for years has been existing as a jargon of specific professional environments has become the subject of scientific researches (Smith, 2007). Initially, psychology considered that concept as very detached and not quite serious, not having enough essential foundations to undertake any detailed analysis. Basically, the problem of inability to deal with professional aspect of life and a very wide influence of its debilitating effects on many other areas of human life have forced contemporary psychology to look into the problem of burnout (Anczewska, Edwards, Roszczyńska, 2005). It has been a quite bumpy road to achieve the scientific psychology acceptance of the fact of the burnout phenomenon. Substantially, that was partially caused by the "victims" themselves. That would be embarrassing for stockbrokers or lawyers to shout out loud their tiredness and fatigue. Such behavior could have a negative influence on their professionalism and might significantly diminish the rank of their position. Moreover, even nowadays such a recognition of human frailties is considered to be inappropriate and socially denuding or unacceptable in certain professional groups (Maslach, 2001).

Whereas the first reliable descriptions and analysis of the stress effects and the use of the concept of burnout appear in the second half of the 20th century. They were concurrently, but independently of each other introduced to the scientific terminology by a psychiatrist Herbert Freudenberg and social psychologist Christina Maslach in America in the early 1970s. First time, Burnout Syndrome was described by Freudenberger in 1974. While he was working with juvenile drug addicts at New York facility with a group of committed and idealistic volunteers recruited from young Americans, he observed gradual loss of their charisma, motivation and charity commitment leading to the presence of many psychosomatic symptoms. Such a very dynamic and strong dedication to work for the entire year within that specific environment led them to apparent exhaustion, which he called a "burnout". This term was commonly (but highly accurately) used there to describe functioning of people who have been addicted for a long time (Freudenberger, 1983).

Maslach has explored the phenomenon of burnout in slightly different way. While working together with her colleagues from the University of Berkeley and conducting extensive research among working in stressful occupations people (including social workers, psychiatric nurses, lawyers providing legal advice and assistance to the poor, clinical psychologists, psychiatrists, prisons' employees), she tried to determine how they deal with their work related emotional tension. She was interested in the types of techniques they were using to successfully distance themselves from their clients' or patients' problems, and what were the personal and social consequences of applying those techniques (Maslach, 1993). Collected data revealed that many people – by analyzing their own professional experience – reported their emotional exhaustion and weakened feelings, increase of negative perception and patient misconduct and, as a result of those emotional tensions, apparent signs of professional competence crisis. Many of them suggested the reduction or gradual loss of empathy towards others. During the presentation of the study outcomes one of the lawyers has called this specific phenomenon a "burnout". The term has been picked up by other participants, and then – not without the mentioned above obstacles – introduced to the psychological literature (Maslach, Schaufeli, 1993).

Today, the burnout occurs commonly in modern organizations, although most often is not considered to be an organizational problem at the workplace. Common thinking about the professional burnout is focused on employee and his weaknesses related to dealing with his psychological difficulties. Whereas, the burnout syndrome is strongly associated with the stress inducing place of work and the chronic emotional burden experienced by the employee. People working under such a long lasting, permanent stress begin to experience a lack of harmony between themselves and organization, what leads to losing their motivation to continue working with the previous commitment. The effects in the form of symptoms of burnout are not only the entity's personal problem, but they cause some measurable costs for the organization, thus the phenomenon of burnout becomes a major social problem. Therefore, the issue of burnout, in the context of organizational pressure, demands some broad researches and practical advices for the modern working environments. The past decade has brought a dynamic scientific, academic progress in the broad concept of the burnout occurence. We have already known that term does not apply to all occupational groups. There are certain conditions that must exist to initiate the process of burnout. The truth is that there are no "secure" professions free from the problems of stress, but definitely, it was found that certain groups of professions are almost doomed to a constant rubbing risk of the burning out. The group of professional health care workers has become a basis for hundreds of studies conducted and initiated by Maslach. They have been conducted on physicians of all specialties as well as nurses, paramedics and physical therapists. Studies have proven that they belong to a high-risk group of people particularly susceptible to a work-related stress, what is a specificity of their profession. So let's stop for a moment and take a closer look at the problems concerning people who are saving others' health or lives, but more often, in an uncontrolled way, force themselve to reduce the quality of their own lives at the expense of both their physical and mental health. There should be implemented an analitic method of studying the origin of the burnout syndrome formation in order to understand the threat resulting from the job-related stress or unnatural, excessive involvement at the work life. In my opinion, the most reliable model in this matter is the one developed by Christina Marslach, which is the most exact, illustrative and, at the same time, the most refined.

It includes three basic dimensions: (1) emotional exhaustion; (2) depersonalisation (3) decreased satisfaction from the achievements.

1. **The Emotional Exhaustion:** A feeling of excessive fatigue and emotional exhaustion of resources. Characteristics for this dimension are: a sense of general fatigue, a lack of natural energy and zeal to act, no joy of life, increased irritability and impulsiveness. There are some signs of the need of greater efforts to perform professional tasks. Thera are also many other psychosomatic symptoms. The main the causes of exhaustion are: an excess of duties and conflicts at work. On the professional level, a person feels exploited and exhausted, and at the same time, does not see the possibility of recuperation. He most often complains of the lack of energy to start a new day and meet people, whom he is supposed to help. In the psychological aspect, it is observed the loosening of emotional bonds with his mentee, which often is demonstrated by a loss of attachment and intimacy.
2. **Depersonalisation:** This term has a different meaning from the one accepted in psychiatry. It defines the specific attitude towards other people, which is expressed by the negative, cynical, excessive interpersonal dissociation, and often the loss of idealism. Relationships with others lose their previous personal character, become impersonal, de-identified. Depersonalisation is derivative of an excessive emotional exhaustion. It can be seen as a form of self-defense by creating emotional indifference buffer to protect himself from any interactions. However, there is a risk that the attitude of indifference can lead to an apersonal attitude toward others and dehumanization.

3. **Diminished Satisfaction From the Professional Achievements:** Manifested by decrease of the sense of competence and work productivity. This reduction of the sense of self-efficacy and effectiveness may be associated with one's depressiveness and difficulties in dealing with the job requirements, and the stress associated with performing the professional duties.

The situation may be worsened by the lack or insufficient support from the environment, as well as neglecting the improvement of professionalism and competence. The existing state of professional apathy can be associated with a sense of meaninglessness and resignation attitude. The employee demonstrates the increased feeling of inadequacy and the lack of skills which are necessary to assist his customers. As a result, that may lead to erroneous beliefs in his own worthlessness.

All mentioned above symptoms in conjunction with the circumstances of their occurrence create a distinctive syndrome of bad adaptation at work. On its grounds is the exhaustion caused by excessive burden of the employee. It is noted that the advantage of the three-dimensional model is the appropriate expounding the sources of experienced stress in the weave of social conditions, which allows you to distinguish the burnout from other, non-work related unpleasant experience and stress. The main interpersonal relations at work, including relationships with patients, colleagues and managers, are the most important in the process of burning out. However, please note, that they can be both a source of emotional tension and gratification or motivation. In the latter case, they become helpful (especially if they carry a positive aspect) in dealing with job related stress and the effects of the burnout. Maslach (1982) emphasizes that, if the examination of the phenomenon of burnout is limited only to emotional exhaustion – bypassing the depersonalization and the job dissatisfaction-it will lose the full picture of socially important phenomenon. A 3D model of the burnout, proposed by Maslach, is widely accepted and the adopted dimensions have become widely used by different specialists in various polemics about the job-related stress. Maslach points out that even in a situation which does not clearly refers to this model, the established terminology is used in many discussions and scientific works or is synonymous to what she has proposed. However, the source and effect remain the same. For example, the exhaustion sometimes is known as an attrition, loss of energy, fatigue, weakness. Depersonalization is a negative or inappropriate attitude to patients, loss of idealism, annoyance, and lack of professional satisfaction shall be replaced by terms: decreased productivity or capacity, lowering morale, withdrawal or inability to deal with work responsibilities (Maslach C. 1997).

Analysis of the latest research, taking up the issue of the burnout structure, points out a tendency to describe the three-extracted basic dimension of burnout in more general terms than it was done in the original version. The sole emotional exhaustion is not talked about, but is generally about exhaustion, which applies to both aspects, emotional and physical condition.

Depersonalisation-expressed by an unfavorable change in attitudes towards patients-is replaced by the designation ‘ cynicism ‘, pointing to the coolness, distance and indifference attitude towards their own work, and also towards their students or clients. The lack of professional satisfaction is replaced by the designation of the inefficiencies of what connects the notion of professional inadequacy and loss of confidence in their own abilities. This change in terminology, in a large extent, is dictated by an attempt to develop a more general concept of burnout, and of not restricting it only to the competition, which took place in the initial period of this phenomenon studies.

In fact, there is no ordinarily accepted definition of burnout. In general, we can say that it is an extended reaction to some prolonged active emotional and interpersonal work stressors (Maslach 2001). Freudenberger and Richelson defines the burnout as a state of fatigue or frustration resulting from dedication to some matters, way of life or to a relationship, which did not bring the expected rewards (Pines, 2000). The multidimensional concept of Maslach is the most popular. According to the author burnout is a psychological syndrome of emotional exhaustion, depersonalization, and diminished sense of personal achievements, which can occur in people who working with others in a specific way (Maslach, 2000). The emotional exhaustion is the feeling of excessive emotional load, tiredness, emotional emptiness, the lack of mental and physical energy. It is the most striking symptom of the syndrome. The term depersonalization, unlike the one in the psychiatric tradition, refers to negative attitudes towards patients, clients, students, alumni, tendency to treat children in a neutral, impersonal, cynical or contemptuous way. Perhaps, in order to avoid confusion, it could be better to use the term depersonalization in Polish or to propose the term dehumanization. Depersonalization in the psychopathological sense is a condition, while in the case of a dimension of burnout it means the dynamic defense process of standoff towards recipients. This dimension of the team in a special way, emphasizes its interpersonal aspect. The third component of burnout is the tendency to evaluate their own work in a negative way, professional skills and accomplishments. The English term a reduced personal accomplishment is usually translated as reduced sense of personal achievements, however, it sometimes is used in the context of the reduction of the personal job involvement, a diminishment of personal achievements or reduced satisfaction. Sęk believes that the present state of knowledge does not allow for a rigid use of one term (Sęk, 2001). According to Maslach athe burnout affects mainly the specific occupations representatives, w providing social services and requiring a close direct work with people, personal involvement in the interpersonal contacts, which are often associated with helping others, and in which their social skills are the essential tools. These are the jobs subscribed in English as human services or helping professions. They include doctors, nurses, psychologists, social workers, teachers, educators.

An alternative understanding of the burnout was proposed by Pines and Aronson. According to them it is a state of physical, emotional and mental exhaustion, caused by prolonged involvement in various burdensome emotional situations. The authors mention about three dimensions of this syndrome, however, all come down to one, the exhaustion. Discussion becomes The separation of understood that way the burnout syndrome from the exhaustion strongly related stress becomes controversial (Schufelli. 1998). According to Pines and Aronson the burning out also occurs in professions that are not targeted to working with people, as well as in situations unrelated to work. For example, it may apply to the marriage or long term aquaintance and friendship. The following definitions of Burnout vary in the scope of their concepts and amount of the marked dimensions. Some include dynamical burnout, rather as the process of burning out (such as a three-step Chernissa's model) (Burke, 1995). Schaufeli and Enzmann (1998) proposed the following definition: Burnout is persistent, negative work-related condition, occurring in persons generally healthy. It is characterized mostly by exhaustion, accompanied by psychological and physical discomfort, a sense of reduced efficiency, diminished motivation and dysfunctional attitudes and behaviors at work. This condition develops gradually. and comes from the discrepancy between the intentions and the realities of the profession. The burnout often is a self-reinforcing process due to inadequate coping strategies. This definition captures the most important aspects of the syndrome, sums up the content of the definitions by other authors and some therapeutic implications. Difficulties in determining the order of appearance of individual expressions of the burnout and their correlations are partially related to a small number of studies. The prevailing view, where the necessary factor to initiate an adverse phenomenon leading to a burnout is work related stress resulting from the lack of balance between the work requirements and the human capabilities, and especially with the load the problems and also resulting from patients, students, pupils, interpersonal work expectations. The crucial sense might have a feeling of the great discrepancy between the expected work-related ideals and the true requirements, the reality of the profession. In this case, the burn out would mostly affect the most motivated and idealistic newcomers at the beginning of his career, sucriphising way too much energy to fulfill their unrealistic expectations. Freudenberger notes, for example, that the burnout occurs about one year after the start of work (Freudenberg, 1974). An alternative approach assumes the burnout is a final result of chronic exposure to stressors at work, and appears later. The empirical researches show that indicators of the burnout are fairly stable in course of time, what supports the latter concept. Stress is necessary, but it is not a sufficient condition for the burnout development. According to Sęk, the burnout is not as much a direct result of chronic stress as it derives from an non-modified stress of your own proactive activity (Sęk, 2000). The basis for the burnout development is the widespread experience of failure in dealing with stress. In the classic model of burnout, proposed by Maslach and Leiter, in case of a staff member whose adaptability in dealing with stress have collapsed, initially there is an emotional exhaustion development. Being unable to cope with this status the employee begins to resist some of the too close, meaningful relationships with his recipients by increasing emotional distance, demonstrating more and more callous, indifferent treatment and their depersonalization. The consequence of this unreliable defensive strategy is the lack of job satisfaction, the tendency to negatively assess their own performance and diminished commitment. This is a sequential model, in which the individual dimensions of the burnout appear in a specific order, are interrelated, mutually reinforcing. Golembiewski proposed the model called phase (Golembiewski, 1998). At the beginning the agitation appears, followed by a reduction of the sense of personal achievements, and emotional exhaustion. The author also suggests that the three dimensions of the burnout can develop at the same time, but independently of each other, giving, as a result, eight patterns or phases of the burnout. Perhaps the relationship between dimensions of the burnout vary in each group. In Sęk's study there is a sequential, selfstrengthening structure with an emotional exhaustion at first, leading then to the depersonalization and consequently to reduced sense of personal achievements among nurses, while in the group of the surveyed teachers the individual elements of the syndrome are independent of each other.

There still is a remaining open question about the separation of the burnout syndrome and the types of connection with other status and mental disorders. The subject of controversy is especially a differentiation of the burnout and stress, depression, reduced work satisfaction and chronic fatigue syndrome (Bakker A.B. 2000). Current researches do not allow for a clear resolution of this issue. Burnout is usually seen as a specific form of response to stress. However, it seems that these are separate phenomenon, because: Burnout is a long lasting process, emerging as a result of a work related stress with the collapse of adaptability, and the strength of that emotional exhaustion highly correlates with stress, however, depersonalization and reduced sense of personal achievements are not listed among common stress reactions and show only little or moderate correlation with the stress, the burnout depends on the original motivation and high job expectations, while stress can be experienced by each individual regardless of the motivation level. Therefore, the burnout is rather a chronic, multi-dimensional response to the stress, which especially the second and the third dimension are specific. Many of the burnout symptoms can also occur in depression. Like in the stress, there is a quite a strong correlation between depression and emotional exhaustion, and the other two dimensions are much weaker (Schaufeli in 1998). Probably they are congenial, but separate states. However, the stronger are signs of burnout, the greater the resemblance to depressive symptomatology. It's also possible that similar personality factors promote both states (Iacovides. 2003). The main difference between them is that depression penetrates all aspects of life, whereas the burnout is limited to the job, leaving the functioning in other areas of life unchanged, at least in the initial period. The symptoms of chronic fatigue syndrome might be similar to the burnout, but in the clinical picture they are dominated by physical ailments and mental accompany them. As in the previously mentioned states, the similarity of burning refers primarily to emotional exhaustion, the other two dimensions do not exist in the chronic fatigue syndrome. Satisfaction is a congenial term and it has a longer history than the burnout. It negatively correlates in a moderate way with emotional exhaustion, slightly negatively with depersonalization, and positively, though insignificantly with a personal commitment. So, these are the concepts related to each other, but the interpretation of the mutual dependencies remains contentious so far. It is not known whether smoking is the cause of the lack of professional satisfaction, or a reduction job satisfaction contributes to the onset of burnout. It is possible that both burnout and reduction of work satisfaction are caused by a common factor, for example, bad working conditions. The burnout, and especially its dimension of personal commitment, needs to be distinguished from the original lack of engagement, as both the states might be similar in their external manifestations. According to Sęk, the knowledge about burnout sometimes might be a specifically cognitive overbuilt defensive pattern against the original lack of professional engagement. It is believed that the burnout might develop only in people with high levels of their initial motivation. The term exhaustion assumes prior state of high arousal. To burn out, you have to first burn. There are some present discussions on the issue of the inclusion of burnout syndrome to the international classification of diseases and related health problems. Wiesmuller and his associates postulate to include the burnout syndrome to a somatic group of disorders (Somatoform Disorders). In the classification of the Diagnostic and Statistical Manual of Mental Disorders (DSM-IV) it is the category designed phenomena that does not meet the criteria of mental disorders, however, require attention and treatment. It describes many job-related problems: lack of job satisfaction and uncertainty concerning the choice of career. The ICD-10 of mental and behavioral disorders places the burnout among some factors affecting the overall health status and contact with health services (Vesalius 2000). The developed to date tools allow us to compare the level of the burnout to different study groups. However, except the arbitrarily adopted statistical criteria of objective standards, there is no specific criteria taking into account some national and cultural specificities, that would allow to properly diagnose it. The presumption is that cultural factors play a significant role, because the hitherto conducted studies reported significant differences in burnout terminology in various countries (Turnipseed DL. 1997). In general, studies conducted in the United States reported a higher average level of emotional exhaustion and depersonalization than the one conducted in Western European countries.

The results obtained from the study of population of Polish nurses were closer to American indicators, which are higher than in most of the studies conducted in Western Europe (Schaufeli in 1994). At the present stage of knowledge, the MBI questionnaire or any other tool are not suitable for diagnostic purposes. To change that it is necessary to determine clinically relevant border points, by comparing the results of self descriptive questionnaires with an independent assessment of psychologists or psychiatrists. Some studies confirm the usability of the MBI questionnaire in an individual assessment of burnout.

Some temporary, requiring further verification, diagnostic criteria were elaborated only in the Netherlands. The preliminary estimates show that about 4% of the Dutch working population suffers from the clinical burnout syndrome.

WORK-RELATED AND THE INSTITUTION ORGANIZATIONAL STRUCTURE FACTORS

In this group there are included some work requirements and resources: their deficiency or absence (Bakker AB 2003). The lack of comfort and free access to the tools necessary to obtain the proper working effect is very significant. Extremely important is an employee's feeling, that with appropriate equipped technical and substantive support he can sustain the quality of his work. This is one element of this group. However, it is also important the sole work demand as it relates to the colloquial sense of being useful, being a part of a whole.

The Job Requirements

Among the job requirements there are work-related stressors and also stressors arising from the peculiarities of working with people. This distinction is important for theories of burnout, because if it is to be specific for the social service professions, the second group of factors should play a greater role. The stressors associated with the profession are: workload, time pressure, which is too much work to do in a too short time, role conflict and role ambiguity. Role conflict occurs when you meet at work, contrary to the requirements of, put up with for example. the role of educational and disciplinary action. The ambiguity of roles associated with the lack of necessary for performance of work information and lack of clarity as to the purpose of work and responsibilities. Workload and time pressure are strongly related to emotional exhaustion, with depersonalization and a sense of personal achievements. The physical exhaustion is often an inflammatory factor of diminished emotional performance. In addition, the conviction about performing this job on a regular basis, periodically working for another person or performing duties that go beyond his competence can be demotivating. This leads to the very troublesome situation and confirms the fact that role conflict and role ambiguity exhibit moderate or strong relationship with burning out. Among the arising from the peculiarities of working with people stressors are listed those usually in direct contact with customers, patients, students, their number, the load of their problems, the confrontation with suffering, death and with aggression. A lot of research, contrary to the intent of the theoretical, not confirmed by stronger depending on the burn from this group of factors (Schultz, 1995).

The Lack of Resources

Resources include such factors as support, feedback, autonomy at work, participation in decision-making, control of their own work, remuneration, career opportunities. The most common tested of these factors is the support from his superiors, colleagues or other people (Halbesleben., 2004). Support, especially from his superiors, is negatively correlated with burning out, however, much less than the requirements of the work. Other factors included in the resources also correlate (as expected) with all the dimensions of burnout, the strength of these compounds in the various studies is often small. Some authors suggest that the work requirements are stronger related to emotional exhaustion and the resources mainly with depersonalization and a sense of personal achievements, however, the results of research are not always clear and in this respect not always confirm assumed findings (Leiter MP. 1996).

Individual Factors, Demographic

As regards age, more burnout cases are observed among younger individuals. Perhaps this is related to a painful confrontation between dreams and expectations with reality, or with lack of experience. That cannot be excluded that your burned out employees just abandon profession quickly, so in an older group remain those who know how to develop the adaptive mechanisms. Conflicting test results regarding a gender (Leiter MP., 1996). In part the study women gain higher scores on a scale of emotional exhaustion, and the men on the scale of depersonalization. In some studies, single people have higher indicators of the burnout than the ones living in relationships. Slightly higher levels of the burnout can be observed frequently in people with higher education. Perhaps people better educated have higher expectations and take up a position with bigger responsibility. In a substantial part of the research, however, do not seem to be any significant relationships between demographic variables and indicators of Burnout (Maslach, 2001).

Personality Factors

The impact of personality factors was less studied than situational factors, however, certain dependencies are described in the literature fairly consistently. People with low levels of so-called mental resistance are more vulnerable to the burnout process. People mentally resistant are characterized by a tendency to strongly engage in what they do, openness to changes, interpreting stressful events as challenges, and a sense of having a full control of different events and their own lives (Heszen-Niejodek, 2000). Burnout rates are usually higher in people with an external location of source control, coping with their stress in a passive way. The self-esteem correlated with all dimensions of the burnout is low, but it's hard to tell if it is a disposing factor to burnout or rather its consistency. The researchers quite often studied five factors of personality called the big five by Costa and McCrae. These studies show that the burnout promotes mainly high level of neuroticism.

This dimention includes: anxiety, hostility, depression, impulsiveness, sensitivity and shyness (Leiter MP., 1996). According to Sęk's studies the symptoms of conditions predisposition to burn are: the tendency to judge the situation in terms of risks, a mechanism to avoid the difficulties and irrational beliefs, while the immunizing are: general sense of self-efficacy and cognitive control based on the positive experiences focused on the individual's changes. Correlations between burnout and a sense of coherence or sense of meaning in life has been studied relatively rare (Söderfeldt M 2000).

Work Related Attitudes

High, unrealistic expectations to work were very often cited as one of the main factors conducive to the burnout. Conceptual confusion and methodological differences may be the reason of the lack of conclusive research results. In fact, not always legible is to distinguish whether the expectations relate to the characteristics of the sole work to be enjoyable, interesting, or to the results of the learning progress of students, the recovery of patients, or the possibility of success, achieve significant (Schaufeli in 1998).

An attempt to systematize the issue Burnout is important. It allows to capture the problem in the most figurative way. However, it is essential to know the causes of pressure which yields an individual, which uncontrolled and not eliminated on time lead to psychological and physical breakdown, loss of balance and necessity to change the present life and way of thinking. The most common reason is stress. In any form, in any quantity, especially the long-lasting.

The phenomenon of stress is currently one of the most popular topics of both conversational considerations as well as scientific researches. Therefore, the term stress is no longer just scientific, though undoubtedly calls for the scientific description and precise clarification, as it is responsible for a variety of disorders of human functioning. Research on stress shall be taken in such disciplines as psychology, sociology, anthropology or widely understood medical science.

In accordance with the recognition of the term, stress means "the state of the burdening of the system of psychological adjustment, occuring in dangerous situations, hindering or inability to implement the individual's important objectives, targets, values." Many scientists understand the phenomenon of stress just as the situation that arises when the individual's challenges and external circumstances exceed its ability to cope with perceptual stresogenic situation.

In a variety of approaches, however, slightly different emphasized the importance of the selected aspects of stress. One of the first considerations on stress was run by H. Selye, focusing on the physiological meaning of stress and specifying this phenomenon as a status of the body, with a non-specifc physiological changes that respond to certain body challenges. In this approach, the stress is a part of Cannon's concept, developing the idea of homeostasis or balance, and acknowledging that stress is the result of internal disorders of homeostasis, and resistance to stress is associated with the ability to maintain the stability of the internal environment (homeostasis) conditions being subject to different stimuli. The author has used the concept of stress for the determination of the reactions of the body as a kind of fight, search methods, defense or escape from the unfriendly elements of sterss builders. All that in order to restore the balance of the body to minimize or eliminate the operation of various factors of pressure.

In another sterss research they clearly expanded scientific studies on the psychological aspect, what started the stage of understanding stress as a psychological category. In that approach they have studied the different emotional disorders experienced by anindividual in some life-threatening conditions or experienced difficulties in interpersonal relationships and tasks. It was noted that situations do not have to be especially threatening to worsen the mental functioning of the human being. The problem occurs in everyday life, in fact, is associated with various factors, which arouse in each individual. Often there are situations, in spite of all its (assumed) destruction, very effective, stimulant, constructive, forcing the above-average activity.

Stress was also featured as a result of the difficult situation in which there was a discrepancy between the tasks or the needs of man and the possibilities to perform these tasks or meet the demanding the needs fulfilment.

In the classical approach to stress there should also be brought up the trading model developed by R.S. Lazarus and s. Folkmana, who put emphasis on individual's interaction with the environment, a subjective rating this interaction by the individual and following the type of activities undertaken by the individual acting in a stressful situation.

In analyzing the phenomenon of stress you should also pay attention to the approaches attempting to reconcile different perspectives, in order to fully and multifaceted characterize this phenomenon. This way, J. Strelau developed definition of stress reconciling the physiological approach (centered around ^physical response to the stress) and the interactive approach (stressing the body's reactions to external stimuli). The author suggested to define stress as "the state consisting of strong negative emotions and the accompanying by some physiological and biochemical changes, excessing the normal state of arousal".

It should also be taken for consideration the definition of stress proposed by P. G. Zimbardo and F. Rucha who in their analysis of stress have noted that the causes can varied, and most importantly, both in a pleasant and an unpleasant way. Their essence is that they all require changes, and consequently re-adapt to the situation. The authors stress that, regardless of the source of stress biological body's reactions are always the same, and therefore an individual throughout his life span will face the stress and its consequences, whenever he has to confront some new requirements.

Based on various observations of people behaviour in stressful situations Lazarus pointed out three significances of this phenomenon:

- **Load:** Understood as the external stimulus;
- **The Pressure:** Referred as an internal reaction triggered by a stimulus;
- **Voltage:** Understood as a disorder.

This way, the author has defined stress as a highly subjective phenomenon, because the variety of stimuli stressors and subjective evaluation of the events by the individual makes stress something strongly individualized and difficult to determine. It is important, however, that in their mutual interactions between the individual and the environment take into account both the requirements of the environment, as well as individual people deal with committing events (Lazarus, 1999).

The last consideration on stress popularity won the concept stress Hobfolla, referred to as the theory of behavior resources (COR). In this approach, the author is looking for general principles that guide the deliberate human behavior. Defines them as the desire of individuals to maintain, protect and contribute their own resources. To create for them the enclave of untouchability and controlled. Resources and are understood as valued by the items, personal property or the circumstances, experiences. According to the author the man continuously tries to acquire resources, which does not have yet, keeps the ones he already has got, and protects those who for some reason are subject of risk. And therefore, the source of stress is an imbalance in the exchange of resources between the individual and the environment (Hobfoll, 1998).

As you can see, the evolution within the meaning of the phenomenon of stress is associated with multidisciplinary approaches. However, regardless of the differences in this matter, today's psychologists understand stress as a result of any stimuli, both positive and negative, that might be the cause of the disorders and psychosomatic diseases, but they can also mobilize the body and provide an opportunity for human development.

Work is natural for man and desired activity. However, since ancient times, there have aroused very ambivalent emotions, positive or negative. Depending on the circumstances and of the purposes can be used, to support the development and provide satisfaction, but it can also be a pathogenic agent, be a source of tension the emotional illness, disorders in social and family functioning of the human being. Work-related stress (stress professional) is a very serious problem not only for individuals experiencing stress, but also for organizations and society as a whole. The results many studies are very disturbing, because professional stress is a phenomenon very common, but also indicators of work-related stress are constantly on the rise. It indicates the fact that, over the past several decades of professional stress levels alarmingly increased. This applies mainly to industrialized countries, and manifests itself in the rapidly growing indicators of sickness and incapacity for work caused by stress. Each work may be a place where the employee comes into contact with stressors causing the state a strong tension. Thus, each work can be a source of stress. Stress factors related to work are classified in many ways. Synthetic cap ture proposed by Stranks (Stranks J. 2005), groups professional stressors into three categories:

- **Environmental Factors:** The conditions under which a given unit came to work, for example noise or air temperature;
- **Professional Factors:** For the same work, responsibilities and requirements, the amount of work and the scope of control over the tasks;
- **Social Factors:** Contacts with other people, your colleagues, but also with your friends, your loved ones outside of the organization.

David Fontana also has identified three groups of work-related stressors, subjecting them to more detailed split (Fontana, 1991):

1. **Organizational Problems:**
    a. Lack of support for the employee,
    b. Long and inconvenient working hours
    c. Low prestige, wages and promotion prospects,
    d. Unnecessary rituals and procedures
    e. The uncertainty and lack of a sense of constancy
2. **Work-Related Problems:**
    a. Difficult customers or employees/colleagues
    b. Inadequate preparation
    c. The liability associated with the work
    d. Inability to efficient operation of or the provision of assistance to another,
    e. Work overload or underload
3. **Specific Causes of Stress:**
    a. The ambiguity of roles
    b. Role conflict
    c. perfectionism
    d. There is no impact on the decisions
    e. Frequent conflicts with superiors
    f. Lack of support from colleagues
    g. Monotonous work
    h. Poor communication
    i. Inappropriate targeting
    j. Conflicts among workers

Organize work-related stressors can be shot n. hop, in which the author clearly presents their categories. This is the content of the work, work conditions and social relations at work. The table shows the most important stressors, belonging to each of these categories. Based on this statement, and earlier, for example, cited the classification, it can be concluded that the source of stress may be factors from different areas of the functioning of the professional man. Literature review, we can conclude that most of the studies on stress has been focused on the content of the work and working conditions. Today, while the plane relevant search becomes an area of human relationships.

Regardless of the category of the stimulus may show different types of physiological and emotional response to stress. In people who experience high levels of stress. There are many symptoms of psychosomatic and stress relieving capacity of the disorder and rest from work. In a number of studies have demonstrated that the greater stress professional experience, this has less satisfaction with work, and greater dissatisfaction with its implementation. Often feel also a sense of failure and incompetence, leading to a reduction in self-esteem (Hops n. 2007).

So for many people, work is a source of stress is the cause of ailments-physical and mental health. At the same time, professional stress is a phenomenon the inevitable, what more is increasing as a result of structural change and economic. One of the serious consequences of experiencing the stress of work, especially long-term, chronic becomes a Burnout, which is today a serious organizational problem and obstacle in building environmentally friendly jobs.

The phenomenon of the burnout can be defined as a psychological syndrome emotional exhaustion, depersonalization, and reduced sense of personal achievements. These three components are therefore about burnout and distinguish it from other psychological States such as stress, fatigue or feeling of alienation (social alienation). Emotional exhaustion means a sense of the person, that is excessively charged emotionally in the work. It is often described as fatigue, loss of energy, weakness or fatigue. Depersonalisation is revealed in the form of a question, respond to other people, who are the recipients of the services of the person concerned, and so for example. customers or clients. Most frequently manifested in the adoption of neutral posture, soulless or even negative, in contrast to irritability, dislike and low level of interest. In turn, the reduced sense of personal achievements means a decline in the sense of one's own competence and success in professional life. Is associated with the belief of the person about their own nieproduktywności, reduced the possibilities of the implementation of the tasks and the inability to cope with difficult situations at the level of working life.

Maslach and Leiter have six main areas, in the context of which the can be considered a source of Burnout:

- Excessive workload (too many assigned tasks, exhaustion, excessive availability, time pressure)
- The lack of a sense of control (lack of participation in the decisions, ineffective leadership)
- A sense of they underestimated and lack of job satisfaction (too low salaries, lack of discretion)
- Interpersonal problems in the workplace in terms of communication and obtain support
- A sense of injustice/unequal treatment of employees
- The discrepancy between personal values and the values of the organization.

Each of the above-mentioned areas can be individually and subjectively experienced and will require another direction changes. Always, however, reactions of Burnout will have a similar symptomatologię, regardless of the specific area, generating signs of burnout.

The phenomenon of Burnout is characterized by five stages:

1. **Physiological Stage:** This is a phase of the physiological symptoms, IE. pain, malaise, loss of appetite, exhaustion, difficulty in sleeping.
2. **Stages of Social:** This is the stage for which are characteristic: irritability, isolating to uncertainty in human relationships, grievances and grief to others.

3. **Intellectual Stage:** In this phase comes to disorders of cognitive processes, What is revealed difficulties in adopting and communicating information, and delighting in the errors in thinking.
4. **Psychoemotional Stage:** At this stage appear behavioral changes, i.e.. the abuse of alcohol, tobacco, drugs, drug, disregard of its obligations, decrease in liability and risk.
5. **Stage of the Spiritual:** This phase is associated with loss of faith in the fundamental principles and values, reveals the inner emptiness and lack of interest in other people.

It should be noted that the transition from one stage to another is unstable and often takes place outside of individual's wareness. Always, however, the person affected by Burnout Syndrome experience the exhaustion of physical, emotional, the intellectual and spiritual. Importantly, these problems occur both at working life and leisure time. Therefore, the influence on behavior the unit not only in the workplace, but also have their transfer to family and social environment. Burnout is a complex process, which builds up slowly. Does not appear Suddenly and unexpectedly, but is distributed in time and is usually measured in years. The state of Burnout is the result of prolonged and repeated stress load. Most frequently as a result of years of very intense work, usually associated with intensive operation contacts unfortunately. As a consequence of human functioning in conditions of prolonged stress becomes a factor triggering processes of exasperation, listlessness, discouragement and exhaustion. This collection of symptoms over the months or years to effect what is burnout.

Burnout syndrome is the result of chronic mental exhaustion and sense of the lack of meaning in the action taken. An important factor in the level of Burnout are both stress factors, working conditions, and individual properties of an entity. It is observed, after all, a person, which, despite the unpredictable workloads are still just as involved, charismatic and well know methods for dealing with stressogenic situations. However and unfortunately, most of the public responds to the workload (in each dimension) think ourselves showing: fatigue on many levels of life. Full involvement in work, close contact and the desire to be interpersonal being a professional in their professional activities make you see symptoms of burn-out. Affected people realize a decrease in strength, the sense of the reduction or lack of competence, low self-efficacy and belief about the lack of ability to control events in your life both professional and private. Among the features people particularly susceptible to Burnout instance is given by:

- A strong commitment to work
- Big expectations for their own people
- Denying your own load limits
- Offset by the wayside to your needs and interests
- Willing to accept new responsibilities and tasks
- The imbalance between workload and life satisfaction.

According to the international classification of diseases and related health problems ICD-10 Burnout belongs to the category of problems related to the difficulties in life. Thus, the burnout is related to vulnerability to drift unit loads psychological, and it can be assumed that it is personal experience stress in the social context of work. According to the C. Maslach emotional exhaustion is this component Burnout vocational training, which is most closely associated with stress, which confirms the relevance of the Locate the phenomenon of burn-in stress (personal immunity to stress). At the same time, the author stresses that personality variables and individual differences are less important in the emergence of a burn-out from the social factors. In this way, C. Maslach assigns a special role factors-and as a key source of Burnout indicates the functioning of the organization.

In-depth analysis of the phenomenon of burnout and the results of numerous studies require sacrifice. Special attention needs sytuacyjnemu in startup process of burnout. According to the C. Maslach and Leiter P.M. causes Burnout can be traced in six areas: excessive workloads, lack of a sense of control, insufficient reward, the collapse of the community, the lack of fair treatment and conflict of values. Organizational irregularities in these areas contribute to a work overload, a sense of being undervalued, the loss of the joy of work and the breakdown of relationships. Consequently, the talented, committed and full of good intentions, employees begin to experience difficulties in the relationship with the work (Maslach C. 2001). Chronic burnout seems to be an unavoidable consequence of the lack of response organizational environment for people. Employees working in the state of long-term, permanent stress begin to experience a lack of harmony between your person and the organization. A sense of lack of fit, in effect, provides a starting point for an instance of the burnout. You can therefore be made by Maslach, that causes Burnout should be increasingly sought in the work environment than in the properties of the people.

Nurses

This burnout risk group includes: doctors, nurses, social workers, teachers, police officers, emergency service workers. Among them, a nurse profession holds a special place. Many authors claim that in this profession there is many elements relevant to the development team burnout. These include: personality traits, which are the most desirable image of the role of the professional nurse, beliefs and values that govern the choice of profession, work tremendously demanding emotionally and the structure and organization of work.

Therefore, the occupational group of nurses from the beginning research on burning was the focus of investigators. Studies have helped define this phenomenon, have provided knowledge about its structure and dynamics, there are many theoretical models, which in turn have pointed out how can you prevent the formation and the development of burnout. Burnout can be a huge obstacle in working life and personal people that perform the profession of nurse. Therefore, no investment in prevention of occupational burnout among nurses may not be misconceived. The more that people working in occupations exposed to burn can specify, at least in general, the phenomenon of burnout, it is their awareness of the causes of and capabilities to counter burning is already greatly reduced and falsified. When Freudenberger described for the first time, Burnout, described it as a drop in energy levels that occurs in the employee due to overload other problems. This situation may take place when work is based on the relationships, interpersonal skills, requiring emotional. The author pointed out that the drop in energy results in impaired mental and physical man, which, in turn, negatively affect his professional life and private. For Aronson Burnout is slowly following cessation.

A man in this state has a sense of emotional exhaustion, mental and physical, feels helpless, cannot see in front of you, the work no longer, and integrated tsearch loses also the joy of living. Maslach, a forerunner of research on burning, and the author of basic publications on this topic, she attributed this phenomenon to people carrying out social events in which work with people is on caring relationships. Research carried out among representatives of these professions have resulted in the development by Maslach and Jackson three-material model of burnout, according to which it is defined as a "psychological exhaustion syndrome emotional, depersonalization, and reduced sense of personal achievements, which can occur among people, working with other people in a certain way ". Emotional exhaustion applies to the sense of the person concerned, that the emotional load, which experiencing, beyond its capabilities, that no longer has sufficient resources of emotions, in order to meet the expectations of other people and act as the existing roles. Depersonalisation specifies the ratio of the unit to the other, expressing the excessive isolation, relevant, and even indifferent response to clients or recipients of services. Reduced sense of personal achievements applies against a unit to itself, the deterioration of her sense of competence and efficiency at work.

Nursing belongs to a group of professions of trust society, whose role and social roles are infiltrating, and their representatives are expected to professionalism and conduct by higher ethical-moral standards than those which generally apply to the rest of society. People deciding to practise the profession expect will draw from work satisfaction and satisfaction, that giving of yourself to others will be a source of energy for their own life drive. Work in this profession is associated with experiencing stress on many levels, which, in the absence of effective ways of coping, can lead to a sense of discouragement, load and loss of professional satisfaction. Daily contact with the disease, suffering and death forces the nurse to frequent confrontation with the nieodwołalnością loss of life and health. The provision of nursing care is based on establishing and maintaining a close relationship with a patient symptoms and his loved ones, cooperation with other members of the team of therapeutic and other health professionals and non-medical. The entire surrounding nurse or nurse the world professional also consists of people. Each of them have their psychosocial considerations, set out the views and habits, and each of them is the daily briefs-, which often have their reflection in contact with another human being. This specific type of stress generated by the working relationship with another human being, it makes the profession of nurse one of the most exposed to burnout. Although the commitment, high sensitivity and a sense of responsibility for others, as well as resourcefulness and reliability are the characteristics of a very desirable, because it allow you to be a good nurse, is very conducive to emotional overload. The susceptibility to burn predisposes also multi-purpose nature of the work and its complex structure and organization. Occupational requirements in relation to the nurses continually grow to meet them, it is necessary to increase the level of knowledge and professional qualifications and social skills. The nominated social can be for nursing staff a heavy load. The society believes that nurses profession is a very responsible job and often expresses itself in dealing with staff. It is not always done in a glorious and often a nurse as a direct contact with the patient experiencing unpleasant situation, and claim-in its meaning of degrading its dignity and giving seed of guilt and discomfort.

In the course of being carried out repeatedly for research on the burnout phenomenon on nurses, there were burdensome and negatively perceived characteristics of the profession, which are grouped into specific categories.

Requirements related to the specificity of the profession (they can be analysed before the decision on the selection of the profession because they are predictable, but impossible to eliminate), irregular lifestyle caused by work on the shifts, particularly at night. The lack of regularity in the functioning of the body, collapsing circadian rhythm with the need to sleep during periods for physiological sleep is seen by the nurses as a very big disadvantage. After decades of mixing on the same night the body goes (many people) in the phase of the rebellion with often severe psychosomatic symptoms. Often, women bringing up young children complain of terrible fatigue when after a few months or even weeks of his notorious Act by your child at night are finished and chronically tired. The same problem applies to people from the circadian rhythm in case of frequent travel, especially with the change of time. Adjusting and reverting to hemostasis is not simple and requires always the time. We are at the stage of evolution of the accustomed to regularity you dictate by the Sun, the light and the pineal gland. It allows us to organize our existence in a certain framework and allows the cyclical reset. Unfortunately, even the regular participation in the disturbed, but reversed rhythm of life does not cause organic habit. This includes, inter alia, the duty of health care professionals. Because continuous exposure to currency fluctuations in this topic might be for those inconvenient or even harmful.

The possibility of being infected through close physical contact with the sick, contact with secretions, feces and dirt-is another aspect that was extracted as a factor stimulating a sense of inconvenience. Uncertainty concerning the contact with another human being, limited confidence as to his sincerity, integrity in a situation when the US obligation to provide him with the necessary assistance can be applied. Continuous vigilance procedures and rapid assessment of the situation in order to obtain the maximum safety for health and life not only the patient, but also his, is always at the expense of emotional. Especially in the case of contact with the patient difficult, aggressive, bet live as Newcastle try. Always, after all, there are somewhere in the US care for coming and for their safety. Sick, or the transfer of disease to family members is something undesirable, it's obvious. The element of risk is also seen very unfavorably inclined not only incidentally by the nurses.

The cumbersome lists also the elements of physical work accompanying the implementation of treatment steps and nurturing. To perform the difficult and complicated medical procedures with the patient is picked up by a nurse as a big minus in the performance of professional activities. Despite the technical facilities and the specific rules and procedures many times reality put nursing staff before the ruthless reality. Heavy patients, helping with daily activities or monotone each step does not allow you to find here comfortable conditions of work. Nurse, by participating in the many hours of interdisciplinary operations with a huge amount of equipment wysokospecjalistycznego, must force your body to long hours of inconvenient and niefizjologicznych body position. Preparation of equipment, tools and material completed in weighing several kilograms's also is entered in the roles of nurses working in operating room. Many times it has been shown that physical exhaustion factor or systemic diseases (diseases of the spine, heart disease) are link inflammation to begin a process of frustration ending multi-clip tray of the burnout syndrome. Symptom of disability, infirmity of his own body in the case of nursing personnel is reflected in the thinking about reduced fitness in your profession. This is a very sad, but but very real picture.

To the mental stress include (reasonably foreseeable, but their effort makes itself felt only in the course of work) a huge responsibility with which involves medication and treatment and the awareness that the mistake may be worsening of the patient's health or even death. Aggravating also need to maintain vigilance and control to frequent contact with pain, suffering, disability and death. Experience with human suffering, including suffering (sufferers often associate in nurses who accompanied in the healing process) is an amazing emotional baggage for this occupational group. The emotional considerations, which should be equipped with a nurse, although so very desirable, are often shot in the knee. Unconditional empathy can improve, refine the process of treatment, thanks to the wczuciu the role of the patient. Allows you to visualize your needs. However, the excess emotional border integration with the patient can be an emotional suicide for medical staff. Especially if the final effect of the treatment process, very different from the initial assumptions and perceptions. There are known cases when the death or disability of a patient, despite all efforts, wyryły in so destructive in the personality of the employee, that caused the collapse of his own professional values, led to rebellion and abandon the profession. An important element contributing to the determination of this criterion are also normal, everyday interpersonal relations. It is important who we work with, we exchange views and who listens to us, especially if we are in the process of treating another human being. The most difficult are the relationships in times of high tension associated with the performance obligations. Often, the dynamics of the treatment process-which include unplanned phrases in the healing process of the patient as a cardiac arrest patient, massive bleeding during the operation or totally unexpected reactions of the organism – cause no self-control of some co-workers. Surgical nurses adept to the profession, as the biggest stress determine deposited operator. The lack of the basic principles of social interaction, lack of manners and aggressive ignorance represent a major challenge to maintain emotional balance and often and activities of nurses. To pass on mutual professional liability or official blame incompetence (often not scratch) only for the release of your own emotions for example. the doctor is not at all uncommon. Although that offended by the nurse is aware of your own values and refuted such accusations, however, it is always associated with huge interpersonal discomfort and at rozchwianiem. Difficult subject is also alienation and lack of acceptance in the environment. Is a very serious matter, and many employee, not only in health care, forced to change career plans.

The lack of conditions for the treatment of (elements that hinder or prevent the process of treatment and nursing care, and nurses have no effect on their occurrence): instrumental deficiencies (e.g., lack of medicines, bandages, disposable equipment, medical equipment), some general (for example, for an insufficient nursing staff in relation to the number of patients, architectural barriers, bad liked) and system deficiencies (e.g. obsolete provisions, storage meltdowns, organisation of medical care). To the wider comfort nursing also contributes in no small degree of technical facilities. For educated and experienced nurses lack of comprehensiveness in the treatment of the patient is very disruptive and clearly this is marked in the form of various surveys and forms when examining the problem of burnout or evaluating of the quality of working conditions. Is a very important element of a sense of safety in the workplace. Very depressed for nursing environment fact simultaneous contact with the responsibility of compliance with defined and imposed top medical procedures in the collision with the lack of physical (hardware, lekowym, human resources) the completion of these formalities. It reminds the situation if we wanted to write a book, we know the spelling rules, we know what will be its title and plot but ... we have no paper or have only a pen and a twist on what to start writing. Sad but true and unfortunately very common. As previously mentioned the nurses most often do not have this effect, and it's even more compounded by frustration in them which is a vector to burnout. The lack of any manoeuvres, impotency and often forcing the overriding quality standards makeshift solutions gives nurses a feeling of flimsiness of their hard work. This peculiar and painful despair, Inc. in their working lives of nurses. Due to the expansion of the scope of the rights of the patient and the number of lawsuits for not done medical procedures-this situation is planned to improve it but it is still an element of stressful work of health protection.

Low wages, that is, whether the remuneration of nurses to professional requirements and individual effort expended by the nurses in its execution, is also unfavorable for nurses disparity in salary compared to other professional groups. Becoming a nurse in the whole world is with very very difficult multi-stage education. In the field of higher education in many countries over the last 30 years a huge transformation and expanded the level of teaching in the training of nursing personnel. In addition to the graduate medical universities is also required continuous training to postgraduate. Also because of the quite understandable breakdown of the specialties in nursing (dictated by the dynamic development of the Departments of Medicine) is required to have the title of specialist in the active field of nursing. It is therefore the obligation of continuing education for nurses and broaden his knowledge. If we add to these values responsibilities per nurse, her kompetencyjność and responsibility, we have before us a highly qualified provider of security services society health needs. So why to continue this profession if they cannot look forward to an appropriate financial gratification for their work? Dissatisfaction with the salary is not a whim or unelegant nudge. It is a response to discomfort. For centuries, it is known that one of the strongest motivators to action is money and ethical consideration for the work. In many countries it is a very controversial topic and although low salaries of nurses are a matter of indisputable unfortunately are field continuing battles with the dignity of this group financial professional. Referring to the burnout it is not difficult to understand that this issue is a very important element influencing negative perceptions of their profession through the prism of financial attractiveness. The lack of opportunities for a dignified existence received salary or work in several hospitals to go on holiday are an effective intimidation to perform the profession and factor effectively lowering your own ego. Hence, the simple way to burnout.

Low professional status, which is manifested by lack of real social recognition for easy work of nurses, lack of legal acts governing the position of nurses in the functioning of the health system. Still, the role of nurses in society is unclear, not clearly identified and conflict. There are people who regard nurses for wise and competent person, trustworthy and socially necessary. However, still and too often, this occupational group is considered from the point of view of its servile function. Crushed by centuries of belief may not enjoy the concept of nurses as independent skilled professions that the profession of public confidence and the necessary to the proper functioning of health care at a high level. Nurses are today members of the treatment team, the leading independent responsible processes of patient care. Often, the nurse is a source of knowledge about the patient and often first takes important first steps in the healing process. The enormity of the knowledge and skills required to have a nurse puts them to a high degree in the hierarchy of professions, not just medical. Very unfair is the treatment of these people only as a medical and social assessment this low contributes to very bad emotional sentiment among nursing staff. Nurse pay duties, overwhelmed by the vastness of knowledge and unappreciated for inserted in their work efforts and commitment have the right to be frustrated, has the right not to feel satisfaction from the way they chose. The base to the very conflicting, warring emotions between vocation and pure regret to ... yourself, to your colleagues and also for the patient.

The evil team cooperation to healing, the most important are the problems resulting from the hierarchical structure of the profession, such as: receiving conflicting instructions from supervisors at different levels and dumping responsibility for the effects of the therapy for nurses. The cumbersome lists also difficulty in interpersonal relations with people involved in the same issue, for example. with medical staff, technical, secondary, employees of the administration. This category lists also demote work nurses by people directly working with them, in a situation when the presentation of recognition would be for them an important gratification. In principle, this category is something like the previous problem with low respect for the nursing profession. As previously mentioned, it is difficult to break, change ingrained social position on the status of this group. Any produced no balance of competence or the correctness of the interpersonal relationship on different lines: the superior-nurse, doctor-nurse, the patient-nurse are the consequence of too low a recognition of this profession. This is reflected in the many aspects, not only about personal dignity but also to promote.

Bad cooperation with patients and their families: the difficulties in building correct relationships caused by personality traits and the wrong understanding by them of the role of nurses, the instrumental treatment of nurses, lack of respect, excessive requirements and requests of the sick, the lack of feedback from patients about the satisfaction with the work of nurses, which deprives them of one of the most important gratification in this profession, namely recognition in the eyes of the patient and his family. For real, involved nurse patient is the meaning of her work. Every action and every think that performs on the professional field is dedicated to the patient. The real nail in the coffin in the course of professional work, unimaginable defeat and a very unpleasant experience for nurse is the patient's dissatisfaction and lack of therapeutic effect, even though the wearer effort and dedication. It is often lightly tossed, misplaced. Often, malice caused by frustration of the patient or his family. However, it is always a painful kick that remains in the minds and prompts to the destructive analysis and ask questions: what I did wrong? You may need to be different?, And so on. Such events definitely reduce the value of self-assessment of nurses, subject under question the meaning of her dedication and sacrifice.

Illustration of the above categories on the burnout clearly shows that the causes are very complex. Many authors agree that overall, Burnout is the result of chronic stresowego the nature of the interaction that occurs between the person and the situation. Repeatability of certain hostile events, fear them or their consequences are the engine for progressive, most often the slow evolution of burnout syndrome.

Paramedics

Medical emergency is an area, where the source of stress is the second, the stranger and the situation which led to interference with emergency services. Sometimes it is the same patient, and sometimes the people with whom you interact in providing aid. Paramedic is a qualified health care professional who participates in the immediate life-saving interventions or human health. For him the situations or the average, but not devoid of large dose of stress. Is a member of a small team, working with doctors, nurses, emergency response personnel from other ambulances and hospital Emergency Room workers. Is in direct contact with the family of the patient, which can be particularly difficult in a situation of sudden illness or accident of a child when it needs to alleviate the fear and panic of his parents. The rescuer often passes through a thin barrier of privacy of the patient, and even his intimacy. Enters into his apartment, he finds it in moments of greatest weakness, not only physical, but also mental and social. The patient expects from the rescuer fast and professionally, alleviate suffering, his focus and commitment. This situation is stressful for the rescuer, and the same patient for which lifeguard is still a foreign person, often decisive to its fate (Cydulka R.K. 2008).

There are some common factors in the work of the paramedic, who are the primary source of stress. These include a sense of lack of control-as a lifeguard is a variety of factors, which it influences and such that are outside of its control. As a result of the complicated and very elaborate apprenticeships in the course of education and training-is a conscious situation and predict events that may arise in the course of its activities and current circumstances. Is prepared for a rapid response and to prevent unwanted effects. However, despite a solid preparation, you may receive a number of inconveniences and unconventional situations, which may come as a surprise to the rescuer, and at the same time to become a source of stress. The latter situations when rescuer meets with violence on the part of the patient or his family, which especially happens when they are under the influence of alcohol or other drugs (Popa f. 2010) Sometimes also known by paramedic is the body's response to the deployed treatment-positive or negative, sometimes despite the efforts of the terminating in death. Next a stressor is a sense of uncertainty – it may arise from doubts about the rightness of choices, as well as doubt their own abilities. When the rescuer takes professional activities to help the patient his knowledge about the patient is quite limited. Not always to the end of the spectrum is able to obtain information about his health status, lifestyle, recent activities or medicines. Follow specific tailored to the situation of the procedures, however, the choice of the proper procedure may be initially it works, a huge dose of stress. Everyday work in a medical emergency is the need to make tough decisions in a short period of time. When you are not certain your wrong, which may depend on a human life, there is uncertainty as one of the biggest stressors that can lead to burnout syndrome. As in the case of nurses, eternal fiancee fights with uncertainty and stress of taken decisions is a great field to the development of burnout syndrome.

To paramedic are high requirements. The specificity of work in emergency services undoubtedly involves the exposure of their situations dangerous to life. They are related to the high voltage przeplatanym long periods of relative calm, or routine. Negative interpersonal relationships, the excess duties are sources of stress in the emergency services and the nature of traumatic events with which the rescuers come together every day to increase work-related tensions. The threat of physical harm to health, participation in situations requiring rapid and difficult medical decisions, frequent confrontation with life threatening and the sheer scale of the death and a sense of helplessness during the rescue process, causes massive emotional tension and mental exhaustion. Where the magnitude of the maximum concentration and emotional involvement with the use of manual, physical skills wieńczony is a poor result or the death of a patient before a lifeguard stands tall internal skill understanding and come to terms with it.

It is understandable, therefore, that this work requires special predisposition and high resistance. In the relationship with the patient lifespan is based on its competence and trust, which must get in the eyes of the victim in a very short period of time. Typically, the contact with the patient is short-lived, and the opinion that creates the situations is persistent. Therefore, it is essential to have a good psychological paramedic preparation for some undesirable patient relationship did not become a source of emotional discomfort in a lifeguard.

In particularly difficult situations, paramedic must be prepared to make a decision not or the cessation of rescue intervention. This applies to patients able to extremely severe, Terminal, or if the action to restore vital functions exceeds the time specified procedurally. Decisions “do not resuscitate” are also part of ethics and moral in the relationship with the patient and his family. These moments of rescuers describe as exceptionally difficult and dangerous to your psyche. Tangible contact with death and accompanied by her circumstances (despair of loved ones) is always a huge experience and long stays in memory. Many rescue workers shall be loose talks that several relatives were abandoning the profession because of the trauma of a failed rescue action.

Stress also has an impact on the take by paramedic yet difficult decisions in emergency mass, epidemics or disasters. Sense of responsibility for a lot of people in conjunction with stress-can run be paralysing for a person with low adaptive capacity. As a rule, adrenaline makes the increase in activity and physical mobilization. However, the repeated experience of such situations leads to the gradual burnout, indifference and fatigue. A symptom is also addiction to adrenaline and desire to participate in such events is made only for a specific boost having no connection with the empathy and the desire to help. However, these are isolated cases.

Another source of stress may be the feeling of failure to meet expectations - every man from the people, which to some extent deliberately helps counts on gratitude or though a good word, which is the simple word “thank you”. Similar expectations, often unconscious, has a paramedic in relation to the people that care, helps in difficult circumstances, sometimes even saves lives. However, at the time of the threat to his health or life the patient focused on yourself and do not mean that at this point, to show gratitude to someone. All of this can cause the rescuer feeling that more gives you from each other than an instead. An important and always found a stressor is paramedic work stress of shift work. Problem discussed in the case of group discussion in this nursing profession have similar consequences. It results mainly from the natural circadian cycle disorders, or work during the day and sleep at night. However, it is a part of their job description, because the health service providers must be constantly available, and the quality of their action must be the same at any time of the day. Shift work entails adverse effects for the body, such as sleep disorders, chronic fatigue, which leads to a deflection and dysfunction in family life and society. It contributes to the severity of the negative feelings, the deterioration of the health and physical and mental. It lowers the sense of satisfaction, causes increased tension, the deterioration of self-esteem and decrease efficiency. For employers, this means a decrease in performance and safety and increased sickness absence.

Too long exposure to stress at work can have irreversible health effects, directly affects the reduction of efficiency, lack of compassion for the victims and the existence of negative feelings to yourself such as lowering self-esteem or self-worth. All of these factors can result in reduced ability to overcome stress and consequently move away from the profession.

In the activities of the paramedics there is also the problem of injuries and exposure to infection to pathogenic organic material. Lifting heavy patients and transporting them to the vehicle contributes to later problems with their bones and muscles injuries. The scale of paramedic workers problems is huge and often disqualifies a person to practise this profession.

The profession of paramedic is a job in which exposure to stress is high and where there is a risk of the burnout syndrome. In an Israeli study of a group of paramedics, the burnout occurred in 35% of the polled individuals(Nirel N. 2008). A similar result can be observed in the study, in which 35% of respondents noticed to feel tired at home exhausted all day, what is considered to be a symptom of the burnout. In addition, most of the surveyed people considered their work to be too stressful, and noted the presence of the selected symptoms of the burnout.

Most incriminating factor at work in the light of the results obtained is the remuneration system. However, the most common sign of the burnout was a signifficant tiredness after work. Most of tested individuals have confirmed the use of some constructive ways to deal with stress, but also the unconstructive ones, such as the use of stimulants (including caffeine and nicotine), where consumption increased in difficult situations. Although the vast majority of paramedics have recognized his work as valuable and would have chosen a job in this profession again. There was a moderate and high level of job satisfaction among the responders, what is similar to the results of the research done among American doctors of emergency medicine specialties, where, despite the high level of the burnout, 65% of physicians found their work to be satisfying. Based on the research it can be concluded that among working in Krakow and the surrounding area paramedics there is a dangerously many symptoms of the burnout. This shows the employers the need for creation and implementation some activities to reduce stress levels among employees and to prevent the occurrence of the burnout. Early action, such as a minimalization of the excessive stress or reduction of early symptoms of the burn-out, would prevent the progress of a full-blown intrathecal burnout syndrome (Dudek B. 2004). It is very important that the effects of stress and burnout are experienced not only by employees, but also by the paramedics' employers, who have got among their staff members many worse burnout cases than some of the patients, who consequently receive lower quality care. Nevertheles, there are many effective interventions helping to build a resistance to stress, lower the tension during especially difficult situations (death of the patient, the mass event, etc.), such as providing psychological support and training, relaxation techniques, promoting physical activity and maintenance of appropriate rest periods between their work shifts.

One of the popular methods implemented by employers should be the hiring of psychologist, who helps the paramedics in difficult situations. Particularly important aspect of this form of support is working with rescuers immediately after a particularly traumatic experiences, so called debriefing. The importance of this method was asknowledged by an international practice, since the lack of a suitable psychological action after such an event can lead to post-traumatic stress disorder and serious risk of the rapid burnout (Regel S. 2007). In addition, some employers promote active leisure time as a form of coping with stress and finanse employees tickets to the gym, swimming pool, etc., which is an important element in supporting psychological interventions. So far, however, there haven't done any research studies to analyze the effects of these interventions on the level of work-related burningout among paramedics (at least in Poland).

The analysis of these two occupational groups provides a good illustration of the causality of the onset of the burnout symptoms. In recent years the scale of the problem is so large and growing that it has become the subject of verification and observation in each group. Modern psychology very seriously treats this phenomenon and continues working on developing some ways of minimizing its prevalence.

Therefore, the measures taken to prevent burn-out are associated directly with the antistress activities. Primary prevention concerns the work environment. It should consist of the assessment of the psychological risk and elimination or modification of those risk factors that put stress upon employees in order to minimize their amount and eventually to avoid the occurance of the tension. Secondary prevention relates to people. Its mission is to teach the employee how they can effectively deal with the existing stressful situations. Secondary prevention relates to an individual, not to the work environment. Tertiary prevention also applies to a person, but it is to treat the health consequences experienced by the stressed out employee.

According to H. Sęk, the burnout counteracting factors are: a sense of cognitive control, which comes from some positive self-esteem experiences and willingness to make certain personal changes; general acceptance of the own job effectiveness as a positive feeling of resoursefulness. Therefore, the measures to prevent the burnout symptoms development should include the improvement of employee's self-esteem, mainly by increasing his sense of professional competence; strengthening the initial challenge assessment, which is assessing the employee's situation as a challenge. According to H.Sęk, the prevention of burnout should find both the positive and negative strategies. Positive strategies aim at strengthening environmental resources. With regard to the nursing profession, positive approach would be equipping medical field professionalists and students of nursing with the general skills to deal with their stress. The social skills improvement and the proper use of the commitment decks and empathy are as important as professional preparation. It is also crucial to develop the skills to use the positive life experiences and evolution of realistic professional beliefs. The negative strategies are adjusted to minimize risk factors. They consist of reducing and eliminating job nuisance, especially at the macro-social level, for example, by changing the salaries, strengthening the social status of the profession, reducing financial and organisational deficits. The intensity and duration of the stress impact stress can be also decreased by some individual's activities, for example by an appropriate rest, relaxation, maintaining work-life balance. The negative strategy should also modify favorable burnout attitudes and personality traits and the completion of the actual shortage of professional competence. Most of the authors suggests that preventive efforts and countermeasures to Burnout took place at several levels: individual, institutional and institutional indywidualno.

Action at the individual level are based on the use of personal resources of the unit to prevent the negative effects of stress. Most commonly used strategies for samopoznaniu and strategies on reducing the effects of stress.

The first consists of employee learning techniques of self-observation, self metric using professional measuring tools to detect signs of burnout, stress control by passive and active knowledge on this topic. To strategies to reduce the effects of stress include: promoting a healthy lifestyle (regular physical activity, proper nutrition, a sufficient number of hours of sleep, to comply with naprzemienności of work and rest, smoking tobacco), the use of different relaxation techniques (in order to remove unwanted, physiological stress response), cognitive behavioral techniques notes the erroneous and harmful beliefs about work to be done. Action at the level of the relationship – the unit is addressed mainly to increase the resilience of the employee's work-related stressors. The task of the intervention in this area is: increased employee knowledge about its own capabilities and limitations, developing effective strategies to handle deal with problems and negative emotions, emotional, instrumental and support in the workplace, the availability of treatment for people at risk of burning and rehabilitation for people "shred". Among the possible to take preventive actions at the level of the employee-company work include: the implementation of educational programmes on stress and burnout, organizing training interpersonal skills, communication and conflict resolution, coping with stress, training, management of own time and the proper use of working time, promoting realistic knowledge of the profession and "professional life". An important element in the prevention of stress and burnout on the level of intervention is to organise in the workplace social support system. Employee support groups would create the appropriate social climate in the environment work, give the possibility of emotional odreagowania issues and get advice from people more experienced. Social support obtained by other team action than formal support groups led by trained leaders also fully protective function before burning. Especially the involvement of associates in creating the atmosphere of camaraderieand kindness, help in the adaptation of the professional staff, common to discuss issues of care, the possibility of exchanging professional experience, showing itself by associates of mutual respect and recognition of [1]. Measures to prevent the development of symptoms of Burnout at the level of the institutions are targeted to increase quality and reduce costs. To this end, it is proposed to carry out regular staff, anonymous testing, allowing to estimate problem of stress and the risk of burnout. Employees in addition to the mandatory health examinations, should be able to carry out a voluntary survey assessing the symptoms of burn-out. Workplace can and should strive to improve the work environment by removing or modifying the stressors, improve mutual communication workers, prevention of buiding up theconflicts at work, the introduction of additional holidays or breaks to enable a more efficient recuperation, to enable employees to participate in internal and external training. Other suggestions relate to the introduction of flexible work plan, adequate to the contribution of the reward system, establish clear and fair principles of management, a clear determination of professional obligations, the inclusion of employees in planning professional development. Reasonable is considered also the creation of the Department of Health Care Services, which would provide a professional guidance for people at risk of burning out and implement prevention programs. As you can see the possibilities of preventing burnout among professional nurses is much. The burnout prevention strategy should already begin at the stage of medical training and last throughout the period of individual's career. It seems that the implementation of a preventive measure system would help to reduce this negative phenomena among nurses.

CONCLUSION

In the face of numerous studies on the working environment, the concept of professional burnout is not new. Around the world, almost every civilized country is home to organizations and institutions that research the working environment. Establishing and accepting that the working environment, the type of activity performed, and any inconveniences that may be a part of the psychophysical state of an employee, actually took years. Several decades of work, primarily psychologists and sociologists, have resulted in the systematization of the notion of professional burnout. While already observing such a phenomenon among the professional community can be regarded as undoubted success in the field of health and safety at work, implementation and public recognition is not always easy and achievable. In many countries, this topic is still very controversial or is not very serious. The phenomenon that disturbs the assumption of efficient and effective work in which an employee is merely a source or income vector is by no means undesirable. The concept of professional burnout after lichen in many communities does not work. This is primarily a topic that concerns certain professions. The isolation of particular occupational groups, particularly those exposed to professional burnout, contributed to the analysis of the working conditions of the people who performed the occupations. It has confirmed the socio-psychological assumption that all our human actions leave us unmovable, often very lasting. Once again it was proved this time on the professional canvas that man is an integrated psychophysical whole. Working, carrying out daily duties is a huge part of life for the vast majority of mankind. For many it is the meaning and the driving force of life. A force that can not be rid of or separated from everyday life. But there are some people for whom work is not a passion and a source of satisfaction. The conditions under which they have to perform the imposed duties are so unfriendly and in many respects contradictory to the correct rules of work hygiene, ethics and social cohesion that are rather a substitute for discomfort and perception of work as necessary evil.

Medical staff is a special occupational group. Mental involvement in contact with another person, the individual treatment of each patient through the lens of empathy and compassion in connection with severe technical conditions (such as patient lifting, exposure to injury and infection) is a cocktail that translates into many aspects of a medical worker's life. Not without reason the nurses are included in the results of many studies as workers are exceptionally exploited and are particularly exposed to the windshield and short working life. Also, medical staff life expectancy does not reach long periods of time. The embarrassing "professional burnout" is primarily a worker's performance problem. However, few employers analyze the working conditions that their employees provide. The ignorance of the problem and noticing the needs of subordinates, not perceiving the "human element" in them, leads most often to lowering the quality of their services. In the case of public health, it is a very risky practice to take care of the health and life of the public. Balancing on the border of safety and responsibility. Lack of decisive, wisely developed and above all the stubbornness of the implemented methods of preventing this phenomenon. Although employers' awareness and work culture evolve, however, the prevention of this topic is very low. Young people who start medical studies in the fields of nursing or medical rescue of the "second face" of the profession are not anticipated. Nobody prepares them and does not realize how to handle the tremendous amount of stress they will face in professional life. They are not aware that, as a result of total sacrifice and lack of separation skills from private life, they may "burn" and that the risk of burnout is so great. They learn about it accidentally or when they feel discouraged for work, fall into depression or have a full spectrum of psychosomatic symptoms. Only the enormous involvement of occupational psychologists, even greater popularization of the issue, and top-notch recognition of occupational burnout as a rational threat to health and disease - will gradually increase our self-awareness as employees as contributors to the proper functioning of our communities.

REFERENCES

Anczewska, M., Switaj, P., & Roszczyńska, J. (2005). *Professional burnout.* In Phases of Psychiatry and Neurology.

Bytnar, B. (2010). *Quality of life of instrumentalists working in shifts.* Rzeszów: Przegląd Medyczny Uniwersytetu Rzeszowskiego.

Cydulka, R. K., & Korte, R. (2008). Career satisfaction in EM: The ABEM longitudinal study of Emergency Physicians. *Annals of Emergency Medicine, 51*(6), 714–722. doi:10.1016/j.annemergmed.2008.01.005 PMID:18395936

Czerniak, J. (2012). Accidental bumps. *Magazyn Pielęgniarki i Położnej*, 7-8.

Debrand-Passard, A., & Luce-Wunderle, G. (2010). *Operational nursing.* Wroclaw: Urban & Partner.

Dębska, G., Pasek, M., & Wilczek-Rużyczka, E. (2014). *Psychological burden and professional burnout among nurses working in various occupational specializations.* Poland: Hygeia Public Healt.

Dłużewska, M. (2012). Exploration of conditions in the formation of the burnout process - analysis based on own research. *Pielęgniarstwo Polskie, 2*(44), 63–72.

Dudek, B., Waszkowska, M., Merecz, D., & Hanke, W. (2004). Protection of workers' health from the effects of occupational stress. Institute of Occupational Medicine, Łódź.

Erenkfeit, K., Dudzińska, L. & Indyk, A. (2012). The impact of the working environment on the emergence of professional burnout. *Medycyna Środowiskowa* [Enviromental Medicine], *15*(3), 121-128.

Fengler, J. (2000). *Helping to tire-burn in work.* Gdansk: Gdańskie Wydawnictwo Psychologiczne.

Florkowski, M. (2009). *Working nights. Work and Health.* Warszawa: Unimedia.

Freudenberger, H. J. (1974). Staff burn-out. *The Journal of Social Issues, 30*(1), 159–165. doi:10.1111/j.1540-4560.1974.tb00706.x

Freudenberger, H. J. (1983). *Burnout: Contemporary issues, trends and concerns. Stress and burnout in the human service professions.* New York: Pergamon.

Golembiewski, R. T., Boudreau, R. A., Sun, B. C., & Luo, H. (1998). *Estimates of burnout in public agencies.* Public Administr Rev.

Iwanowicz-Palus, G. (2005). *Valuing work. Management in nursing.* Lublin. Czelej, Iwanowicz- Palus, G. J. & Kicia, M. (2005). *To burn must be on fire - stress and professional burnout in nurses and midwives.* Poland. *Pielęgniarstwo, XXI*, 25–27.

Kaducakova, H., & Lehotska, M. (2010). *Factors influencing the work of nurses in social welfare centers* (pp. 176–183). Cracow: AFM.

Ksykiewicz-Dorota, A. (2005). *Ergonomic analysis of the work. Management in nursing.* Lublin: Czelej.

Kuriata, E., Felińczak, A., Grzebieluch, J., & Szachniewicz, M. (2011). Detrimental factors and workload of nurses employed in the hospital. Part II. Nursing. *Public Health*, 269–273.

Lewandowska, A., & Litwin, B. (2009). Professional burnout as a threat to nursing work. In Yearbook of the Pomeranian Medical Academy in Szczecin.

Łuczak, A. (2011). *Standardization work on mental workload* (pp. 105–115). Kraków: PAN.

Maslach, C. (2001). What have we learned about burnout and health? *Psychology & Health.*

Maslach, C., & Leiter, M. (1997). *The truth about burnout.* San Francisco, CA: Jossey-Bass.

Maslach, C., & Schaufeli, W. B. (1993). *Historical and conceptual development of burnout. Professional burnout: Recent developments in theory and research.* Washington, DC: Taylor and Francis.

Maslach, C. A. (1998). Multidimensional theory of burnout. Theories of organizational stress. Oxford University Press 68-85, New York.

Maslach, C. & Jackson, S. (1982). Burnout in health professions: A social psychological analysis. Social psychology of health and illness. New York: Erlbaum.

Nirel, N., Goldwag, R., Feigenberg, Z., Abadi, D., & Halpern, P. (2008). Stress, work overload, burnout, and satisfaction among paramedics in Israel. *Prehospital and Disaster Medicine, 23*(06), 537–546. doi:10.1017/S1049023X00006385 PMID:19557971

Popa, F., & Arafat, R. (2010). Occupational Burnout levels in Emergency Medicine – a nationwide study and analysis. *Journal of Medicine and Life, 3*(3), 207–215. PMID:20945809

Ramuszewicz, M., Krajewska-Kułak, E., Rolka, H., Łukaszuk, C., & Kułak, K. (2005). Problem of professional burnout among operative nurses. *Surgery Poland, VII*, 244–251.

Regel, S. (2007). Post-trauma support in the workplace: The current status and practice of critical incident stress management (CISM) and psychological debriefing (PD) within organizations in the UK. *Occupational Medicine (Philadelphia, Pa.), 57*(6), 411–416. PMID:17728314

Schaufeli, W., & Enzmann, D. (1998). *The burnout companion to study and practice: A Critical Analysis.* London: Taylor & Francis.

Sęk, H. (2012). *Professional burnout. Reasons and prevention.* Warsaw: PWN.

Wrońska, I., & Krajewska-Kułak, E. (2007). Selected issues in European nursing. Czelej, Lublin.

Chapter 5
The Patient/Provider Relationship in Emergency Medicine:
Organization, Communication, and Understanding

Julita Soczywko
Nicolaus Copernicus University, Poland

Dorota Rutkowska
Nicolaus Copernicus University, Poland

ABSTRACT

Emergency medicine is a rapidly developing medical specialty which focuses on the diagnostic process, initial stabilization, and the treatment of patients suffering from acute illnesses or injuries. Emergency care can be provided in prehospital settings by emergency medical services, as well as in emergency departments. The primary providers of emergency care are: emergency medicine physicians, emergency nurses, and paramedics. Emergency medical personnel are required to be prepared to take decisive action at any time of day or night. It is essential for them to possess basic knowledge relating to psychology and an ability to utilize interpersonal communication skills. A critical role of medical workers in emergency settings is to provide a patient with emotional support coupled with medical assistance. Interpersonal communication skills depend on the personal abilities of an individual, however, these skills can be also enhanced through training and work experience.

INTRODUCTION

In this occupation, emergency medical staff frequently confront human tragedy. It is essential for them to possess basic knowledge relating to psychology and an ability to utilize interpersonal communication skills. Emergency medical personnel trained in the practice of interpersonal communication and

DOI: 10.4018/978-1-5225-3946-9.ch005

psychology are able to establish a relationship with a patient based on trust. This type of bond helps to build a relationship between the patient and the medical professional that creates a level of comfort between the two parties. This level of comfort creates a situation where the taking of a patient's history, performing a physical examination, or the starting of treatment, all become easier for both the patient, and the medical professional.

Working long shifts under difficult circumstances, frequent emotional involvement at work along with exposure to chronic stress, can lead to the emotional and physical exhaustion of emergency medical personnel. All these factors can be the cause of the development of professional burnout syndrome. Depending on the level of the advancement of burnout syndrome, proper steps should be taken by an employee, in order to regain a physical and mental balance. Treatment of burnout syndrome is based on rest and the establishment of the proper work/life balance. When an individual has reached the most advanced stage of this condition, professional counseling is required.

Due to exposure to chronic stress, resulting in burnout syndrome, many changes occur in the body's physiological pathways. These changes can ultimately lead to a deterioration of an individual's general health and the development of a number of serious diseases. The diagnosis of burnout syndrome involves psychological questionnaires and laboratory tests.

The diagnosis and prevention of burnout syndrome plays a crucial role in highly demanding professions, such as emergency medicine physician, emergency nurse or paramedic. In order to promote the prevention of this syndrome, it requires regular access to counseling, training in coping with difficult situations, and learning to maintain a work/life balance. The prevention of burnout syndrome should be the result of mutual cooperation between an employer and his/her employees.

Emergency medicine plays a vital role in the field of health promotion. Emergency medical personnel because of their education and training, are well equipped to provide the general public with basic information regarding first aid in case of emergencies. These educational programs are frequently organized for children in schools, employees in their workplaces, or among volunteers interested in this matter. Educational programs in first aid and basic life support aim to provide the general public with medical knowledge, which may now, or in the future prove useful in saving lives.

Emergency Medicine in Poland: How It Started

In November of 1999, a government program entitled, "Integrated Emergency Medical Services", began in Poland. The program primarily included the creation, as well as, the formation of the organizational structures of the emergency departments including the training and development of specialized medical personnel. Simultaneously, new structures pertaining to prehospital emergency medical services were developed. These developments initiated the creation of a new wide-ranging emergency medicine system.

The state emergency medical services law (Ustawa, 1868) was adopted in 2006, and it altered both Polish emergency medicine and the emergency medical services system of the country. The law defined, in a straightforward manner, the composition of the system which included the emergency departments and prehospital emergency medical teams.

Structurally, the law's goals were the integration of the units within the emergency medical services system, and the continuing educational and professional development of the specialized groups of medical staff working in the system. Another objective was to establish the positions of emergency medicine specialist (physician), emergency medicine nurse, and licensed paramedic. The last of these professions, licensed paramedic, was a new position which required the establishment of a new set of qualifications as per the new law.

The Main Objectives of Emergency Medicine in Poland

The undeniable right of every human being is access to healthcare, and in life threatening situations, access to specialized, highly qualified medical attention as soon as possible. The main goals are to stabilize the patient, relieve pain and suffering, as well as to provide guidance regarding further specialist care and treatment if needed. Every person in society is entitled to a healthcare system that complies with basic human rights.

Beginning in 1999, Poland's commitment to the above-mentioned healthcare objectives demonstrated the country's growing maturity, and strongly indicated the importance of the healthcare agenda. It also provided evidence of the country's attention to its citizens' health safety. As a result, emergency medicine became a rapidly developing branch of medicine. The organization of emergency medicine focused on delivering rapid and highly effective prehospital care, as well as the treatment of patients with immediate threats to their health. Improvements in emergency medicine training were also developed with an emphasis placed on research, clinical work, graduate and postgraduate studies.

Emergency medicine as a clinical discipline has several core goals. The most important being the basic human right to the guarantee of quality medical care particularly during a life threatening or emergency situation. Additionally, emergency medicine is held in high esteem in the society, and simultaneously has become an indicator of the quality of health care and the effectiveness of the country's delivery systems.

Emergency medicine is characterized by its constant organizational readiness and highly educated specialists who work within its structures while always prepared to react rapidly in emergency settings. The specialized services of emergency medicine, particularly clinical procedures, are intended to mitigate health threats, regardless of the type, or place and time of their occurrence. A patient's lack of insurance, or inability to pay for services, should not be a consideration (Brennan et al., 2005).

The values described above placed particularly high demands on emergency medicine specialists, emergency nurses, and paramedics. Emergency medicine professionals are required to perform in highly stressful situations. Their actions in these situations require them to be highly qualified, and for them to maintain these qualifications in order to perform their duties. Medical decisions must be made quickly, and at times, with limited sources of diagnostic information. These decisions place great demands on emergency medicine specialists.

Members of the emergency medical services system are required to have excellent clinical preparation. As a result, their clinical knowledge gives them the ability to make quick decisions in order to undertake numerous lifesaving procedures. Their concrete actions are determined by a patient's health. Consequently, a patient's well-being or even possible survival depend on these actions.

The main intention of the overall emergency medical community (providers, teaching institutions, ministers, medical centers, professional organizations, etc.) is to provide the professionals with the "tools" necessary to effectively fulfil their responsibilities. Ongoing government support, the creation of medical and ethical guidelines, and access to continuing high quality emergency medicine education, are examples of these "tools". It is extremely important to emphasize that the strategic objectives of the emergency medical community are not only patient centered, but also need to address the working conditions that emergency medical staff encounter.

The Role of Ethics in Emergency Medicine

Although there are no written or codified ethical guidelines pertaining directly to emergency medicine, over time an unwritten code of ethics has evolved. One of this unwritten code's most important elements is the creation of a bond between the patient and the emergency medicine professional. In this patient/medical professional relationship, the emergency medical services worker recognizes and acknowledges the patient's needs.

A patient's fundamental right is unlimited access to high quality emergency medical services as needed. Therefore, it is forbidden to restrict or delay emergency treatment based on race, ethnicity, religious beliefs, a patient's social status, sexual orientation, or a patient's illness or injury. Under no circumstances, is it allowed to not provide emergency medical care based upon a patient's financial situation. Greater social awareness has significantly strengthened the requirement to guarantee these rights to all citizens.

One of the consequences of this increasing civic and social awareness is a systematic growth in the number of patient emergency department visits. As a result, an escalation occurs in the number of medical and ethical issues that arise in the patient/emergency physician relationship. Undeniably, a patient often arrives at the emergency department with urgent complaints or even life-threatening disorders. In these situations, medical decisions and their disposition must readily be made. There is very little time to take a detailed patient history, order the necessary diagnostic tests and consults, and to consider all treatment options. Emergency medicine personnel, even under the most difficult situations, are always expected to work quickly and efficiently.

Additionally, many times a patient in the emergency department has a limited capability to provide added information needed to help assess the situation. A patient's ability to take part in the decision-making process may be restricted due to his/her medical issues. For example, a patient may be unconscious. In these cases, the patient must fully rely on the skills, experience, and capabilities of the emergency medicine specialist, nurse and paramedic. Therefore, the emergency medicine physician must entirely assume responsibility not only on his/her own behalf, but on behalf of the patient as well. This can be extremely difficult, especially when there is frequently limited knowledge about a patient's past health issues and previous treatments. On the other hand, at times emergency medicine personnel face a situation when their patient rejects proposed treatment despite indications otherwise. It is extremely important to determine whether the patient is making a rational decision. It is necessary to maintain a balance between respecting a patient's decision, and the responsibility of the health care professional providing the recommended treatment given the circumstances. In other words, it is essential for the individual health care provider to not only draw upon their experience, but to take ethical actions in accordance with professional standards. Each individual case should be governed by the ethics of the patient/medical provider relationship.

In terms of patient care, emergency medical personnel are required to possess the relevant communication skills including the use of a bit of psychology with their patients.

Principles of Communication Between Emergency Personnel and Patients

Words can sometimes carry ambiguous information, and can be delivered in ambiguous ways. We have all experienced a situation where a person's statement can be interpreted differently by another person. Misinterpretation can take place depending upon the individual who is speaking, his/her tone, and the given circumstances. Many times, words are unnecessary: a clear look or a facial expression is enough to communicate a message. On the other hand, at times, the message to be delivered does not match the individual's body language: their gestures contradict their words, and their eyes communicate mixed feelings. A contradictory message can be sent or received and thus, can become a source of anxiety, disorientation, or confusion. Consequently, this can lead to an individual's withdrawal from the interaction. It is important to recognize the three factors involved in the communication process: provider – the person who is sending a message, recipient – the person who is receiving the information, and the means of delivery – the specific way of supplying the information (e.g. gestures, words, visuals). Skillful communication requires: active listening, the verbal transmission of information, and non-verbal signals, for example, body language including gestures, facial expressions, etc. Communications between individuals or groups that promote mutual agreement and the achievement of common goals, are known as parallel or complementary interactions. These types of communicative interactions are clear to both the provider of the information and the receiver. As a result, there is no misinterpretation between the two parties (Benien et al. 2005).

A less effective type of communication is known as intersecting interactions. These interactions create a discrepancy between the provider's intentions and the recipient's interpretation. A good example is when a doctor does not answer a patient's question because the doctor is busy reading the patient's medical records and therefore, has not heard the question. The patient may interpret this situation as a sign of hostility.

A third, and the least effective type of communication, is an interaction with a double intention: one open and the other one hidden. These kinds of interactions lead to a "game" of manipulation, which can ultimately result in confrontation or breaking off the interaction. The verbal content of each conversation is open, but the body language communicates a hidden message. An example of a commonly used "game" is called "yes, but ...". In this case, an open message communicates a willingness to help, but a hidden message signals refusal because of an excuse (Mayerscough P.R. et al. 2003). Patients and medical personnel use manipulation games to cope with difficult medical situations. For example, a patient expresses dissatisfaction with their medical care by falsely reporting a deterioration of his/her condition, despite ongoing treatment. A similar behavioral mechanism can be demonstrated by a family member, or by the medical staff who face the reality of having to inform a patient about his lethal or extremely severe disease. This manipulation game is frequently expressed in words, "he will not be able to take it". In this case, the open intention is to protect the patient from a devastating emotional reaction resulting from the life-changing news. The hidden intention, which represents the only true message, is used to avoid upsetting a patient emotionally due to the medical personnel's and/or the family's reluctance to cope with the patient's reaction. Ultimately, manipulation games lead to a weakening of relationships, avoidance of interactions, and a sense of isolation for all the parties involved. However, there are some cases when manipulation games prove to be a valuable tool. Manipulation games can be more useful than open communications in lifting a patient's spirits and attitude. Clear and straightforward open communication is recommended as the most effective and proven way of interacting. If the provider of the information knows the receiver well, including his/her expectations, cognitive abilities and situational context, it is easier for the provider to select the most appropriate words and gestures, in order to facilitate the proper interpretation of the message by the receiver (Mayerscough et al., 2003).

The intentions of the message and its relational aspect, which are mainly included in non-verbal communication, are significant elements of social communication as well. Sometimes, the relational aspect dominates, and can interrupt the interaction. Non-verbal signals are extremely important. The content of non-verbal information is trusted more than a message expressed with words.

According to the above, interpersonal skills, sensitivity and empathy are as equally needed for employment in the field of emergency medicine, as one's medical qualifications. Emergency physicians, emergency nurses, and paramedics not only deal with cases on a clinical level, but on a human level as well. Their patients are diverse and complex individuals. In the field of emergency medicine, the treatment process requires significant social skills. All this requires some psychological skills, such as: empathy, active listening, therapeutic conversation, reading of the nonverbal signals, etc. Therefore, the issue of communication between emergency medical personnel and a patient, has already found its place in the curriculum of medical education in Poland (Kliszcz et al. 2012).

In order to grow in their professional development, emergency physicians, emergency nurses and paramedics, are required to expand their knowledge and practical skills related to interpersonal communications. It is undeniable that self-improvement in this area obviously benefits the work of emergency medicine personnel. In order to maintain the principles of effective communication, it is also extremely important to draw upon mistakes that may have been made in the past. Speaking too fast, using jargon or vague expressions, and a misplaced focus on selected facts instead of on the whole content of a statement, are examples of mistakes that can hinder effective communication. The impaired psychophysical condition of a patient can also present difficulty in the patient/medical personnel communication process in emergency medicine. Examples of other critical barriers to effective communication are: guessing and assuming, selective listening, and judging. Criticizing and placing blame on the patient, interrupting him, or overwhelming him with information should also be avoided.

Interactions between a patient and emergency medical staff can be divided into two influential methods: instrumental actions - closely related to emergency procedures, and expressive actions – directed toward a patient's psychological needs. If instrumental actions, such as invasive procedures, disturb a patient psychologically, emotionally oriented expressive actions can help to restore a patient's psychological balance. Thus, in many cases the expressive actions of emergency medical staff may be desired by a patient even more than instrumental actions. Expressive actions include susceptibility to a patient's emotions, as well as an ability of expressing and understanding an emergency medical worker's own emotions. It is impossible to provide emotional support to a patient, if emergency personnel do not maintain their own emotional balance. It is important to remember that anxiety or irritability can be projected onto other people because of various interactions. In order to assess a patient's emotional state, it is essential to analyze both verbal and non-verbal expressions, including tone of voice, eye contact and body language.

The main principles for proper communication with a patient include:

- Reliability and professionalism
- An individual's approach
- Listening skills
- Compatibility of verbal and non-verbal communications
- Clear and simple messaging
- Encouragement of patient responses
- Recognition of a patient's needs and ability of fulfilling them
- Asking open-ended questions to encourage a patient to give a complete response
- Obtaining information regarding both somatic complaints and emotional issues
- Focusing on problematic issues which were only vaguely referenced by a patient
- Effective utilization of silence

Emergency medical personnel with communication skills gained through professional experience will be able to complete difficult work tasks more efficiently. The skills mentioned above include empathy and assertiveness. Empathy helps an emergency medical worker to recognize and understand a patient's situation. However, medical personnel should avoid excessive and unrestricted emotional involvement due to the risk of professional burnout. Assertiveness is defined as a friendly and gentle firmness devoid of aggression and submissiveness. This assertiveness allows an individual to establish a work-life balance by maintaining a distance from issues beyond their control as well as utilizing stress-reduction techniques, and psychological rest through active participation in other areas of life. The parallel aims of both the emergency medical personnel and the patients is the fulfillment of their needs, including avoiding manipulation, protecting emotional boundaries, and keeping control of the interaction. Some individuals possess a positive predisposition regarding empathy and assertiveness, and for other individuals these qualities can be learned and developed over time. It is possible to continually strengthen these attributes through experience and added practice. Constant self-improvement regarding empathy and assertiveness is effectively reinforced by practicing these skills in every day work. Empathy can help provide access to the mind-set and emotions of a patient while helping to assess if full disclosure of a patient's condition is required and necessary (Kliszcz et al., 2012).

In communicating with a patient, it is especially important not to overwhelm him/her with excess data, but to deliver the necessary vital information. Effective communication between medical personnel and patients can be established by implementing the use of a common "communication dictionary" which consists of simple words and avoids professional terminology or jargon. Aristotle once said, "Express yourself like the common people, but think like a wise man".

Delivering bad news to a patient is one of the most challenging responsibilities of emergency physicians. There are certain fundamental rules that should be followed. First, it is necessary to always tell the truth, and the truth only. However, it is important not to completely take away a patient's hope. Each emergency physician should make arrangements to allow for the time needed to be part of a difficult conversation while making certain this conversation takes place in the proper environment and respects a patient's privacy.

When summarizing all the conditions needed for effective interpersonal communication discussed above, it is recommended that emergency services personnel practice the following rules:

- Communicate in a clear and understandable way
- Actively listen
- Repeat the most important information
- Demonstrate understanding and acceptance
- Explain, ask, and answer questions
- Be sensitive to the recipient
- Avoid dishonesty
- Treat each patient as an individual
- Show interest in the patient, not just his/her illness
- Take into account the situational context
- Do not abandon the patient in difficult moments
- Maintain rational hope, offer emotional support

The most desirable attributes of emergency medical personnel can be described as follows: being ready to listen, while maintaining a calm attitude and allowing a patient to express his/her various emotions. This approach facilitates the recording of a patient's history and the implementation of the proper treatment. The patient/medical worker interaction should be the source of mutual satisfaction. A friendly and nonthreatening approach taken towards the patient always compensates for any shortcomings in communication skills.

Psychology in the Work of Emergency Services

On a daily basis, emergency medical employees face high demands and expectations placed on them. The everyday work of emergency professionals involves making quick and difficult medical decisions while confronting life threatening situations. The frequent proximity of death may create a feeling of helplessness in the face of human mortality. As a result, enormous tension and mental exhaustion may occur. Thus, the work of emergency medical services personnel requires individuals who possess certain professional and emotional predispositions and qualifications.

As mentioned before, emergency services worker should build a relationship with a patient based on trust. This trust will consequently reinforce a patient's confidence in the competence of the medical professional. The establishment of a strong patient/medical personnel relationship right away is even more important in emergency settings because this is usually a brief interaction. However, in the eyes of a patient even this short interaction with emergency medicine will leave a permanent impression. In order to maintain trust, a patient should be fully informed about his/her health situation, as well as the needed procedures and treatments. This process should be undertaken with the goal of preserving a patient's dignity and respecting his/her rights. The patient should be fully aware of treatment options, as well as their possible consequences. At times, extremely difficult decisions must be made. An example of such a decision is saving a patient's life at the expense of his/her limb which requires amputation. Another particularly difficult situation arises when the emergency medicine physician must decide whether to discontinue or to not even initiate therapeutic measures in patients who are in very severe or terminal condition. A "Do not resuscitate" (DNR) order can be the result of the ethical and moral obligations of the physician after consulting with a patient and respecting the wishes of a patient's family (Kliszcz et al., 2012).

The constant progression and development of emergency medicine creates new treatment opportunities and improved medical technologies. However, these new technological achievements used in life-saving procedures generate an increase in financial commitments. Although the emergency physician is obliged to utilize the most recent advances in the field of medicine, including technologically advanced diagnostic procedures and treatments, the escalating costs of these procedures must be taken into consideration as well. Therefore, new ethical dilemmas arise. Where is the line between the costs generated by emergency procedures and the measurable benefits for the patient? The practice of emergency medicine can be drastically diminished because of significant financial constraints. Nevertheless, this possible dilemma should never be part of the decision-making process regarding a patient in an emergency setting. The patient should receive all the necessary assistance and have access to the available resources. In this situation the physician must represent a patient's needs and expectations in a definitive way. Discussions regarding financial issues of health care in emergencies cannot take place in front of the suffering patient and should be transferred to the management or political level.

Another extreme scenario which emergency medicine professionals can encounter in their practice is an accident with mass casualties, epidemic, or catastrophe. In these situations, there is a substantial disproportion between the availability of medical resources and the number of patients requiring medical assistance. Consequently, it is necessary to initiate the medical segregation (triage) process. During triage, casualties are divided into several groups, depending on their injuries and possible treatment. Under these circumstances, it is essential to give priority to patients who can benefit the most from the limited use of available medical resources. Victims with fatal injuries as a result of a mass casualties event do not take priority in triage due to highly limited resources. Patients with minor complaints, who are able to wait, are given low priority as well, and they will be provided with medical assistance at a later time.

The ethical and moral responsibility for decisions made during a catastrophe cannot lay solely on the shoulders of the emergency physician. Individuals responsible for the organization of the health care system, as well as the creation of operational plans in the event of mass injuries and catastrophes, should be held most accountable.

In the practice of emergency medicine another difficult decision to make is one regarding not initiating or discontinuing medical procedures in cases where there is a lack of effectiveness, and which results in the death of the patient. It is even more problematic in prehospital conditions. At the scene of an event an emergency physician must make decisions independently without any additional help, for example, no consults are available.

In the field of emergency medicine there are a number of factors which increase stress on an individual, including:

- Long and difficult shifts
- Responsibility for making quick decisions, including life-threatening situations
- Constant fear of making mistakes
- Frequent interactions with death bed patients and their families
- Triage decisions during catastrophic events
- Loss of team members during rescue operations
- Being the focus of public and media attention

Helping a family cope with the pain and loss of a family member is one of the toughest tasks of the emergency physician. A psychologist, counselor, or therapist should be available, but in reality, this is often not the case. Under these circumstances the emergency physician should proceed with empathy, calmness, and rely on his/her professional experience.

All of the above factors may contribute to burnout syndrome which is a potential condition faced by emergency medical services personnel. The identification and diagnosis of burnout syndrome will be detailed in a later section of this chapter.

Job related stress and burnout of emergency services employees are very serious threats to the profession. Under difficult working conditions, such as poor work place organization or financial limitations, an increase in stress and/or burnout can occur. These factors can frequently hinder the development of emergency medicine.

Human Responses to Life-Threatening Situations

Emotional and somatic symptoms can occur in emergency medical personnel as a response to severe stress. In addition, psychological reactions are activated by the body. The function of these reactions, is adapting to the current situation and preparing for expected consequences. Psychological reactions lead to the reduction of emotional and somatic symptoms (Kępiński A. et al.2003).

Main reactions to stress include:

- **Emotional:** Fear, anxiety, mental tension, nervousness
- **Somatic:** Increased heart rate and muscle tone, dry mouth
- **Psychological:** Seeking solutions to a problem, searching for helpful information and support. Keeping "cool" leads to effective problem-solving

Acute Stress Reaction

A strong emotional response to stress can have a debilitating effect on an individual's ability to work. This diminished ability to work efficiently is known as acute stress reaction or acute stress disorder. The symptoms may be varied and mixed. At the outset of this reaction to stress an initial state of stupefaction occurs, characterized by a diminished attention span, an inability to comprehend surrounding events, and a sense of confusion. Later, reactions can include increased agitation, and withdrawal including totally "escaping" from the stressful situation. Usually, vegetative symptoms, such as increased heart rate, sweating or blushing coexist with anxiety. These symptoms usually appear within a few minutes of the stressful events and disappear after a short period of time (few hours to two or three days). Memory impairment caused by a reaction to acute stress may occur (Kępiński et al., 2003).

Diagnostic criteria related to acute stress reaction include:

- Witnessing or experiencing a serious health or life-threatening event, which generate intense fear, a sense of helplessness or horror;
- Dissociative symptoms: sense of paralysis, apathy, stupefaction, disorientation, sense of an altered environment, disruption in memory;
- Recurring memories of the painful event;
- Avoidance of anything that resembles the painful event;
- Severe symptoms of anxiety, and panic attacks;
- Diminished general performance.

Reactions to Stress: General Mechanisms

An intermediate state of reaction can exist between an individual's initial reaction and the serious acute reactions to stress. Some general patterns can be identified during various reactions to stress. The main symptoms include:

- **Anxiety:** Stress is triggered by a threatening situation
- **Depression:** Caused by the loss of someone close or something valuable, including loss of opportunity, hope, beliefs or dreams

Many times, mixed anxiety-depressive symptoms are observed. An example can be a car accident which is a life-threatening situation, or results in a loss of independence because of injuries.

The typical response to stress involves a coping mechanism of avoidance. The individual avoids situations and people associated with stressful events. The most common defense mechanism is denial. This mechanism is characterized by the downplaying of the seriousness of the situation and includes difficulty in recalling the details of the painful event. Ultimately, denial leads to relieve of anxiety. These reactions to stress described above, subside gradually, due to "working it over" and adapting to consequences of traumatic experience. Nevertheless, difficulties with remembering some of the details may persist. In some cases, stress is relieved by utilization of improper methods, which delay the process of "working it over" and extend time of the stress reaction. Examples of such methods are:

- Alcohol or drug abuse
- An unintentional use of immature defense mechanisms, such as: projection (involuntary transfer of one's own anger to another person, who is perceived as a cause of tragedy), or regression (child-like helplessness in the face of stress)

Delayed Consequences of Stress

Emergency medical personnel, in addition to training involving proceedings with patients suffering from acute stress disorder, should be also aware of late reactions, which may present as a result of extremely tragic events. Emergency medicine employees, similarly to victims, may be subjected to late stages of stress reaction, natural stages of the response to death, and post-traumatic stress disorder (PTSD).

Stress is a natural reaction. Two types of stress can be distinguished: constructive and excessive. Constructive stress is beneficial and improves efficiency. Excessive stress, also known as distress, causes severe disruption in an individual's ability to function. Symptoms of excessive reaction to stress include: irritability in interactions with other people, attention deficit problems, sleep disorders (difficulty falling asleep or nightmares), anxiety, difficulty with making decisions, unreasonable guilt, loss of appetite, loss of sexual interest, isolation, and a disinterest in work. If someone exhibits these symptoms, it is recommended that steps be taken in order to relieve the effects of stress. These steps should lead to an improvement in an individual's overall lifestyle. Examples of these changes include: more time dedicated to leisure and family life, regular physical activity and healthy nutrition, better management of their work time, reduced consumption of cigarettes and alcohol, as well as practicing relaxation techniques (e.g. hobbies, relaxation exercises, travel). If these actions are ineffective, one should seek professional help (e.g. from a psychologist, counselor or therapist).

Death: Stages of Reaction

On a regular basis, emergency medical professionals are exposed to death, and they interact with many grieving individuals who have lost a close friend, or a family member. Consequently, it is essential for them to possess knowledge regarding the common reactions to death. The reaction to death involves four stages:

- In the beginning, numbness, denial, despair, and a sense of disbelief present
- The second stage is dominated by personal thoughts and memories of the deceased

- next, a lack of focus, insomnia, lack of appetite, decreased ability to work, and the feeling that "life has lost its meaning" may appear
- In the final stage of the reorganization, painful feelings subside gradually and a return to a normal state takes place; remembering happy memories involving the deceased becomes possible

More intense reactions, such as guilt ("it is me, not him, who should die") may also occur. In the second stage, thoughts of the deceased may be so intense, that sometimes delusions of his/her presence appear (normally these are recognized as unreal). Excessive reaction to death requires psychotherapeutic help (Kępiński et al., 2003).

Post-Traumatic Stress Disorder (PTSD)

Post-traumatic stress disorder, or PTSD, is defined as a delayed (often by several weeks), or a prolonged (a month or longer) reaction to an extremely stressful experience. Characteristic symptoms include involuntary and repetitive recurrence of traumas as persistent undesired memories, dreams or nightmares. Furthermore, apathy, rejection of contacts with other people, and diminished interest in the surrounding environment may be observed. Moreover, a person suffering from PTSD is unable to experience pleasure any more. Those who suffer from PTSD avoid activities and situations which remind them of past traumatic events. Excessive vigilance and over-sensitivity to stimuli are also observed. In many cases, sleep disorder, anxiety, and depression occur as a result of PTSD (Wciórka et al., 2012).

Stress-Related Consequences: Prevention

In order to prevent a diminished work performance of emergency medicine personnel due to acute stress reaction, it is highly recommended to discuss with a professional one's typical response to stressful situations. Participating in several rescue actions as an observer and analyzing these experiences can be also advisable. Moreover, all emergency medicine professionals should be familiar with proper relaxation techniques. A medical team's fitness and ability to perform their difficult duties depends highly on their ability to get rest and relaxation including:

- Balancing work with the need for proper rest
- Learning ways to cope with constant stress
- Understanding and utilizing familiar relaxation techniques

Victims of Highly Stressful Events: Recommended Procedures

For emergency personnel, the primary guiding principles when treating victims of highly stressful catastrophic events are based on establishing a relationship with the affected person while also providing moral support. These principles facilitate the process of collecting the essential information necessary for the continuation of an effective rescue. Furthermore, the victim's recovery will be easier and quicker. In order to provide support to a victim, interpersonal interactions should include:

- **Avoidance of Hasty and Impulsive Actions:** Patience and keeping calm raise trust and provide sense of security

- **Proactivity and Determination:** Help to find a solution to the problem
- **Willingness to Understand:** Being ready to hear the patient out
- **Attempting to Understand:** Becoming aware of a victim's emotional state
- consideration of a victim's behavior as a reaction to stress, not as a manifestation of ill will (Wciórka et al., 2010)

When interacting with a person experiencing emotional distress, a variety of reactions may be triggered, serving to protect one from becoming overly involved. There are three main mistakes that hamper gaining trust and establishing a relationship with a patient: patronizing the patient, disrespecting him/her, or being judgmental and looking for guilty parties. Although every accident requires an individual assessment and approach, in most circumstances the following principles can be applied:

- It is important to accommodate a victim in the most comfortable conditions available, the place should be calm, possibly quiet and safe
- A victim should not be left alone and must be able to have the opportunity to stay in direct contact with another individual; if several people were affected by the same tragedy they can be placed together in one area
- Offering a victim something to drink or eat may be relevant, also on a symbolic level
- It is essential to encourage a victim to express his/her feelings regarding the experience
- Providing the possibility to communicate with family and loved ones is necessary
- Offering assistance in solving current problems resulting from the unplanned event, for example providing childcare and notifying the employer about the reason for absence from work
- It is essential to realize that victims may sometimes express very strong emotions which may seem unjustified and unclear, examples are: denial of obvious facts (claiming that the tragedy did not happen), a sense of guilt, feeling threatened, or blaming the deceased person for the tragedy (Wciórka et al., 2012).

Emergency medicine professionals are at risk of experiencing similar reactions to stress to those of victims and witnesses of accidents. Consequently, an individual needs the appropriate training to work under stressful conditions. This training should include:

- Education in the area of stress responses
- Getting familiar with one's own reaction to stress
- Mastering relaxation techniques
- Participation in courses which aim at lessening the consequences of work related stress

In addition to the actions mentioned above, it is extremely important to provide systematic counseling support in a workplace, e.g. by creating psychological support programs with the participation of other co-workers. In these programs professional psychological help is accompanied by the testimony of co-workers, who understand this specific nature of their profession. An emergency physician, emergency nurse or paramedic, who is going through professional difficulties, may feel a natural closeness to people with similar experiences. Developing this natural support system within a work place may contribute to the reduction of work-related stress and help to create a healthy and effective work environment for emergency medical services personnel (Kliszcz et al., 2012).

Although employee assistance programs may increase the availability of support, in order for them to be successful, a common understanding regarding their limitations is necessary. Psychological support from co-workers is extremely valuable, however, in many cases, it cannot replace professional help of specialists. The functioning of the support system described above must be based on clearly defined rules pertaining to the recruitment, supervision and evaluation of the participants. The program, as well as the emergency medicine employees who provide support to their co-workers must be supervised by a team of professional psychologists and therapists. This professional supervision is usually provided by employee focused health and social services within a work place, external support programs, or a combination of both. The combined option is the most effective.

Initiatives undertaken by employers, such as the formation of carefully constructed support programs, are examples of fulfilling their responsibility to care for their employees' mental health and to protect those same employees from the negative impact of constant involvement in traumatic events. Integral components of an effective employees' support program are regular training sessions, which provide information regarding the effects of occupational and post-traumatic stress, and removal of the stigma of these reactions as being "abnormal" (Kliszcz J. et al. 2012). Creation of the programs described above serves to promote a work culture, which does not criticize one's need for support. Proper counseling and mental health care provided to employees at the right time, can be extremely beneficial to both the employee and the employer. These measures lead to a heightening of an employee's job satisfaction, enhanced work performance and effectiveness, commitment, and overall mental well-being.

Diagnosis of Burnout Syndrome

Professional burnout syndrome is defined as the physical, emotional and psychological reactions of the human mind and body in response to workplace stress (Cassella C. 2010, Felton 1998, Głębocka and Lisowska, 2007; Kamrowska, 2007; Maslach and Jackson, 1981). Burnout syndrome can also be described as physical and mental exhaustion caused by prolonged activities, or by excessive tension associated with dissatisfaction with one's professional duties (Felton, 1998; Kamrowska and Kamrowski, 2010; Maslach and Jackson, 1981; Montero-Marin et al., 2009). Professionals who work with the public trust, who are required to be extremely involved in their duties, such as: emergency physicians, emergency nurses, paramedics or teachers, are frequently diagnosed with burnout syndrome (Felton, 1998; Maslach and Jackson, 1981; Montero-Marin et al., 2009; Popa et al., 2010; Siemińska et al., 2007). The above-mentioned professionals constantly interact with particular groups of people (e.g. patients). Thus, it is imperative for them to be professional as they perform their required procedures, to possess a wide-range of knowledge regarding their subject, and to treat their patients as individuals. Another important feature of working with the public is to care for one's appearance and presence (Kamrowska and Kamrowski, 2010; Maslach and Jackson, 1981; Montero-Marin et al., 2009; Siemińska et al., 2007).

The most common source of dissatisfaction associated with the professional duties of emergency medicine personnel are: an over involvement in certain individual cases, high expectations with limited perceptible results, along with prolonged exposure to intense physical and mental stress (Kamrowska and Kamrowski, 2010; Maslach and Jackson, 1981; Siemińska et al., 2001). The initial symptoms of professional burnout syndrome are associated with a deterioration of a person's general disposition, and a lack of quality in their work. Examples of these symptoms are: headaches, fatigue/tiredness, irritability, problems with concentration, frequent colds, impotency and insomnia. No changes in laboratory parameters are observed at this stage. A few days of rest is generally sufficient to regain an equilibrium (Maslach and Jackson, 1981; Montero-Marin et al., 2009; Siemińska et al., 2007; Salch and Shapiro, 2008).

During the second stage of burnout syndrome, an increase in the intensity of the symptoms described above takes place. In addition, an employee becomes abusive and/or contemptuous in interactions with others (e.g. co-workers, patients, students, family members). In this stage, changes of laboratory parameters can be observed, and these changes can affect bodily functions. In order to return to a state of "balance", patients require at least several weeks of rest. Moreover, a change of attitude regarding their performed professional duties is necessary (Felton, 1998; Kamrowska, 2007; Montero-Marin et al., 2011).

The third stage of professional burnout syndrome is associated with the full and permanent physical and emotional exhaustion of the employee. Consequently, his/her work performance is drastically diminished. Additionally, the risk of health issues, such as: hypertension or peptic ulcer disease, is increased. The patient experiences a lack of understanding from others, alienation, anxiety, and ultimately depression (Popa et al., 2010; Kamrowska, 2007). The third stage of burnout syndrome is a result of exposure to chronic stress. Their bodily functions are out of balance, and changes in some laboratory parameters described as stress markers are noted. Their levels stay out of normal values long after the stress has ceased. Exposure to chronic stress changes the employee's life completely. His/her work and family problems pile up and start to overlap with other issues. At this stage, falling into addiction is often observed, which additionally exaggerates the problems (Felton, 1998; Kamrowska, 2007; Maslach and Jackson, 1981). In order to recover, professional help and assistance is necessary, for example sessions with an experienced psychologist or psychiatrist (Fernandez et al., 2010; Maslach and Jackson, 1981).

The basic diagnostics of burnout syndrome begins with the completion of a questionnaire known as the Maslach Burnout Inventory (MBI). The questionnaire was developed in 1981 by Christina Maslach. Test questions are divided into three parts which pertain to: emotional exhaustion, dissatisfaction in regard to performed work, and depersonalization which is also defined as cynicism (Maslach and Jackson, 1981). A patient answers the questions, and a summary of these answers aids in making a proper diagnosis. The MBI questionnaire is the most frequently used and recognized tool in the diagnostic process of burnout syndrome (Feston 1998, Głębocka and Lisowska, 2007; Kamrowska, 2007; Kamrowska and Kamrowski, 2010; Kitaoka-Higashiguchi et al., 2009; Okamoto et al., 2008; Mommersteeg et al., 2006; Montero-Marin et al., 2009; Popa et al., 2010; Salch and Shapiro, 2008).

The Burnout Clinical Subtype Questionnaire (BCSQ) is a more advanced test that allows the psychologist to provide more specific and individual therapy to patients suffering from burnout syndrome (Montero-Marin et al., 2009, 2011; Popa et al., 2010).

By implementing the proper treatment of an individual with burnout syndrome, a final stage can be achieved. At this stage regeneration begins with the healing of wounds and a sense of satisfaction regarding work can be experienced again (Felton, 1998; Kamrowska, 2007).

Professional Burnout Syndrome: Physical Changes

Research regarding stress response involves the measurement of certain laboratory parameters and the detailed analysis of the results (Clow et al., 2010; Preuessner, 1999; Salch and Shapiro, 2008). Psychological research, however, is focused on the evaluation of the patient's behavior and emotional engagement. The human response to stress consists of three components: psychological factor - associated with behavioral changes, metabolic factor – related to a stimulation of the hypothalamic-pituitary-adrenal axis, and the occurrence of hypertension – connected to the autonomic nervous system. Therefore, it seems reasonable to combine psychological studies (MBI questionnaire) with biochemical tests in the diagnostic process of burnout syndrome (Noble, 2002; Sertoz et al., 2008). The type and strength of the bodily response to stress depends on the individual, e.g. genetic characteristics (Brosschot, 2010; Kamrowska, 2007; Sertoz et al., 2008).

The basic response to stress depends on the autonomic nervous system, which regulates blood pressure, affects the adrenal axis, and stimulates secretion of stress hormones: adrenaline, noradrenaline, cortisol, and prolactin (Noble, 2002; Brosschot, 2010). Health complications in the course of burnout syndrome are dependent on each patient's individual response. The intensity and the sequence of symptoms occurring in each patient will be different depending on the strength and type of stimulus (Brosschot, 2010; Fernandez et al., 2010; McEwen and Kalia, 2010; Salch and Shapiro, 2008; Xu et al., 2009). For example, hypertension and increased heart rate can be caused by stimulation of the nervous system and/or excessive secretion of adrenaline and cortisol. Consequently, the patient will be at higher risk for cardiovascular and renal diseases (Xu et al. 2009).

Cortisol

The cortisol level is the best indicator of hypothalamic-pituitary-adrenal axis function (Chida and Steptoe, 2009; Foley and Kirschbaum, 2010; McEwan and Kalia, 2010; Sertoz et al., 2008). Ten to twenty milligrams of cortisol a day are secreted in a physiological state. Cortisol secretion is characterized by a physiological daily rhythm. This rhythm can be disturbed, e.g. by stress exposure and/or in the case of Cushing's syndrome. The highest secretion of cortisol occurs in the morning, twenty to forty-five minutes after waking up. The lowest levels of this hormone occur at night. The levels of cortisol increase approximately ten minutes after the stimulating event, and its highest levels occur ten to thirty minutes later. This heighten concentration level gradually decreases. Ninety percent of the secreted hormone's excess is buffered by a specific corticosteroid-binding protein (CBG), albumin, and finally by erythrocytes which have a lower affinity to cortisol. Exogenous cortisol is primarily bound by albumins (Foley and Kirchbaum, 2010; McEwan and Kalia, 2010).

Only an unbounded form of cortisol has the ability to penetrate biological membranes and activate receptors. The hormone's action can be described in three levels: energy metabolism of the body, cardiovascular system function, and influence on the immune system (Chandola et al., 2010; Rohleder et al., 2010; Sertoz et al., 2008). Cortisol receptors are located in the cytoplasm of all cell types. Two types of these receptors have been described: mineralocorticoid (MR) and glucocorticoid (GR). MRs are characterized by greater affinity to cortisol and have relevant functions in the nervous and immune systems. GRs have lower affinity to cortisol, and affect metabolism and blood vessels (Rohleder et al., 2010).

Only free cortisol can affect the cells. Thus, the concentration of free cortisol in blood and saliva has the best correlation with the human body's response to stress. Total cortisol concentration is affected by stress as well, however, it also depends on the amount of corticosteroid-binding proteins (CBGs) and albumins. CBGs levels depend on liver function and on the concentration of estrogens. (Foley and Kirchbaum, 2010; Hansen et al., 2009). In women, any variation in estrogen levels, such as menstruation, pregnancy, hormonal contraception, is strongly connected to changes in total cortisol level. However, the correlation with free cortisol fraction's levels is much weaker (Preuessner et al., 2008; Foley and Kirchbaum, 2020). Changes in the cortisol levels of females depend on many factors, however stress is one of the most important. In males, strong similarities were observed between the early reactions to stress stimulus, and those resulting from exposure to chronic stress (Chandola et al., 2010; Pruessner et al., 1999, 2008).

In addition to cortisol measurements in basic conditions, it is well advised to perform multiple tests over a 24-hour period. The routine testing of cortisol secretion consists of measurements taken in the morning (up to forty minutes after waking up), during the day, the evening, and at night. Modifications of this test are encountered, and they are comprised of three measurements: the highest concentration is recorded in the morning, lower - during the day, and the lowest before falling asleep. Long-term stress exposure disturbs the daily rhythm of cortisol secretion, and consequently, the highest hormone concentrations are observed during working hours (Clow et al., 2010; Preuessner et al., 1999; Rohleder et al., 2010).

Cortisol Awakening Response (CAR)

The measuring of free cortisol levels in saliva and urine were also found to be useful in the diagnostic procedures related to burnout syndrome. These tests are used to assess the activity of the hypothalamic-pituitary-adrenal axis, and are related to changes in the free cortisol levels of the blood (Chida and Steptoe, 2009; Melamed et al., 1999; Preuessner et al., 1999; Sertoz et al., 2008).

The measurement of the cortisol concentration in saliva is a non-invasive test used in the assessment of cortisol awakening response (CAR). Saliva collection is relatively simple, can be done by oneself, and the sample can be conveniently delivered to the laboratory. Patients are instructed to collect saliva up to thirty minutes after waking up, and before their first meal, before brushing their teeth, drinking or smoking (Chida and Steptoe, 2009; Preuessner et al., 2008).

In the diagnostic process of burnout syndrome cortisol level measurement in saliva provides an alternative option to blood tests. Cortisol level changes in saliva and blood are very similar and correlate directly to the stress response. In control groups, there were no significant changes observed in the basic hormone concentration between men and women (Chida and Steptoe, 2009; Melamed et al., 1999; Preuessner et al., 1999, 2008). However, after stress stimulation cortisol levels measured in the female study group were significantly higher than in the male group. Researchers suggest that fluctuations in the daily rhythm of cortisol excretion are even more pronounced for CAR than for a standard blood test. These reported fluctuations in CAR appear before the occurrence of the final stage of burnout syndrome, i.e. during the reversal phase with no changes of blood markers, when a few days of rest can help to ease the tension. Increased cortisol levels in the CAR test are observed only after one day of the stress factor occurrence. Whereas, in the case of chronic stress in patients with symptomatic burnout syndrome, the concentration of cortisol in the CAR test drops (Chida and Steptoe, 2009; Melamed et al., 1999; Tops et al., 2006). This phenomenon can be explained by the slower adrenal cortex response, its depletion, or lack of ACTH shortly before waking up. Changes in ACTH levels are associated with reduced corticoliberin secretion due to the negative effects of stress on the hypothalamus (e.g. changes in the production of liberins and statins occur due to the disturbance of the sleep phases REM-nREM rhythm). The cortisol levels after awakening may also decrease in people who have problems falling asleep, or suffer from insomnia (Brosschot, 2010; Clow et al., 2010; Salch and Shapiro, 2008). This is particularly important because employees at risk of suffering from burnout syndrome frequently complain of problems falling asleep and a lack of regenerative sleep (Brosschot, 2010; Clow et al., 2020).

Deviations from the baseline of cortisol levels can be observed in other diseases, including: schizophrenia, posttraumatic stress disorder or hippocampal injuries. The measurement of the cortisol levels of saliva may be useful in the diagnosis and evaluation of the progress of the treatment in patients suffering from these disorders (Preuessner et al., 2008; Rohleder et al., 2010).

Urine Cortisol (UC)

The urine cortisol levels measurement is characterized by a sensitivity similar to blood and saliva tests (Hansen et al., 2009; Noble, 2002; Vogelzangs et al., 2010). In order to determine the level of cortisol in urine a standard 24-hour urine collection is necessary, and requires a great deal of effort from the patient. The results should be evaluated in relation to creatinine clearance (calculations based on 24-hour urine collection and blood levels). The result of a cortisol concentration measurement from a single urine sample is significant only if its level exceeds the range of accepted reference values. However, if the result is within normal limits, changes in blood cortisol levels cannot be ruled out based on this single urine sample test. Many of the deficiencies of the cortisol blood test do not apply to the urine cortisol test. The latter reflects the average amount of cortisol which is released into the plasma and filtered throughout the day (Hansen et al., 2009; Vogelzangs et al., 2010). Currently, this assessment is used as a supplement to a blood cortisol level test, in case the laboratory does not acquire a method for measurement of the hormone's free fraction. The analysis of the results should include a comparison of the values in blood and urine. Individuals suffering from burnout syndrome will have high levels of cortisol in both blood and urine. When the hormone production stops the levels in both bodily fluids will begin to decrease (Vogelzangs et al., 2010).

Adrenocorticotropic Hormone (ACTH)

ACTH (adrenocorticotropin) is another hormone used in the assessment of the function of the hypothalamic-pituitary-adrenal axis. The measurement of the concentration of ACTH is used to determine the origin of the increased cortisol level. The amount of adrenocorticotropin increases rapidly just before, or at the moment of wakening. It stimulates the adrenal cortex to produce and release cortisol resulting in an increase in cortisol for ten to thirty minutes after ACTH ejection. The secretion of ACTH, similar to cortisol, is related to the circadian rhythm, however, it begins about ten minutes earlier. The lowest concentrations are noted in the evening and at night (Clow et al., 2010; Preuessner et al., 1999).

Over the course of burnout syndrome, all the components of the hypothalamic-pituitary-adrenal axis are usually stimulated. Higher values of ACTH are noted following the appearance of stress stimulus. During work the amount of adrenocorticotropin does not change or increase. The described condition persists until the patient moves to the third stage of burnout syndrome. This stage is associated with severe and persistent changes in emotion and health. It is possible that among this group of patients the levels of ACTH and cortisol will decrease, most likely due to depletion of the producing cells and/or when the threshold of hypothalamic sensitivity to the stress factor rises (Clow et al., 2010; Foley and Kirchbaum, 2010; Preuessner et al., 1999; Tops et al., 2006).

Corticotropin-Releasing Hormone (CRH)

Another hormone used to evaluate the function of the hypothalamic-pituitary-adrenal axis is corticotropin-releasing hormone (CRH) or corticoliberin. CRH measurement is not a routine test. Physiologically this hormone is released by the hypothalamus as a result of nervous system stimulation. CRH is secreted in a daily rhythm consistent with the rhythm of ACTH and cortisol excretion. Corticoliberin affects the pituitary cells by stimulating the production and release of corticotropin, whereas cortisol and ACTH inhibit CRH's production (McEwan and Kalia, 2010; Vanltallie, 2002; Wahlberg et al., 2009).

Increased corticoliberin concentrations occur most likely due to stress, and may be attributed to the increased perception of pain stimuli. Patients in pain, with impaired cognitive functions, and elevated CRH levels are reported to have a poorer response to the first-line analgesics. This is explained by a complex mechanism, which includes the influence of liberin on GABA receptors and the binding of the neurotransmitters (e.g. substance P) with the glucocorticoid receptors (McEwan and Kalia, 2010). It has been agreed, that psychological stress in burnout syndrome leads to emotional exhaustion and depersonalization, and is of great importance in CRH elevation. Therefore, it is extremely likely that elevated cortisol levels in burnout syndrome may be caused by the increased activity of the nervous system associated with corticoliberin secretion (Miller and O'Callaghan, 2002; Sertoz et al., 2008; Vanltallie, 2002; Wahlberg et al., 2009).

Suppression Tests

Suppression tests such as: dexamethasone suppression test and dexamethasone/CRH test are also used for the evaluation of the hypothalamic-pituitary-adrenal axis function in burnout syndrome. Orally administered dexamethasone is a synthetic glucocorticoid that inhibits the secretion of ACTH and CRH. Consequently, the administration of dexamethasone causes a reduction in the cortisol level. Dexamethasone acts stronger and longer than natural glucocorticosteroids. In order to diagnose and determine the stage of burnout syndrome, a single dose dexamethasone test can be used, according to the following plan (Preuessner et al., 1999; Sertoz et al., 2008).

1. Blood collection in the morning (7:00 am), before the first meal, cortisol and ACTH levels measurement.
2. Dexamethasone administration 1mg orally, around 11:00 pm.
3. Blood collection in the morning (7:00 am), before the first meal, cortisol and ACTH levels measurement.

Possible modifications to the test described above include increasing the number of dexamethasone doses, or the amount of the drug administered as needed (Preuessner et al., 1999; Sertoz et al., 2008). Dexamethasone inhibits pituitary and hypothalamic cells, and this leads to the discontinuation of corticotropin and corticoliberin production. In healthy individuals with normal blood cortisol and ACTH levels, after the administration of dexamethasone at night, cortisol and ACTH levels decrease below the reference values of the morning. In the case of individuals with cortisol disorders and patients suffering from burnout syndrome, dexamethasone inhibits the activity of the axis, however, morning levels of examined hormones are not as low as in the case of healthy subjects (Preuessner et al., 1999; Sertoz et al., 2008).

The dexamethasone/CRH test is performed as follows (Wahlberg et al., 2009):

1. Blood collection in the morning (7:00 am), before the first meal, cortisol and ACTH levels measurement
2. Dexamethasone administration - 1mg orally, around 11:00 pm
3. Blood collection in the morning (7:00 am), before the first meal, cortisol and ACTH levels measurement
4. CRH administration - 100µg intravenously, around 2 pm
5. Blood collection every fifteen minutes over a three-hour period of CRH administration (seven blood samples)

In healthy individuals, administration of dexamethasone results in a drop in both blood cortisol and ACTH levels. However, CRH affects ACTH, and after ten to thirty minutes, cortisol secretion. As a result, the effect of dexamethasone is neutralized. In patients with burnout syndrome, all tested hormones have elevated values. Although after dexamethasone administration their levels dropped, the dynamics of these changes and their final values were different from those of healthy people. After administration of human corticoliberin, an increase in ACTH and cortisol levels were noted. These changes later appeared when compared with the control group. Therefore, in the diagnosis of burnout syndrome the time of observation after CRH administration should be extended until the levels of both evaluated hormones stop increasing (Wahlberg et al., 2001). Due to stress the adrenal axis may be stimulated. However, after cessation of its activation, returning to a physiological state or re-activation requires more time. This indicates that cells previously affected by stressors have a delayed reaction (McEwan and Kalia, 2010; Sertoz et al., 2008).

The CRH test is most frequently used to diagnose Cushing's syndrome. Despite the hypercortisolemia occurrence, it has not been found useful in the diagnostic process of burnout syndrome (Wahlberg et al., 2009).

17-Hydroxycorticosteroids (17-OHCSs)

17-hydroxycorticosteroids are the main metabolites of adrenal glucocorticoids. The 17-OHCSs level is measured in the urine which is obtained during a 24-hour collection (results must be calculated in relation to creatinine clearance). High basic cortisol level correlates well with the amount of excreted metabolites in the urine. In burnout syndrome diagnostics, it may serve as a supplementary test for individuals with suspected cortisol disturbances. Additionally, renal function is evaluated. After the administration of a suppressing medication to patients with burnout syndrome, a slight decrease in 17-OHCSs levels is observed when compared to the control group (Pruessner et al., 1999).

Adrenaline, Noradrenaline

Determining the levels of catecholamines in blood and urine has been accepted as a measurable element of the bodily response to stress. Increased adrenaline secretion is associated with high blood pressure and cardiac episodes (Brosschot, 2010; Hansen et al., 2009; Lee et al., 2010; Noble, 2002; Vanltallie, 2002). Therefore, it is extremely important to determine the influence of a spectrum of stressful stimuli on the human body's basic functions. Blood samples to be used for burnout syndrome diagnosis should be taken multiple times, under comparable conditions (e.g. in the morning - before the first meal), before, during, and after work. Additionally, blood should be taken after unplanned stressful situations that occur during routine duties.

For a urine test, 24-hour collection is required, and the results should be calculated in relation to creatinine clearance (Noble, 2002). It is also possible to test the levels of adrenaline and noradrenaline in a single sample of urine. The specimen should be collected immediately after the individual finishes work. In case the employee was involved in an extremely stressful situation, the first sample after the incident should be collected (Lee et al., 2010). It has been established that the amount of adrenaline in urine represents about 2% of the total hormone in the blood. In the case of noradrenaline, urine hormone represents around 20% of blood level (Hansen et al., 2009). Discussed neurohormones are metabolized to meta-derivatives, i.e. metanephrine and normetanephrine, which are eventually converted to vanillylmandelic acid (VMA). Subsequently, VMA is excreted in the urine and its concentration correlates well with the total amount of both catecholamines in the body (Noble, 2002; Szelenyi and Vizi, 2007).

In the initial stage of burnout syndrome, when a patient arrives at work, an ejection of catecholamines takes place. The amount of ejected hormones can also escalate because of unplanned events which are not typical for a normal day. During the most extreme stage of burnout syndrome, it is possible to obtain reduced blood and urine concentrations of both discussed hormones even when the patient is subjected to additional stress stimuli (Brosschot, 2010; Hansen et al., 2009; Lee et al., 2010; Vanltallie, 2002).

Adrenaline and noradrenaline are neurotransmitters of the nervous system that affect vascular smooth muscle, stimulate the heart, and increase blood pressure. In addition, they influence the liver, causing breakdown of the stored glycogen, resulting in glucose release into the blood stream. A quick adaptive reaction dependent on catecholamines aims in survival, but when it is inadequate, it causes imbalance of the human organism. It has been noted, that people who are subjected to permanent stress, causing the release of adrenaline and noradrenaline, are at higher risk of developing hypertension and cardiovascular disease which may be followed by life-threatening complications (Dimsdale, 2007; Hansen et al., 2009; Kjedsen et al., 2006; Lee et al., 2010; Noble, 2002; Szelènyi and Vizi, 2007; Vanltallie, 2002).

It has been established that a decrease in dopamine levels may be both a cause and a consequence of acute and chronic stress. The burnout syndrome is characterized by a reduction in the level of self-satisfaction coupled with emotional exhaustion which is associated with a decreased number of dopaminergic receptors (Cassella, 2010; Tops et al., 2007). Glucocorticoids are substances which influence the presence of receptors in neurons, as well (Szelènyi and Vizi, 2007). Another abnormality caused by stress is a drop in the concentration of serotonin and a reduction in the number of serotonin receptors. Similar changes occur in patients with depression which may be also one of the symptoms of chronic stress exposure. Frequently, the employee does not seek help until severe emotional and psychological disorders occur, and at which time a diagnostic process of burnout syndrome commences (Tops et al., 2007).

The Immune Response to Chronic Stress Exposure

Due to the numerous connections between the functions of neurons, hormones, and immunocompetent cells, it is extremely difficult to answer the question: what functions of hormones, neurons, etc. will change in response to stress stimuli? The situation becomes even more complicated in cases where the stress exposure is chronic or intensifies with time (Dimsdale, 2007; Hansen et al., 2010; Vizi, 2007). Neurohormones bind with adrenergic receptors located on the surface of cells. After the connection between the ligand and appropriate receptor occurs, a cascade of reactions begins. The result ultimately is an increase of the cyclic AMP concentration in the cell. Fluctuations in the AMP concentration play an important role in the production of pro- and anti-inflammatory cytokines in the immune cells (Lee et al., 2010; Miller and O'Callaghan, 2002; Vizi, 2007).

It has been observed that workers suffering from burnout syndrome are more susceptible to physical diseases when compared to healthy people (Dimsdale, 2007; Feston, 1998; Fernandez et al., 2010; Hansen et al., 2010; Montero-Marin et al., 2011; Ohlin et al., 2008; Xu et al., 2009). An increased incidence of infectious diseases, circulatory system disorders, mental disorders, autoimmune and allergic diseases have been reported (Dimsdale, 2008; Hansen et al., 2010; Siemińska-Nitka et al., 2007; Tops et al., 2006). Changes in the concentrations of cytokines interfere with cellular interactions and affect the neurons, and elevated cortisol levels strongly influence the immune cells by stimulating and/or inhibiting the production pathways of pro- and anti-inflammatory mediators (Hansen et al., 2010; Tops et al., 2006). The effect of cortisol on immune cells is related more to its effects on glucocorticoid receptors than to the quantity of freely circulating hormones. However, increased receptor production is associated with prolonged elevations in cortisol levels and nervous system stimulation.

In many patients suffering from burnout syndrome, a significant reduction in the number of natural killer cells (NK cells) is observed. The function of NK cells is to destroy the organism's own cells infected with intracellular pathogens, such as viruses. The ability to recognize altered tissues and participation in a specific "race" with infectious agents require from natural killer cells a great efficacy, immunocompetence, and their maintaining stable numbers. A reduction in the amount of NK cells may lead to increased morbidity of the workers. It has been observed that changes in the number of NK cells in women were significantly higher than in men. Both groups were dissatisfied with work, and this dissatisfaction was related to emotional and physical stress. Interestingly, the change in NK cell count was much lower during night shifts. It has been acknowledged that working at night is more stressful compared to working during the day. Moreover, the decrease in the level and cytotoxicity of the NK cells population was observed during the development of chronic inflammation and leukemia (Lee et al., 2010; Nakamura et al., 1999; Okamoto et al., 2008).

Another parameter that may be altered in patients with burnout syndrome is the number of T and B lymphocytes. The total lymphocyte count may be diminished (Okamoto et al. 2008, Rohleder et al., 2009) or changes in the count associated with only one cell population may occur (Nakata et al., 2010). Most studies showed a change in the proportion of T and B cells, which may be associated with a reduction in the number of individual subpopulations (Bellingrath et al., 2010; Hansen et al., 2010; Mommersteeg et al., 2006; Okamoto et al., 2008; van Kanel et al., 2008). Additionally, alterations of T-helper and T-suppressor populations were observed while lymphocytes B manifested decreased activity (Bellingrath et al. 2010, Mommersteeg et al. 2006, Nakata et al., 2010). Patients exposed to chronic stress have an increased incidence of bacterial infections, and during these infections there is a rise in the total number of lymphocytes (Bellingrath et al., 2010; Mommersteeg, 2006; Nakata et al., 2010). However, a diminished response to the activation of lymphocytes T was observed (Szelenyi and Vizi, 2007; Rohleder et al., 2010). Added stress also stimulates plasma cells to produce antibodies (Lee et al., 2010). Particularly, an increased secretion of IgA in the airways (measured in saliva) was noted, despite the drop in the total concentration of antibodies in the blood (Lee et al., 2010).

It is noted that both the rate of cell stimulation, and the cell's ability to produce cytokines are altered in patients subjected to prolonged stress (Bellingrath et al., 2010; Hansen et al., 2009, 2010; Rohleder et al., 2010; Szelènyi and Vizi, 2007). Changes in the production of pro- and anti-inflammatory cytokines begin a cascade of events which lead to immunity disorders in the entire organism. Stress stimulation raises the levels of interleukin 6 (IL-6), interleukin 10 (IL-10) and tumor necrosis factor alpha (TNF-∝). Interleukin 6 is produced by macrophages and lymphocytes B, as well as by other body cells (e.g. adipocytes). It has pro-inflammatory properties, and strongly stimulates liver cells to produce acute phase proteins, including C-reactive protein. There is a rising intensity in the level of this protein only a few hours after the stress stimulus occurrence. The alterations of C-reactive protein levels in blood may be an extremely reliable parameter when assessing the body's response to stress. It is especially relevant in relation to burnout syndrome, that an increased CRP level correlates with higher morbidity and mortality due to cardiovascular disease (Bellingrath et al., 2010; Hansen et al., 2010; van Kanel et al., 2008). Anti-inflammatory cytokine – interleukin 10 is released as a reaction to the ejection of inflammatory factors, and is a specific control system of the immune response of the body. TNF-∝, however, is excreted by macrophages and lymphocytes B during the initial phase of inflammation as a response to stimulation. Individual cytokines may affect the body's cells by changing their sensitivity to circulating mediators, transmitters and hormones (Bellingrath et al., 2010; Hansen et al., 2010; Rohleder et al., 2010; Szelènyi and Vizi, 2007; van Kanel et al., 2008). For patients with burnout syndrome, interferon gamma (INF-γ) levels may decrease, since it is produced by macrophages, B lymphocytes and NK cells. The drop in the amount of these particular cells was observed in patients suffering from the mentioned disease (Hansen et al., 2010).

Other Studies

The diagnosis of burnout syndrome is a complicated process. Despite the large number of tests available, it is extremely difficult to obtain an unequivocal diagnosis. Every organism responds to stress in a different way. An excellent example is a change in an individual's weight. After a stressful situation one may experience an increase in hunger, or on the contrary, a total lack of appetite. Chronic exposure to stress at work may lead to a patient's weight gain (Fernandez et al., 2010; Kjeldsen et al, 2006; Wirtz et al. 2008; Xu et al., 2009), or to weight loss (Fernandez et al. 2010, Kjeldsen et al. 2006). Any rapid change in one's body mass index (BMI) should be carefully monitored (Fernandez et al., 2010; Kjeldsen et al., 2006; Wirtz et al., 2008).

Hypercortisolemia causes a rise in the blood's glucose level which consequently leads to the stimulation of insulin secretion. Increased levels of adrenaline, noradrenaline and cortisol connected with hyperglycemia lead to impaired pancreatic function and insulin resistance, which ultimately results in the development of type 2 diabetes (Kitaocha-Higashiguchi et al., 2009; Miller and O'Callaghan, 2002; Rohleder et al., 2010). In overweight and/or obese patients, elevated glucose levels may be evaluated by utilizing glycated hemoglobin (HbA1c) measurements (Hansen et al. 2009, Kitaocha-Higashiguchi et al., 2009).

Lipids and lipoproteins are other parameters altered due to chronic stress. People suffering from burnout syndrome are more likely to have an abnormal lipid profile, significantly increasing their risk for atherosclerosis (Kitaocha-Higashiguchi et al., 2009). Vascular changes and high blood pressure can ultimately lead to life-threatening cardiac episodes (Dimsdale, 2008; Kitaocha-Higashiguchi et al., 2009; McEwan, 2002; Rjedsen et al., 2006).

For women, chronic exposure to stress may lead to hyperprolactinemia, and as a consequence to menstrual disturbances, lactorrhea, behavioral changes, and emotional problems (Miller and O'Callaghan, 2002; Tops et al., 2007).

Table 1. Tests results in burnout syndrome

Parameter	Normal Values	Burnout Syndrome
Blood cortisol level	15 – 700 nmol/l	↑ initially, ↓ (Chandola et al. 2010, Chida and Steptoe 2008, Clow et al. 2010, Foley and Kirchbaum 2010, Hansen et al. 2009, McEwen and Kalia 2010, Miller and O'Callaghan 2002, Mommersteeg et al. 2006, Tops et al. 2006, Wahlberg et al. 2009)
Urinary free cortisol level	30 – 300 nmol/24 h	↑ (Hansen et al. 2009, Vogelzangs et al. 2010)
Salivary cortisol level (CAR)	3,6 – 35,1 nmol/l	↑ initially, ↓ (Bellingrath et al. 2010, Clow et al. 2009, Melamed et al. 1999, Pruessner et al. 2008, Sertoz et al. 2008, Wirtz et al. 2008)
Blood cortisol level, depending on time of the day	150 – 700 nmol/l (morning) 55 – 250 nmol/l (afternoon) 30 – 120 nmol/l (evening)	disturbed (Chandola et al. 2010, Chida and Steptoe 2008, Sertoz et al. 2008, Wahlberg et al. 2009)
17-OHKS	2-8 mg/24 h	↑ initially, ↓ (Preuessner et al. 1999)
ACTH	< 22 pmol/l	↑ (Bellingrath et al. 2010, Clow et al. 2009, Foley and Kirchbaum 2010, McEwen and Kalia 2010, Miller and O'Callaghan 2002, Preuessner et al. 1999, Wahlberg et al. 2009)
CRH	0 – 10 pg/ml	↑ (McEwen and Kalia 2010, Miller and O'Callaghan 2002, Preuessner et al. 1999, Wahlberg et al. 2009)
Adrenaline, noradrenaline in blood	< 0,69, < 3,55 nmol/l	↑ (Chandola et al. 2010, Hansen et al. 2009, Lee et al. 2010, Õhlin et al. 2008)
Adrenaline, noradrenaline in urine	< 110, < 535 nmol/24 h	↑ (Chandola et al. 2010, Hansen et al. 2009, Lee et al. 2010, Õhlin et al. 2008)
Dopamine	< 888 pmol/l	↓ (Cassella 2011, Lee et al. 2010, Tops et al. 2006)
Prolactin	< 20ng/ml	↑ (Tops et al. 2006)
WBC (white blood cell count)	4 – 10 x 10^9 /l	↑, ↓ (Okamoto et al. 2008)
Granulocytes	1,8 – 8,5 x 10^9/l	↑, ↓ (Okamoto et al. 2008)
Lymphocytes Th	0,3 – 1,4 x 10^9/l	Change of the proportion (Bellingrath et al. 2010, Lee et al. 2010, Mommersteeg et al. 2006, Nakata et al. 2010, Okamoto et al. 2008)
NK cells	0,09 – 0,6 x 10^9/l	↓ (Bellingrath et al. 2010, Lee et al. 2010, Okamoto et al. 2008, Nakamura et al. 1999, Nakata et al. 2010)
CRP	0,1 – 3,0 mg/l	↑, ↓ (Lee et al. 2010, van Kanel et al. 2008)
IgA	70 – 310 mg/dl	↑, ↓ (Lee et al. 2010)

continued on following page

Table 1. Continued

Parameter	Normal Values	Burnout Syndrome
IgG	640 – 1350 mg/dl	↑ (Lee et al. 2010)
Il-6	3,13 – 12,5 pg/ml	↑ (Lee et al. 2010, Nakata et al. 2010)
Cholesterol	< 4,5 mmol/l	↑ (Kitaocha-Higashiguchi et al. 2009, Xu et al. 2009)
Cholesterol LDL	< 2,6 mmol/l	↑ (Kitaocha-Higashiguchi et al. 2009)
Cholesterol HDL	> 1,3 mmol/l, > 1,0 mmol/l	↓ (Kitaocha-Higashiguchi et al. 2009)
Triglycerides	< 1,7 mmol/l	↑ (Kitaocha-Higashiguchi et al. 2009)
Fasting blood glucose level	3,4 – 5,5 mmol/l	↑ (Kitaocha-Higashiguchi et al. 2009 Xu et al. 2009)
BMI	19 – 24,9 kg/m^2	↓ < 18,9; ↑ > 25 (Fernandez et al. 2010, Kitaocha-Higashiguchi et al. 2009, Kjeldsen et al. 2006, Wirtz et al. 2008, Xu et al. 2009)
Blood pressure	120/80 mm Hg	↑ (Chandola et al. 2010, Dimsdale 2008, Kitaocha-Higashiguchi et al. 2009, Kjeldsen et al. 2006, Lee et al. 2010, Melamed et al. 1999, Őhlin et al. 2008, Xu et al. 2009)

In summary, the number of people suffering from burnout syndrome is constantly increasing (Kamrowska 2007, Kamrowska and Kamrowski 2020, Popa et al. 2010). As a result, there are more and more days when an employee is unable to fulfill his/her duties. Even rest does not bring relief, and health problems can begin. Gradually, there is an increase in the number and length of medical absences, placing added burdens on co-workers. This situation can be a source of conflict because a lack of rest and an increase in responsibilities are another source of stress and possible first steps towards professional burnout. These circumstances can shortly lead to serious health issues affecting more workers (Felton 1998, Maslach and Jackson 1981, Montero-Marin et al. 2011, Pines and Keinan 2005, Siemińska-Nitka et al. 2007). Bodily responses to changes in one's environment can vary depending on the strength and type of stimuli (McEwen 2002, Tops et al. 2007, Vanltallie 2002). Some of these undesired changes can be revealed during a medical examination, and others can be revealed because of a patient's responses to questions in MBI. The choice of laboratory tests is determined by the attending physician, and should be the result of the physician's knowledge and abilities, from an analysis of the patient's medical history, and from the results of a physical examination. The connection between stress and hormone levels is a proven fact which should be recognized in the diagnosis of burnout syndrome (Vanltallie 2002). The treatment depends on the dominate symptoms (Miller and O'Callaghan 2002, Montero-Marin et al. 2011).

In recent years, an emphasis has been placed on the prophylaxis of burnout syndrome. It seems that the best method is to exercise and/or have a hobby. An employee who does not have a private life outside of work is more vulnerable to physical and emotional changes caused by stress (Brosschot 2010, Felton 1998, Montero-Marin et al. 2009, 2011). The ability to rest, both physically and intellectually, is one of the keys to a long and healthy life (Felton 1998, Brosschot 2010).

Health Promotion in Emergency Medicine

In order for society to take full benefit of the emergency medical services system, proper organization and time are required. One of the tasks of emergency medicine is participating in the promotion of health in society.

Health promotion in emergency medicine consists of education regarding organization and functioning of the system and services available for patients in the hospital and pre-hospital settings. Another role of health promotion is to educate the public about what to do in sudden health related, or even life-threatening situations. Knowledge of how to react in these situations empowers individuals to become actively involved in the functioning of the "survival chain".

The survival chain is a specific structure which functions, and is organized, as a series of individual links, all symbolizing life-saving actions. Each link represents a step toward more advanced actions. The first link symbolizes basic life support actions taken by those who randomly witness life or health threatening events. The final link, which is the most advanced, represents the emergency department, where clinical procedures are followed in order to provide the patient with rapid and effective medical assistance. Another role of emergency medicine is the creation of educational programs whose aim is to promote basic life support procedures directed at the general public, including school children and teenagers, or any citizens interested in these issues (Jakubaszko J.et al. 2004).

Another educational function of emergency medicine in Poland is the development of extended first aid programs. These programs are incorporated in the professional development and training of numerous professions (for example police, fire department), and are also regulated according to emergency medicine guidelines (Jakubaszko et al., 2005).

The Foundations of Paramedic Training in Poland: The European Educational System

One of the major issues centering around higher education at the end of the 20th century was a question regarding the value and quality of traditional education, both academic and professional. The debates, which took place mainly at universities, involved issues related to the concept of knowledge society, appearing in the documents of the Bologna Process. An increased emphasis on academics in occupational education where it was not previously required, was given added attention. At the same time, it was also noted, that in a Europe undergoing transformation, merely possessing a university degree does not guarantee employment or a job for life. Employers have also begun to demand that institutes of higher education determine what material and skills their graduates acquire.

Traditional education systems, oriented primarily on teachers, began to transform into systems focused more on students. The process of building the European Higher Education Area (Bologna Process) started in 1999, and created a fundamental change in the perception of the objectives of higher education. The mainstay in the development of curriculums is their future utilization by the graduate in society.

The main goals of higher education, based on Bologna Declaration, are (Narodowa Agencja Programu "Uczenie się przez całe życie" et al., 2008):

1. Preparation of graduates related to the needs and expectations of the job market.
2. Preparation for being an active citizen in the European democratic society.

3. Development and maintenance of advanced knowledge.
4. Professional development of the students.

New Concept of Professional Education of Paramedics

Nowadays, an extremely important issue is maintaining access for paramedics to high quality education. One strategy to reach this lofty goal is both proper pre- and postgraduate training for future paramedics.

There are three very critical areas pertaining to knowledge and skills in the professional educational process: theoretical knowledge, practical skills and social competences. Mastery of these three areas will allow paramedics to attain professional success.

The theoretical aspects of a paramedic's education involve: basic medical disciplines (e.g. anatomy, physiology, biochemistry), preclinical disciplines (e.g. microbiology, pathomorphology) and clinical disciplines (e.g. emergency medicine, internal medicine). This area of study should also emphasize the ability to utilize theoretical knowledge in solving clinical problems (Jakubaszko et al., 2007).

The area of social competences includes foundations and motivations for recognition of patient's emotional problems, understanding their psychological needs and expectations, as well as development of empathy. Perception and the proper understanding of patient's needs should lead the future paramedic to fulfill them. Area of social competences requires basic knowledge of psychology, psychopathology and familiarity psychophysical differences, e.g. in children, pregnant or menopausal women, elderly or terminal cancer patients. Empathy plays an important role in this area. It is defined as a congenital personality trait, which develops in a process of clinical education. Empathy is a cognitive-emotional process that allows to understand patient's emotional state.

The highest level is the area of practical skills, which should be mastered by every medical graduate. These include the ability of a paramedic to react actively to the patient's affective needs (Jakubaszko et al., 2007).

One of the most important aspects of the educational process of a future paramedic, is a development of the communication skills. In order to reach this goal a paramedic student, early in the educational process, should learn to develop the necessary skills required to effectively communicate and bond with a patient during the diagnostic and therapeutic process.

Evaluation of the Educational Process of Future Paramedics

An important, albeit a difficult task for academic professionals, is to evaluate the over-all education of the student. These include: communication skills, abilities of work organization, and development of student's own, but socially acceptable system of values and principles. These features are manifested in team building exercises which are an integral part of a future paramedic's education. Team building is not only about the theoretical, but is also related to a paramedic's level of engagement during times of crisis. The ability to properly assess, adapt, and react to a situation requires organizational and interpersonal skills. A paramedic is part of a team that consists of his colleagues, supervisors and other medical and administrative personnel. Situations taking place in the work of prehospital emergency medical teams and hospital emergency departments often require simultaneous action in several areas. How can it be evaluated?

To assess teamwork, communication skills, and the over-all effectiveness of the educational system is the most difficult part of the evaluation process. It is based primarily on long-term observation of the student in his/her day-to-day activities, and the collection of partial individual evaluations of those involved. Medical documentation can also be an element of this assessment. The reliability of these evaluations depends primarily on the established criteria, which must be generally known and accepted. The proper education of paramedics, and its reliable evaluation, are only possible, when this training involves obligatory clinical classes with a focus on acquiring professional skills (Jakubaszko et al., 2007).

SUMMARY

The state emergency medical services law filled the gap that previously existed in the Polish health care system. To function properly, an emergency medical services system guarantees a patient in need access to a timely assessment of their medical needs, and provides further specialist treatment in prehospital settings and in the emergency department. Therefore, the main responsibility of the health care system is to create the proper conditions for the effective functioning of emergency departments and prehospital emergency medical teams. In global terms, a health care system must create desirable working conditions, encourage professional development, and offer continuing educational opportunities for all emergency medicine physicians, nurses and paramedics. It is extremely important to remember that an emergency medical services system is built on people. These dedicated professionals dictate the system's efficiency, and are the ones who utilize all the modern rescue equipment available to them.

REFERENCES

Bellingrath, S., Rohleder, N., & Kudielka, B. (2010). Healthly working teachers with high effort-reward-imbalance and overcommitment show increased pro-inflammatory immune activity and a dampened innate immune defence. *Brain, Behavior, and Immunity*, *24*(8), 1332–1339. doi:10.1016/j.bbi.2010.06.011 PMID:20599495

Benien, K. (2005). *Jak prowadzić trudne rozmowy*. Kraków: Wydawnictwo WAM.

Brosschot, J. (2010). Markers of chronic stress: Prolonged physiological activation and (un)conscious perseverative cognition. *Neuroscience and Biobehavioral Reviews*, *35*(1), 46–50. doi:10.1016/j.neubiorev.2010.01.004 PMID:20096302

Cassella, C. (2011). Burnout and the relative value of dopamine. *Anesthesiology*, *114*(1), 213–217. doi:10.1097/ALN.0b013e318201c8cd PMID:21169792

Chandola, T., Heraclides, A., & Kumari, M. (2010). Psychophysiological biomarkers of workplace stressors. *Neuroscience and Biobehavioral Reviews*, *35*(1), 51–57. doi:10.1016/j.neubiorev.2009.11.005 PMID:19914288

Chida, Y., & Steptoe, A. (2009). Cortisol awakening response and psychosocial factors: A systematic review and meta-analysis. *Biological Psychology*, *80*(3), 265–278. doi:10.1016/j.biopsycho.2008.10.004 PMID:19022335

Clow, A., Hucklebridge, F., Stadler, T., Evans, P., & Thorn, L. (2010). The cortisol awakening response: More than a measure of HPA axis function. *Neuroscience and Biobehavioral Reviews*, *35*(1), 97–103. doi:10.1016/j.neubiorev.2009.12.011 PMID:20026350

Deckard, G., Hicks, L., & Hamory, B. (1992). The occurrence and distribution of burnout among infectious diseases physicians. *The Journal of Infectious Diseases*, *165*(2), 224–228. doi:10.1093/infdis/165.2.224 PMID:1730889

Dimsdale, J. (2008). Psychological stress and cardiovascular disease. *Journal of the American College of Cardiology*, *51*(13), 1237–1246. doi:10.1016/j.jacc.2007.12.024 PMID:18371552

Felton, J. (1998). Burnout as a clinical entity – its importance in health care workers; occupational. *Medicine*, *48*(4), 237–250. PMID:9800422

Fernandez, I., Hayan, S., Winters, P., & Liang, H. (2010). Association of workplace chronic and acute stressors with employee weight status: Data from worksites in turmoil. *Journal of Occupational and Environmental Medicine*, *52*(Suppl. 1), s34–s41. doi:10.1097/JOM.0b013e3181c88525 PMID:20061885

Foley, P., & Kirschbaum, C. (2010). Human hypothalamus-pituitary-adrenal axis responses to acute psychosocial stress in laboratory settings. *Neuroscience and Biobehavioral Reviews*, *35*(1), 91–96. doi:10.1016/j.neubiorev.2010.01.010 PMID:20109491

Głębocka, A., & Lisowska, E. (2007). Professional burnout and stress among Polish physicians explained by the Hobfoll resources theory. *Journal of Physiology and Pharmacology*, *58*(Suppl. 5), 243–252. PMID:18204134

Hänsel, A., Hong, S., Cámara, R., & von Känel, R. (2010). Inflammation as a psychophysiological biomarker in chronic psychosocial stress. *Neuroscience and Biobehavioral Reviews*, *35*(1), 115–121. doi:10.1016/j.neubiorev.2009.12.012 PMID:20026349

Hansen, A., Larsen, A., Ragulies, R., Garde, A., & Knudsen, L. (2009). A review of the effect of the psychosocial working environment on physiological changes in blood and urine. *Basis & Clincal Pharmacolgy & Toxicology*, *105*, 73–83. PMID:19563453

Jakubaszko, J. (2004). *Nauczanie pierwszej pomocy. Zalecenia metodyczne*. Wrocław: Biblioteka Polskiego Towarzystwa Medycyny Ratunkowej.

Jakubaszko, J. (2005). *Kwalifikowana pierwsza pomoc. Zalecenia metodyczne*. Wrocław: Biblioteka Polskiego Towarzystwa Medycyny Ratunkowej.

Jakubaszko, J. (2007). *Medical rescue. Undergraduate Course (BSc)*. Wroclaw: Library of Polish Society for Emergency Medicine.

Kamrowska, A. (2007). Wypalenie zawodowe. *Polski Merkuriusz Lekarski*, *23*(136), 317–319. PMID:18293860

Kamrowska, A., & Kamrowski, C. (2010). Wypalenie zawodowe wśród lekarzy psychiatrów. *Polski Merkuriusz Lekarski*, *28*(165), 242–243. PMID:20815178

Kępiński, A. (2005). *Jak leczyć i poznawać człowieka*. Kraków: Wydawnictwo Literackie.

Kitaoka-Higashiguchi, K., Morikawa, Y., Miura, K., Sakaurai, M., Ishizaki, M., Kido, T., & Nakagawa, H. et al. (2009). Burnout risk factors for arteriosclerotic disease: Follow up study. *Journal of Occupational Health*, *51*(2), 123–131. doi:10.1539/joh.L8104 PMID:19212087

Kliszcz, J. (2012). *Psychologia w ratownictwie*. Warszawa: Difin SA.

Lee, K., Yoon, K., Ha, M., Park, J., Cho, S., & Kang, D. (2010). Heart rate variability and urinary catecholamines from job stress in Korean male manufacturing workers according to work seniority. *Industrial Health*, *48*, 331–338.

Maslach, C., & Jackson, S. (1981). The measurement of experienced burnout. *Journal of Occupational Behaviour*, *2*(2), 99113. doi:10.1002/job.4030020205

Mayerscough, P. R., & Ford, M. (2003). *Jak rozmawiać z pacjentem. Podręcznik komunikacji interpersonalnej*. Warszawa: Wydawnictwo Naukowe PWN.

McEvans, B., & Kalia, M. (2010). The role of corticosteroids and stress in chronic pain conditions. *Metabolism: Clinical and Experimental*, *59*(Suppl. 1), s9–s13. PMID:20837196

McEwan, B., & Kalia, M. (2010). The role of corticosteroids and stress in chronic pain conditions. *Metabolism: Clinical and Experimental*, *59*(Suppl. 1), s9–s13. doi:10.1016/j.metabol.2010.07.012 PMID:20837196

Melamed, S., Ugarten, U., Shirom, A., Kahana, L., Lerman, Y., & Froom, P. (1999). Chronic burnout, somatic arousal and elevated salivatory cortisol levels. *Journal of Psychosomatic Research*, *46*(6), 591–598. doi:10.1016/S0022-3999(99)00007-0 PMID:10454175

Miller, D., & O'Callaghan, J. (2002). Neuroendocrine aspects of the response to stress. *Metabolism: Clinical and Experimental*, *51*(6 Suppl. 1), 5–10. doi:10.1053/meta.2002.33184 PMID:12040534

Mommersteeg, P., Heijnen, C., Kavelaars, A., & van Doornen, L. J. P. (2006). Immune and endocrine function in burnout syndrome. *Psychosomatic Medicine*, *68*(6), 879–886. doi:10.1097/01.psy.0000239247.47581.0c PMID:17079708

Montero-Marĭn, J., Garcĭa-Campayo, J., Fayó-Pascual, M., Carrasco, J., Gascón, S., Gili, M., & Mayoral-Cleries, F. (2011). Sociodemographic and occupational risk factors associated with the development of different burnout types: The cross-sectional University of Zaragoza study. *BMC Psychiatry*, *11*(1), 49–62. doi:10.1186/1471-244X-11-49 PMID:21447169

Montero-Marĭn, J., Garcĭa-Campayo, J., Mera, D., & del Hoyo, Y. (2009). A new definition of burnout syndrome based on Farber's proposal. *Journal of Occupational Medicine and Toxicology (London, England)*, *4*(1), 31–48. doi:10.1186/1745-6673-4-31 PMID:19948055

Nakamura, H., Nagase, H., Yoshida, M., & Ogino, K. (1999). Natural killer (NK) cell activity and NK cell subsets in workers with a tendency to burnout. *Journal of Psychosomatic Research*, *46*(6), 569–578. doi:10.1016/S0022-3999(99)00009-4 PMID:10454173

Nakata, A., Takahashi, M., Irie, M., & Swanson, N. (2010). Job satisfaction is associated with elevated natural killer cell immunity among healthy white-collar employees. *Brain, Behavior, and Immunity*, *24*(8), 1268–1275. doi:10.1016/j.bbi.2010.05.004 PMID:20561922

Narodowa Agencja Programu „Uczenie się przez całe życie": Wprowadzenie do projektu Tuning Educational Structures in Europe – Harmonizacja struktur kształcenia w Europie. Wkład uczelni w Proces Boloński. (2008). Warszawa: Fundacja Rozwoju Systemu Edukacji.

Noble, R. (2002). Diagnosis of stress. *Metabolism: Clinical and Experimental*, *51*(6 Suppl. 1), 37–39. doi:10.1053/meta.2002.33190 PMID:12040539

Popa, F., Arafat, R., Purcărea, V. L., Lală, A., Popa–Velea, O., & Bobirnac, G. (2010). Occupational burnout levels in emergency medicine – a stage 2 nationwide study and analysis. *Journal of Medicine and Life*, *3*(4), 449–453. PMID:21254747

Őhlin, B., Berglund, G., Nilsson, P., & Melander, O. (2008). Job strain, job demands and adrenergic beta-1-receptor=polymorphism: A possible interaction affecting blood pressure in men. *Journal of Hypertension*, *26*(8), 1583–1589. doi:10.1097/HJH.0b013e328303df5f PMID:18622236

Okamoto, H., Tsunoda, T., Teruya, K., Takeda, N., Uemura, T., Matsiu, T., & Takashima, Y. et al. (2008). An occupational health study of emergency physicians in Japan: Health assessment by immune variables (CD4, CD8, CD56, and NK cell activity) at the beginning of work. *Journal of Occupational Health*, *50*(2), 136–146. doi:10.1539/joh.L6084 PMID:18403864

Preuessner, J., Hellhammer, D., & Kirschbaum, C. (1999). Burnout, perceived stress, and cortisol responses to awakening. *Psychosomatic Medicine*, *61*(2), 197–204. doi:10.1097/00006842-199903000-00012 PMID:10204973

Brennan, J., & Krohmer, J. (Eds.). (2005). Principles of EMS Systems. Jones and Bartlett Publishers.

Pruessner, M., Boekestyn, L., Bèchard-Evans, L., Abadi, S., Vracotas, N., Joober, R., & Malla, A. et al. (2008). Sex differences in the cortisol response to awakening in recent onset psychosis. *Psychoneuroendocrinology*, *33*(8), 1151–1154. doi:10.1016/j.psyneuen.2008.04.006 PMID:18640785

Rohleder, N., Wolf, J., & Wolf, O. (2010). Glucocorticoid sensitivity of cognitive and inflammatory processes in depression and posttraumatic stress disorders. *Neuroscience and Biobehavioral Reviews*, *35*(1), 104–114. doi:10.1016/j.neubiorev.2009.12.003 PMID:20005894

Salch, P., & Shapiro, C. (2008). Disturbed sleep and burnout: Implications for long-term health [editorial]. *Journal of Psychosomatic Research*, *65*(1), 1–3. doi:10.1016/j.jpsychores.2008.05.028 PMID:18582605

Sertoz, O., Binbay, I., Koylu, E., & Noyan, A. (2008). The role of BDNF and HPA axis in the neurobiology of burnout syndrome. *Progress in Neuro-Psychopharmacology & Biological Psychiatry*, *32*(6), 1459–1465. doi:10.1016/j.pnpbp.2008.05.001 PMID:18541357

Siemiński, M., Nitka-Siemińska, A., & Nyka, W. (2007). Zespół wypalenia. *Centrum Medycyny Rodzinnej*, *1*(1), 45–49.

Szelènyi, J., & Vizi, S. (2007). The catecholamine-cytokine balance interaction between brain and the immune system. *Annals of the New York Academy of Sciences*, *1113*(1), 311–324. doi:10.1196/annals.1391.026 PMID:17584982

Tops, M., Boksem, M., Wijers, A., van Duinen, H., Den Boer, J., Meijman, T., & Korf, J. (2007). The psychobiology of burnout: Are the two different syndromes? *Neuropsychobiology*, *55*(3-4), 143–150. doi:10.1159/000106056 PMID:17641533

Vanltallie, T. (2002). Stress: A risk factor for serious illness. *Metabolism: Clinical and Experimental*, *51*(6 Suppl. 1), 40–45. doi:10.1053/meta.2002.33191 PMID:12040540

Vogelzangs, N., Beekman, A., Milaneschi, Y., Bandinelli, S., Ferrucci, L., & Penninx, B. W. J. H. (2010). Urinary cortisol and six-year risk of all-cause and cardiovascular mortality. *The Journal of Clinical Endocrinology and Metabolism*, *95*(11), 4959–4964. doi:10.1210/jc.2010-0192 PMID:20739384

von Känel, R., Bellingrath, S., & Kudielka, B. (2008). Association between burnout and circulating levels of pro- and anti-inflammatory cytokines in schoolteachers. *Journal of Psychosomatic Research*, *65*(1), 51–59. doi:10.1016/j.jpsychores.2008.02.007 PMID:18582612

Wahlberg, K., Ghatan, P., Modell, S., Nygren, A., Ingvar, M., Åsberg, M., & Heiling, M. (2009). Suppressed neuroendocrine stress response in depressed women on job-stress related long-term sick-leave: A stable marker potentially suggestive of pre-existing vulnerability. *Biological Psychiatry*, *65*(9), 742–747. doi:10.1016/j.biopsych.2008.10.035 PMID:19058782

Wciórka, J. (2010). Psychopatologia: objawy i zespoły zaburzeń psychicznych. In J. Rybakowski, S. Pużyński, & J. Wciórka (Eds.), *Psychiatria. T.1.Podstawy psychiatrii* (pp. 305–398). Wrocław: Elsevier Urban & Partner.

Wciórka, J., Pużyński, S., & Rybakowski, J. (Eds.). (2012). *Psychiatria. T.3. In Metody leczenia. Zagadnienia etyczne, prawne, publiczne, społeczne* (pp. 385–405). Wrocław: Elsevier Urban & Partner.

Wirtz, P., Ehlert, U., Emini, L., & Suter, T. (2008). Higher body mass index (BMI) is associated with reduced glucocorticoid inhibition of inflammatory cytokine production following acute psychosocial stress in men. *Psychoneuroendocrinology*, *33*(8), 1102–1110. doi:10.1016/j.psyneuen.2008.05.002 PMID:18644679

Xu, W., Zhao, Y., Guo, L., Guo, Y., & Gao, W. (2009). Job stress and coronary heart disease: A case-control study using a Chinese population. *Journal of Occupational Health*, *51*(2), 107–113. doi:10.1539/joh.L8060 PMID:19179802

Chapter 6
The Assessment of Actions of the Environment and the Impact of Preventive Medicine for Public Health in Poland

Anna Rosiek
Ross-Medica, Poland

ABSTRACT

This chapter describes how the actions of the medical environment is aiming to improve the health of society can and must be seen on many levels. The author refers to the organizational, ethical, legal and psychological aspects. Also covered are not only patients' education, but also the scope of functioning healthcare organization, which adapts to the needs of the changing environment e.g. requirements of the patient, the development of technology, advances in medicine. Public health problems appear as complex components of the system and cannot be dealt with by a single, simple intervention, whether perceived by the prism of a single feature or element, but must be perceived as influencing factors in the system e.g. several attributes, factors. These together may potentially be used in the future to generate better health outcomes or the functioning of the entire health system in the areas of health sciences, medicine or public health.

INTRODUCTION

Currently, most health problems occur due to the consequences of cardiovascular diseases, cancer, allergies and metabolic disorders. The search for new, more effective methods of solving health problems of the population initiated the creation of a new pro-health movement, as well as contributed to the recognition of the need to take multi-level measures to improve the social, economic and political conditions. This approach resulted in the development of a better health education for the patient on one hand, and the actions taken by organizations and institutions in order to improve healthcare and ensure the "normal" functioning of the society in the event of its loss on the other.

DOI: 10.4018/978-1-5225-3946-9.ch006

It should be noted that the four models of health (clinical, of social roles, adaptive and self-fulfillment), currently existing in the literature, also point to the fact that the currently occurring issues should be considered comprehensively as a whole. Taking into account the issues discussed the definition of health presented here is the one that, is useful in practical use, because of the possibility of relating it to a large group of people who have a history of greater or lesser impairment of health. According to this definition, "health is the ability and willingness of each part of the human body to fulfill, in the normal conditions of micro and macro environment, all the common tasks with sufficient capacity." In the literature, we can find differences in interpretation of health determinants. In this case, there is also an ambiguity as to their determination. However, the most common health determinants by WHO include: lifestyle, genetic and biological factors, environmental (physical and psychosocial), economic, demographic, cultural, political, ecological and social factors types of individual behavior and organization of health care.

Adoption of the health definition and determinants presented above allows for an in-depth understanding of the issue, and will also systematize the existing knowledge about the determinants of health in the light of the study.

The issue of health and its determinants, as well as environmental activities in this field has become the subject of my particular interests, resulting in multi-layered analyzes, the results which were published in the international literature.

Undoubtedly the factors in determining the health of the population are: lifestyle, individual choices and behaviors and health care organization. Individual behaviors such as:

- Sedentary lifestyle, lack of physical activity (Central Statistical Office in Poland, 2015; The National Program, 2015; French, 2005; Sallis & Glanz, 2009)
- Increased consumption of easily accessible and high in calories snacks, (mass- produced junk food) (Central Statistical Office in Poland, 2015; The National Program, 2015; Duffey & Popkin, 2011; Jahns et al., 2001; Zizza et al., 2001; Piernas & Popkin, 2011; Young & Nestle, 2002; Young & Nestle, 2003),

are considered risk behaviors. The processes of globalization, is not only responsible for the change in lifestyles, but also contributes to the development of many diseases including obesity, cardiovascular diseases, respiratory diseases and diabetes. These problems concern equally Polish and European society which means that from the point of view of public health, it is important to know the activities of the environment taken to improve public health.

Although it is important for public health policy to be guided by evidence, if this evidence predominantly supports individual-level interventions that have minimal reach and effect across populations, the benefits of being informed by the existing evidence base might be illusory (Parkhurst & Abeysinghe, 2016). Experience form Poland and other European countries shows, that research on systems needs to provide policy makers and practitioners with robust and relevant evidence that takes adequate account of the real-world circumstances in which people live, policies are made, and interventions are implemented (Rutter et al., 2017; Academy of Medical Sciences, 2016). A complex systems approach uses a broad spectrum of methods to design, implement, and evaluate interventions for changing these systems to improve public health (Diez Roux, 2011). Assessment and describing emergency the properties of a complex system that cannot be directly predicted from the elements within it and are more than just the sum of its parts. For example, the changing distribution of obesity across the population can be conceptualised as an emergent property of the food, employment, transport, economic, and other systems that shape the energy intake and expenditure of individuals. Feedback describes the situation in which a change reinforces or balances further change. For example, if a fast food consumption in public places or consumption fast food in general increase the risk of cardiovascular diseases and media influence on health education makes it fewer young people might then start eating snacking, further reducing its visibility of heart diseases. Adaptation refers to adjustments in behaviour in response to interventions, such as a lowering death by heart disease caused by changing lifestyle and better medical education by media about the consequences of unhealth eating and also standards of gold hour. Rhetoric urging complex systems approaches to public health is only rarely operationalised in ways that generate relevant evidence or effective policies (Academy of Medical Sciences, 2016; AcWutzke et al., 2016; Rutter et al., 2017). Public health problems that emerge as a property of a complex system cannot necessarily be solved with a simple, single intervention, but the interacting factors within the system can potentially be reshaped to generate a more desirable set of outcomes (Finegood, 2011; Rittel & Webber, 1973; Rutter et al., 2017). Author of this paper in complex way analyzed factors within the system of public health in Poland. It should be noted that the determinants of public health are: lifestyle, personal behaviors, and organization of health care. A series of publications (Miller & Page SE, 2007; Petticrew et al., 2013; Moore et al., 2015) and author own research under discussion clearly underlines the strong position of the organization of health care among the determinants of public health. The organization of health care in case of Polish population is just as important as lifestyle and personal behavior of the patient. The results of the analysis indicate that an adequate level of health care organization (using modern technology) not only helps to improve patient's safety, reduces the time required to perform medical intervention, but also helps to improve the quality of medical services and largely prevents premature mortality.

MATERIAL AND METHOD

The study was conducted in Poland. The study was conducted in stages III. In the first stage, the literature was reviewed in terms of current public health problems and a comprehensive approach to their solution. The impact of media and new technologies on human health was analyzed. It was analyzed whether the time spent in front of the monitor and how many hours are harmful to the body and whether the time spent in front of the monitor is related to the development of diseases and what. Then asked the group of women and men in Poland how much time they spend in front of the monitor. At this stage it was found that the time spent in front of the monitor favors the development of cardiovascular diseases, and these diseases are a significant problem for the health of Polish society. The second stage of the study was analyzed does organization of healthcare is a determinant of the health of society on the example of cardiovascular diseases. The study has shown important areas in the functioning of cardiac care, which require improvement in the comprehensive approach to the protection of public health in Poland. An area where the medical environment needs improvement has been identified. In the last stage of the test it was checked that technology and information systems used in health care is as a guarantee patient safety and whether the use of new technologies in treatment contributes to patient satisfaction and hospital recommendations.

The research data was collected from 2011 to 2015 and results were analyzed statistically in 2015. The author used different statistical tests such as: Spearman, Mann-Withney U and also Wilcoxon tests. The Institutional BioMedical Ethics Committee approved this study. Written informed consent for participation in the study was obtained from participants of the study and for publication of this report.

RESEARCH

Discussing the different characteristics related to health improvement efforts, it was necessary to address all the hallmarks of Lalond's health fields. Hence, the presented material touches on the various areas of the presented research problem, showing a comprehensive approach to the health care system. The author with great insight and precision referred to the discussed factors determining the health of Polish society, including in particular the lifestyle, individual behavior of citizens and the organization of health care that has been tested. The environment for improving public health has been multi-faceted, and the results of multidimensional analyzes of the assessment of the medical environment are outlined below.

Characteristics such as lifestyle, individual behavior and organization of health care have a significant impact on the health of Polish society. The material discussed in the chapter clearly emphasizes the strong position of the health care organization, which uses all its resources in the daily functioning of the organization, including: technological, psychological, social (human) factors that contribute to improving the health of Polish society. The organization of health care and its actions in the case of the Polish population are as important as the lifestyle and individual behavior of the patient.

Lifestyle and the Role and Impact of the Media on Changing the Health Behavior of Society

The results of the analyzes have shown that important role in shaping the behavior of individual citizens have actions taken by the media. It is them who influence the shaping of the behavior of individuals, promoting "couch-potato lifestyle", and creating the eating habits of the society. Thus, media also contribute to the development of obesity and diseases caused by it. The amount of time spent watching television or an electronic monitor (computer or tablet) is closely linked to unhealthy behaviors (eating habits). This occurs in all age groups. It is seen in adults, adolescents and children. The risk of cardiovascular disease in adults, regardless of gender, age, education, smoking or medicines they take grows by 8% with each additional hour spent watching television (Wijndaele et al., 2010). An additional two hours per day spent watching TV cause an increased risk of obesity by 23% and the risk of diabetes increased by 14% (Grontved & Hu, 2011; Hu, 2003). In the case of the Polish population, the group that is definitely vulnerable to illnesses (resulting from unhealthy lifestyle) such as cardiovascular disease, type II diabetes, obesity and depression are men. Men spend more time watching television or an electronic monitor than women (Table 1). Therefore, prevention programs should be targeted at this group. As a result, the Polish population statistics show that men live shorter by 10 years than women. As we can see, mass media may cause overweight and obesity in adult men, children, and adolescents. For this reason, preventive programs to combat obesity in Polish society are directed mainly to those target groups.

In conclusion, all illustrated data provide strong evidence that sedentary behaviors, especially prolonged TV watching, are directly related to obesity, diabetes risk, heart diseases, and even increased risk of early death

The actions of the medical environment, in this case are not sufficient. In order to counterbalance the adverse effects on public health resulting from the effects of unhealthy lifestyles, it is necessary to include the media in the activities in the field of public health. Close cooperation of governmental and health sector with the media to develop regulations for promoting only healthy food as well as the inclusion of comprehensive public education on food and promoting physical activity can prevent not only

Table 1. Watching TV/ Screen viewing by sex

Watching TV (Screen Viewing)	Obesity	Diabets Type II	Risk of Cardiovascular Disease	Risk of Cardiovascular Disease (Male/Female)
1 hour	N/A	N/A	8%	N/A
up 2 hours	23%	14%	16%	N/A
Men				
The time spent by men on screen viewing per day in Poland: *Author's own research	10-12 hours			80%-96% (high level of risk); p < 0.05
Women				
The time spent by women on screen viewing per day in Poland: *Author's own research	6-8 hours			48%-64%

Source: Author own study based on literature and own research.

the widespread obesity in Poland and Europe, but can also allow people to change their style of life and will lead to minimizing the risk of advancing of many civilizational diseases.

Organization of Health Care Is a Determinant of the Health of Society on the Example of Cardiovascular Diseases

Individual Behavior of a Patient With Cardiovascular Disease

Cardiovascular diseases have been diagnosed as the biggest public health problem in Poland. Therefore, the ocean of actions taken by the medical community to improve the health of citizens is an important and current issue when assessing a comprehensive approach to the health care system. The results of conducted studies show that the organization of health care is a factor in determining the health of the population, as important as lifestyle. Given that cardiovascular diseases are mainly a consequence of lifestyle, an analysis of health care organizations, was conducted taking into account the target group of patients (patients with acute coronary syndrome). We analyzed the delay in the treatment of patients and its causes. The analysis included patients admitted to hospital in an emergency and classified into cardiac invasive treatment. The conducted study also showed that in the Kujavian-Pomeranian region men are more often treated due to cardiovascular diseases than women and gender difference was statistically significant ($p<0.05$) (Table 2).

Assessing the organization of health care, the delay in access to treatment for the patient, resulting from one- and two-stage transport of the patient to the reference centre was analysed in detail. Included were also delays in access to treatment dependent on the patient himself. Time delays in access to treatment dependent on the patient were calculated from the moment of appearance of chest pain until medical emergencies unit was contacted. These times were significant ($P <0.0001$), and stood in the range from 3 to 720 minutes. The average time delay dependent on the patient was 140 minutes. (Figure 1).

This trend can be observed on a global scale, not only in Poland (Ahmed et al., 2009; Mosley et al., 2007; Moser et al., 2006; Terkelsen et al., 2005). Such long delays suggest, however, insufficient knowledge in patients and the lack of health education in the field of diagnosis of acute coronary syn-

Table 2. Patient demographic data

Two-Stage Transport to a Referral Hospital									
Sex	**STEMI**		**NSTEMI**		**UA**		**Sum**		***p***
	No.	**%**	**No.**	**%**	**No.**	**%**	**No.**	**%**	
Female	10	14.9	10	14.9	2	3.0	22	32.8	$p < 0.05$
Male	21	31.4	23	34.3	1	1.5	45	67.2	
Sum	31	46.3	33	49.2	3	4.5	67	100	
Education Level	**STEMI**		**NSTEMI**		**UA**		**Sum**		***p***
	No.	**%**	**No.**	**%**	**No.**	**%**	**No.**	**%**	
Elementary Level	8	12.0	11	16.4	1	1.5	20	29.9	$p > 0.05$
Basic Technical	16	23.9	13	19.4	2	3.0	31	46.3	
High School	6	8.9	2	3.0	0	0	8	11.9	
University Level	1	1.5	7	10.4	0	0	8	11.9	
Sum	31	46.3	33	49.2	3	4.5	67	100	

Figure 1. The time dependent on the patient—from the beginning of the chest pain until medical help

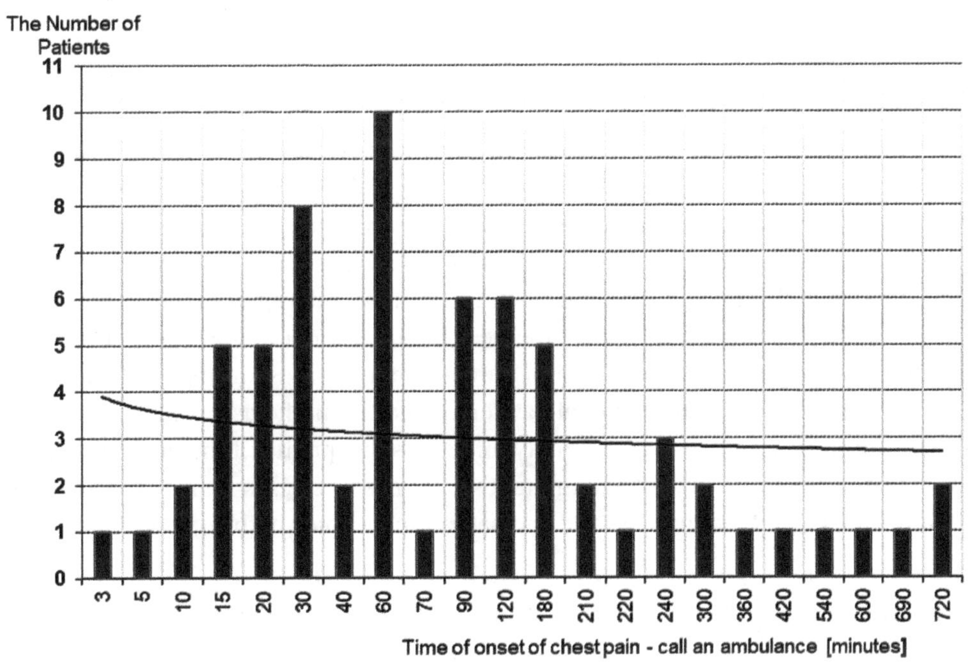

drome. Conducting public education through mass media would increase awareness and knowledge of acute coronary syndrome in society. In the future would help to reduce the time delay dependant on the patient, and education conducted with the participation of the media would allow correct behaviors of people to form in this area.

Emergency the Delay in Access to Treatment for the Patient, Resulting From One and Two-Stage Transport of the Patient to the Hospital

Equally important in the organization of health care for cardiac patients requiring invasive treatment are delays resulting from the two-stage transport to the reference center (Table 3).

Delay times were significant (p<0.0001) and resulted mainly from the fact that the ECG signal was not transmitted to the reference center by the emergency team. The analyzes showed that this fact occurred in case of 53% of patients. In this group time from the admission to hospital to the beginning of the coronary angioplasty was over 90 minutes and was statistically significant (p<0.0001). Given all the time delays occurring in healthcare organization for cardiac patients, it should be noted that the two-stage transport of the patient to the reference center does not meet the standards recommended by the European Society of Cardiology, according to which a patient with acute coronary syndrome should be subjected to therapy within 90 minutes of first medical contact, and in the case of a reference center, within 60 minutes of hospital admission (Steg P.G et al. 2012; O'Gara, P.T et al. 2012). American Heart Association Guidelines for Cardiopulmonary Resuscitation and Emergency Cardiovascular Care from 2010 also suggest that post-cardiac-arrest hospital care has significant potential to reduce early mortality caused by hemodynamic instability and later morbidity and mortality from multi-organ failure and brain injury (Rosiek A et al. 2015; Neumar, R.W. et al. 2008; Peberdy, M.A et al. 2010; Safar, P. 1988).

The analyzes showed that the organization of health care using the single-step transport contributes significantly to the reduction of in-hospital delays. It should be noted, however, that such an organization of health care is only possible with the use of new technologies and telemedicine, which allows the transmission of medical data directly to the reference center. Modern technology used in health care organizations "reduces" geographical distance, which makes it very effective in the treatment of patients from remote areas and rural areas (Buntin, et al. 2011; Spetz & Keane, 2009; Yellowlees et al., 2010) . The development of technology in medicine and its ever wider use that, we can observe recently, increases the number of medical consultations conducted at a distance; it allows for the efficient exchange of medical information and thereby contributes to patient safety and improvement in the quality of medical services, saving the time required to start medical intervention. Organization of health care, using modern technologies allows for the provision of care and equal access to medical services to patients irrespective of social, cultural or geographical barriers. In addition, the use of modern technology leads to a reduction in mortality, improves patient safety, improves the quality of medical services, encourages the patient to play an active role in the healing process and in some cases it also contributes to lowering the cost of health care (e.g. direct transport of the patient to a center with a catheterisation laboratory).

Table 3. Time delays resulting from the two-stage transport to the reference center

Two-Stage Transport to a Referral Hospital	Timedelays Sume (Dependent and Independent)	Group	*p*
		N = 67	
STEMI	95 min	31	<0.0001
NSTEMI	N/A	33	0.2692
UA	140 min	3	<0.0001
Diagnosis with using technology (One-stage transport)	28 min	67	N/A

Source: Author's own study.

The Organization of Health Care for Cardiac Patients Requiring Cardiac Surgery: Lack of Psychological Care on Hospital Wards

An in-depth study of the organization of health care for cardiac patients requiring cardiac surgery showed also that some elements of the organization of medical care can influence the intensity of anxiety and stress before surgery. Stress and anxiety before surgery largely depend on the gender and are more frequent in women ($p < 0.05$). Figure 2.

The stress of the patient's stay in the hospital increases when it is necessary to operate. Literature review shows that waiting for cardiac surgery evokes grater stress response that other types of surgery (Rosiek et al., 2016; Rymaszewska et al., 2003; Krzych, 2009). This phenomenon is disadvantageous, since the additional stress factors may unexpectedly degrade the condition of the patient. Respondents indicated that among the essential elements of the organization of medical care affecting the sense of stress and anxiety are: insufficient contact of medical staff with the patients ($p < 0.05$), the lack of an open attitude of the nursing staff ($p < 0.05$), insufficient psychological support of the patients before treatment ($p < 0.05$), insufficient cardiac patient education before treatment ($p < 0.05$). Table 4.

Improving hospital's organization in these aspects greatly affects the elimination of stress and anxiety in a patient during hospitalization. The analysis showed that factors relating to the organization of medical care have a direct impact on eliminating stress in patients requiring cardiac surgery.

Technology and Information Systems Used in Health Care as a Guarantee Patient Safety

Further analysis of the health care organization has also shown the importance of technology, used in the treatment process and the implementation of new methods of treatment using automated systems (navigation) in health care. Technology and information systems used in health care guarantee patient

Figure 2. Stress distribution by gender in cardiac patients

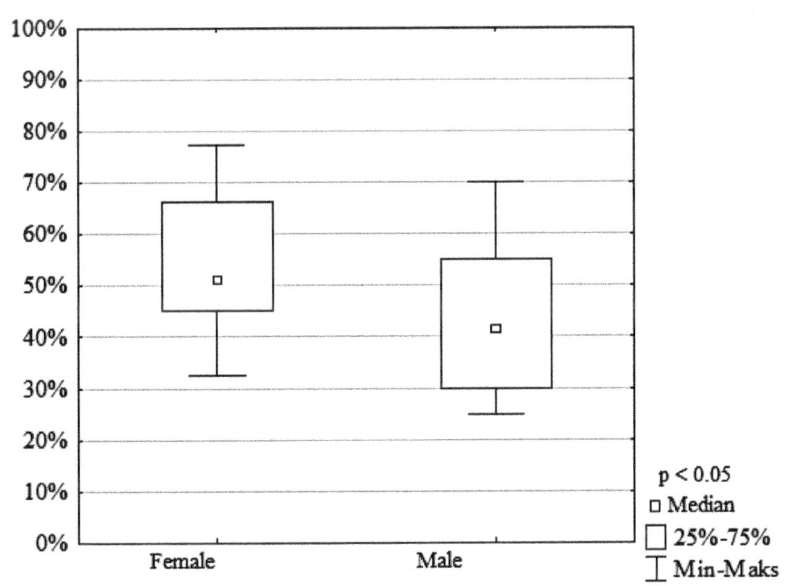

Table 4. Essential elements of the organization of medical care affecting the sense of stress and anxiety

Elements of the Organization of Medical Care	Level p
cardiac patient education conducted on the ward (e.g. on the functioning after surgery)	$p < 0.05$
information on diagnosis provided by medical personnel	$p < 0.05$
interview with a psychologist before surgery	$p < 0.05$
talk with a nurse (before treatment) in whom the patient has confidence	$p < 0.05$
talk with patient's doctor	$p < 0.05$
conversation with a loved one (family member)	$p > 0.05$

Source: Author own study.

safety not only during the emergency medical intervention or surgical interventions, but also during the patient's stay in a hospital. New technologies used in health care organizations improve patient safety ($p < 0.05$), and also contribute to the decline in mortality. Patients (irrespectively of age, sex and education) believe that modern technology and minimally invasive methods used in the treatment are essential to their safety in case of an urgent medical intervention. The relationship between patient's safety and the use of advanced medical technology was statistically significant ($p < 0.05$) in the evaluation of the patients themselves. The conducted analysis showed that 80% of patients in health care facilities using modern technology have a sense of greater security and are likely to recommend the services provided by the medical unit. Table 5.

Patients form both groups are willing to recommend a hospital. In Group I – 79,9% of all patient's and 80% of patients in Group II. As we can see patients appreciated minimal invasive surgery and safety during such procedures which is guaranteed by the technological progress. Advances in surgery have centered on minimizing the invasiveness of surgical procedures as a means to reduce patient morbidity and mortality.

Table 5. Hospital using modern technology (minimal invasive surgery) and patient's willingness to recommend a hospital

Group (Hospitals in Poland Divided by the Number of Beds)	Group I (Hospital With the Number of Beds Above 400)		Group II (Hospitals With the Number of Beds Below 400)		Sum	
Differences	Number	%	Number	%	Number	%
-4	0	0,0	1	1,1	1	0,6
-2	2	2,2	1	1,1	3	1,7
-1	16	17,8	16	17,8	32	17,8
0	49	54,4	61	67,8	110	61,1
1	19	21,1	10	11,1	29	16,1
2	4	4,4	1	1,1	5	2,8

Source: Author own study.

The trend that we can currently observe in health care is the result of globalization of medical services. It points to the need to use modern and advanced technologies for the treatment, which have become the gold standard in the world and reached some areas of health care in Poland. Ensuring patient's treatment with the use of modern technology and automated technological equipment underlines commitment to high-quality patient care while improving patient safety, minimizing the cost of medical care and decrease in mortality in emergencies (Boyd et al., 2002; LaPietra et al., 2000; Cadiere et al., 2001; Silberfein et al., 2007).

DISCUSSION

Comprehensive approach to assessing the health care system has revealed gaps in cardiac health care. Multivariate analysis of environmental actions to improve the health of Polish society has revealed that promoting health through the media can help to reduce delays in the treatment of cardiologic patients for reasons attributable to the patient. From the point of view of the organization of health care in Poland, weaknesses of the functioning of the health care system have emerged. Inadequate psychological care of a cardiologist requiring surgical treatment is the reason for patient dissatisfaction with hospital care. Analysis of technological progress in Poland, in terms of their use in the treatment of cardiovascular disease, has shown that it has improved patient safety, reduced mortality in emergencies, and widely used telemedicine allows for rapid diagnosis of patients even from small towns. (Boyd et al., 2002; LaPietra et al., 2000; Cadiere et al., 2001; Silberfein et al., 2007). Automation and even robotics in medicine have become the cornerstone of health care. It is an integral part of medical services. Hence, by making a comprehensive assessment of the activities of the medical environment, significant technological progress and its role in the health care system in Poland cannot be ignored. The necessity of evaluating the activities in medicine in a complete way, as was done in the present work, is also perceived by other authors (Rutter et al., 2017; Anderson et al., 2013) who also propose in the latest world trends an approach such as discussed in this paper and how they were presented in this study.

SUMMARY

To summarize the undertaken analyses, it should be noted that the determinants of public health are: lifestyle, personal behaviors, and organization of health care. A series of publications under discussion clearly underlines the strong position of the organization of health care among the determinants of public health. The organization of health care in case of Polish population is just as important as lifestyle and personal behavior of the patient. The results of the analysis indicate that an adequate level of health care organization (using modern technology) not only helps to improve patient's safety, reduces the time required to perform medical intervention, but also helps to improve the quality of medical services and largely prevents premature mortality. Undoubtedly an element that contributes significantly to the proper organization of health care is widely understood modern technology, which should become the gold standard in the treatment of diseases resulting from unhealthy lifestyle. Meanwhile, mass media are not sufficiently exploited as a preventive factor in Poland. It seems that a potential increase in media activities aiming at promotion of a healthy lifestyle can bring tangible benefits for public health in Poland. To conclude, the approach to a comprehensive assessment of all determinants of health in the context of the assessment of environmental actions and the impact of preventive medicine on the health of society is a rational justification and points to the innovativeness and relevance of the proposed solution in the field of medicine, health sciences and public health. The approach presented in this chapter is consistent with the latest scientific trend which shows the need of analysis for a complex systems model of evidence for public health (Rutter et al., 2017; Anderson et al., 2013).

REFERENCES

Academy of Medical Sciences. (2016, September). Improving the health of the public by 2040: optimising the research environment for a healthier, fairer future. Retrieved April 26, 2017 from https://acmedsci.ac.uk/policy/policy-projects/health-of-the-public-in-2040

Ahmed, B., Lischke, S., Straight, F., Gogo, P., Leffler, S., Kutler, M., & Dauerman, H. L. et al. (2009). Consistent door-to-balloon times of less than 90 minutes for STEMI patients transferred for primary PCI. *The Journal of Invasive Cardiology*, *21*, 429–433. PMID:19726811

Anderson, L. M., Oliver, S. R., Michie, S., Rehfuess, E., Noyes, J., & Shemilt, I. (2013). Investigating complexity in systematic reviews of interventions by using a spectrum of methods. *Journal of Clinical Epidemiology*, *66*(11), 1223–1229. doi:10.1016/j.jclinepi.2013.06.014 PMID:23953087

Boyd, W. D., Kodera, K., Stahl, K. D., & Rayman, R. (2002). Current status and future directions in computer-enhanced video- and robotic-assisted coronary bypass surgery. *Seminars in Thoracic and Cardiovascular Surgery*, *14*(1), 101–109. doi:10.1053/stcs.2002.31893 PMID:11977023

Buntin, M. B., Burke, M. F., Hoaglin, M. C., & Blumenthal, D. (2011). The benefits of health information technology: A review of the literature shows predominantly positive results. *Health Affairs (Project Hope)*, *30*(3), 464–471. doi:10.1377/hlthaff.2011.0178 PMID:21383365

Cadiere, G. B., Himpens, J., & Germay, O. et al.. (2001). Feasibility of robotic laparoscopic surgery: 146 cases. *World Journal of Surgery*, *25*, 1467–1477. PMID:11760751

Central Statistical Office. (2015). Population Project 2014–2015. Statistical Analyses and Studies, Warsaw 2014, Poland. Retrieved 6 August 2015 from http://www.stat.gov.pl/

Diez Roux, A. V. (2011). Complex systems thinking and current impasses in health disparities research. *American Journal of Public Health*, *101*(9), 1627–1634. doi:10.2105/AJPH.2011.300149 PMID:21778505

Duffey, K. J., & Popkin, B. M. (2011). Energy density, portion size, and eating occasions: Contributions to increased energy intake in the United States, 1977–2006. *PLoS Medicine*, *8*(6). doi:10.1371/journal.pmed.1001050 PMID:21738451

Finegood, D. T. (2011). The complex systems science of obesity. In J. Cawley (Ed.), *The Oxford handbook of the social science of obesity* (pp. 208–236). New York: Oxford University Press.

French, S. A. (2005). Public health strategies for dietary change: Schools and worksites. *The Journal of Nutrition*, *135*, 910–912. PMID:15795458

Grontved, A., & Hu, F. B. (2011). Television viewing and risk of type 2 diabetes, cardiovascular disease, and all-cause mortality: A meta-analysis. *Journal of the American Medical Association*, *305*(23), 2448–2455. doi:10.1001/jama.2011.812 PMID:21673296

Hu, F. B., Li, T. Y., Colditz, G. A., Willett, W. C., & Manson, J. E. (2003). Television watching and other sedentary behaviors in relation to risk of obesity and type 2 diabetes mellitus in women. *Journal of the American Medical Association*, *289*(14), 1785–1791. doi:10.1001/jama.289.14.1785 PMID:12684356

Jahns, L., Siega-Riz, A. M., & Popkin, B. M. (2001). The increasing prevalence of snacking among U.S. children from 1977 to 1996. *Pediatrics*, *138*(4), 493–498. doi:10.1067/mpd.2001.112162 PMID:11295711

Krzych, Ł. J., Pawlak, A., Woźnica, A., Skarysz, J., Eysymontt, Z., Krupka-Matuszczyk, I., & Cisowski, M. et al. (2009). Conditions of severity of anxiety and depression in the perioperative period in the economically active men undergoing coronary artery and cardiopulmonary bypass. *Cardio-Thoracic Surgery Poland*, *6*(3), 238–243.

LaPietra, A., Grossi, E. A., Derivaux, C. C., Applebaum, R. M., Hanjis, C. D., Ribakove, G. H., & Colvin, S. B. et al. (2000). Robotic-assisted instruments enhance minimally invasive mitral valve surgery. *The Annals of Thoracic Surgery*, *70*(3), 835–838. doi:10.1016/S0003-4975(00)01610-6 PMID:11016319

Miller, J. H., & Page, S. E. (Eds.). (2007). *Complex adaptive systems: An introduction to computational models of social life*. Princeton, NJ: Princeton University Press.

Moore, G. F., Audrey, S., & Barker, M. et al.. (2015). Process evaluation of complex interventions: Medical Research Council guidance. *BMJ (Clinical Research Ed.)*, *350*, h1258. PMID:25791983

Moser, D., Kimble, L., Alberts, M., Alonzo, A., Croft, J., & Dracup, K. et al.. (2006). Reducing delay in seeking treatment by patients with acute coronary syndrome and stroke: A scientific statement from the American Heart Association Council on cardiovascular nursing and stroke council. *Circulation*, *114*(2), 168–182. doi:10.1161/CIRCULATIONAHA.106.176040 PMID:16801458

Mosley, I., Nicol, M., Donnan, G., Patrick, I., Kerr, F., & Dewey, H. (2007). The impact of ambulance practice on acute stroke care. *Stroke*, *38*(10), 2765–2770. doi:10.1161/STROKEAHA.107.483446 PMID:17717317

Neumar, R. W., Nolan, J. P., Adrie, C., Aibiki, M., Berg, R. A., Bottiger, B. W., & Vanden Hoek, T. et al. (2008). Post-cardiac arrest syndrome. *Circulation*, *118*(23), 2452–2483. doi:10.1161/CIRCULATIONAHA.108.190652 PMID:18948368

O'Gara, P. T., Kushner, F. G., & Ascheim, D. D. et al.. (2012). ACCF/AHA Guidelines for the management of ST-Elevation of Mycocardial infraction: A report of American College of Cardiology Foundation/American Heart Association task force on practice guidelines. *Circulation*. doi:10.1161/CIR.0b013e3182742cf6

Parkhurst, J. O., & Abeysinghe, S. (2016). What constitutes "good" evidence for public health and social policy-making? From hierarchies to appropriateness. *Social Epistemology*, *30*(5-6), 665–679. doi:10.1080/02691728.2016.1172365

Peberdy, M. A., Callaway, C. W., Neumar, R. W., Geocadin, R. G., Zimmerman, J. L., Donnino, M., & Kronick, S. L. et al. (2010). Part 9: Post–Cardiac Arrest Care 2010 American Heart Association guidelines for cardiopulmonary resuscitation and emergency cardiovascular care. *Circulation*, *122*(18 Suppl. 3), S768–S786. doi:10.1161/CIRCULATIONAHA.110.971002 PMID:20956225

Petticrew, M., Rehfuess, E., Noyes, J., Higgins, J. P. T., Mayhew, A., Pantoja, T., & Sowden, A. et al. (2013). Synthesizing evidence on complex interventions: How meta-analytical, qualitative, and mixed-method approaches can contribute. *Journal of Clinical Epidemiology*, *66*(11), 1230–1243. doi:10.1016/j.jclinepi.2013.06.005 PMID:23953082

Piernas, C., & Popkin, B. M. (2011). Food portion patterns and trends among U.S. children and the relationship to total eating occasion size, 1977–2006. *The Journal of Nutrition*, *141*(6), 1159–1164. doi:10.3945/jn.111.138727 PMID:21525258

Rittel, H. W. J., & Webber, M. M. (1973). Dilemmas in a general theory of planning. *Policy Sciences*, *4*(2), 155–169. doi:10.1007/BF01405730

Rosiek A et al. (2015). A Comparison of Direct and Two-Stage Transportation of Patients to Hospital in Poland. IJERPH.

(2016). Rosiek A et all, Evaluation of stress intensity and anxiety level in preoperative period of cardiac patients. *Biomedical Research*.

Rutter, H., Savona, N., Glonti, K., Bibby, J., Cummins, S., Finegood, D. T., ... & Petticrew, M. (2017). The need for a complex systems model of evidence for public health. doi:10.1016/S0140-6736(17)31267-9

Rymaszewska, J., Kiejna, A., & Hadryś, A. (2003). Depression and anxiety in coronary artery by pass grafting patients. *European Psychologist*, *18*(4), 155–160. doi:10.1016/S0924-9338(03)00052-X PMID:12814847

Safar, P. (1988). Resuscitation from clinical death: Pathophysiologic limits and therapeutic potentials. *Critical Care Medicine*, *16*(10), 923–941. doi:10.1097/00003246-198810000-00003 PMID:3048894

Sallis, J. F., & Glanz, K. (2009). Physical activity and food environments: Solutions to the obesity epidemic. *The Milbank Quarterly*, *87*(1), 123–154. doi:10.1111/j.1468-0009.2009.00550.x PMID:19298418

Silberfein, E. J., Zhou, W., Kougias, P., El Sayed, H. F., Huynh, T. T., Albo, D., & Lin, P. H. et al. (2007). Percutaneous cholecystostomy for acute cholecystitis in high-risk patients: Experience of a surgeon-initiated interventional program. *American Journal of Surgery*, *194*(5), 672–677. doi:10.1016/j.amjsurg.2007.07.019 PMID:17936433

Spetz, J., & Keane, D. (2009). Information technology implementation in a rural hospital: A cautionary tale. *Health Management*, *54*, 337–347, discussion 348. PMID:19831118

Steg, P. G., James, S. K., Atar, D., Badano, L. P., Blomstrom-Lundqvist, C., & Borger, M. A. et al.. (2012). ESC Guidelines for the management of acute mycocardial infraction in patients presenting with ST-segment elevation. *European Heart Journal, 33*(20), 2569–2619. doi:10.1093/eurheartj/ehs215 PMID:22922416

Terkelsen, C. J., Lassen, J. F., Norgaard, B. L., Gerdes, J. C., Poulsen, S. H., Bendix, K., & Andersen, H. R. et al. (2005). Reduction of treatment delay in patients with ST-elevation myocardial infarction: Impact of pre-hospital diagnosis and direct referral to primary percutaneous coronary intervention. *European Heart Journal, 26*(8), 770–777. doi:10.1093/eurheartj/ehi100 PMID:15684279

The National Program. (n.d.). Educational Program—Treatment to Reduce Frequencies. The Prevalence of Overweight and Obesity in Children and Adolescents. Retrieved 6 August 2015 from http://wsd.org.pl/Ogloszenia/

Wijndaele, K., Brage, S., Besson, H., Khaw, K. T., Sharp, S. J., Luben, R., & Ekelund, U. et al. (2010). Increased cardiometabolic risk is associated with increased TV viewing time. *Medicine and Science in Sports and Exercise, 42*(8), 1511–1518. doi:10.1249/MSS.0b013e3181d322ac PMID:20139784

Wutzke, S., Morrice, E., Benton, M., & Wilson, A. (2016). Systems approaches for chronic disease prevention: Sound logic and empirical evidence, but is this view shared outside of academia? *Public Health Research & Practice, 26*(3), e2631632. doi:10.17061/phrp2631632 PMID:27421344

Yellowlees, P. M., Chorba, K., Burke Parish, M., Wynn-Jones, H., & Nafiz, N. (2010). Telemedicine can make healthcare greener. *Telemedicine Journal and e-Health, 16*(2), 229–232. doi:10.1089/tmj.2009.0105 PMID:20156125

Young, L. R., & Nestle, M. (2002). The contribution of expanding portion sizes to the U.S. obesity epidemic. *American Journal of Public Health, 92*(2), 246–249. doi:10.2105/AJPH.92.2.246 PMID:11818300

Young, L. R., & Nestle, M. (2003). Expanding portion sizes in the U.S. marketplace: Implications for nutrition counseling. *Journal of the American Dietetic Association, 103*(2), 231–234. doi:10.1053/jada.2003.50027 PMID:12589331

Zizza, C., Siega-Riz, A. M., & Popkin, B. M. (2001). Significant increase in young adults' snacking between 1977–1978 and 1994–1996 represents a cause for concern! *Preventive Medicine, 32*(4), 303–310. doi:10.1006/pmed.2000.0817 PMID:11304090

Section 2
Ethical Aspects Related to Patient Safety and Involvement in the Treatment Process

Chapter 7
The Involvement of the Patient and his Perspective Evaluation of the Quality of Healthcare

Aleksandra Rosiek-Kryszewska
Nicolaus Copernicus University, Poland

Anna Rosiek
Ross-Medica, Poland

ABSTRACT

This chapter describes how the complexity of the process of satisfying health needs is in providing different type of services at the same time. It is associated with both the qualifications of the staff and the complexity of the procedures. High-quality healthcare is a priority, because it provides trust, safety and health of patients. Engaging a patient in assessing the quality of healthcare contributes to the change in the way people think about healthcare system. In the chapter, the authors point out the role of patient engagement in the quality assessment of healthcare. The quality of medical services is one of the fundamental problems of healthcare. Providing good quality services at the right price - this is the challenge healthcare institutions are facing to stay ahead of the increasingly competitive healthcare market. The hard market demands healthcare units pay attention to the quality of healthcare, seeing the patient's perspective, and gaining greater credibility in the healthcare market.

INTRODUCTION

Currently healthcare systems around the world are facing many problems, like infrastructure gaps and insufficient medical staff. The opportunity to improve and develop the healthcare system is to emphasize the role of the patient and to develop a concept of patient empowerment (Bridges, Loukanova & Carreva, 2017). This concept increases the patient's health awareness, based on knowledge and willingness to cooperate with medical staff to improve the safety and quality of healthcare (Castro, Regenmortel & Vanhaecht, 2016). Patient engagement brings potential benefits not only to himself but also to his surroundings (Cevasco, 2011). It is important to realize that an educated and cooperating patient is the

DOI: 10.4018/978-1-5225-3946-9.ch007

foundation of any well-functioning healthcare system. It is important to place great emphasis on health education not only within the health system, but also within the framework of the functioning of the state as a whole. The benefits of such a solution are unimaginable. In the long run, the benefits provide an opportunity to improve the quality of the health system and to improve the health of the population. The concept of patient empowerment is, however, a long-term process. Noticeable effects can only be seen in the perspective of several dozen years. That is why the earliest education of the whole society is important.

However, in order to properly implement the idea, the activities of governmental and non-governmental institutions should be focused on that task, also at the local levels.

The idea of patient empowerment puts the patients at the center of attention and allows them to take control of their health needs, while designing health services to meet the needs of the beneficiaries (Aujoulat, 2007; Bravo, 2015; Makoult, 2006).

Patient perspective is essential in assessing and improving the quality of healthcare. Concentrating a wide range of activities on the provision of patient-oriented services and respecting their rights allows for faster, more effective action and better adapting to the changing needs of the beneficiaries.

The expectations of patients towards medical services are constantly growing. Patients pay attention not only to the availability of a GP but also a specialist. They focus primarily on the factors that affect the quality of service. Patient treatment, communication skills, time and attention given to the patient and safety during treatment are just some of the factors that contribute to patient satisfaction and improve the efficiency of healthcare facilities. The process of introducing constructive changes in an organization is complex and long-lasting. Employee behavior is often the main barrier to building the efficient management of a hospital (Piercy & Morgan, 1994). In the process of providing services not only knowledge and specialized skills, but also the level of involvement of employees and patients is important (Rogoziński, 2000).

Patient Engagement in Decision-Making Processes

Patient engagement is essential to improve safety and should be a key element in the reorganization of medical procedures (Vahdat, 2014; Hawley, 2017; James, 2013). In recent years discussions have been conducted on how to involve the patient in the decision-making processes. The answer to this question is not straightforward, as the term "patient engagement" was not understood by all in the same way. There are many definitions of patient engagement. Often this concept combined a healthy lifestyle with responsibility for one's own health. For physicians and patients it meant following medical advices. The involved patient was also seen as a person providing health information to medical personnel. But true patient engagement is not just about education or communication. True patient engagement is based on a five-step strategy:

- Defining a patient's engagement in healthcare entities
- The willingness of patients to manage their own healthcare and acquire knowledge and skills
- Active co-operation between patients and medical providers for the design and management of medical care to achieve positive health outcomes
- Culture of the healthcare organization, with priority being patient support (engagement culture)
- Willingness to change the organization in connection with patient engagement

The concept of the five steps is illustrated in Figure 1.

1. Define a Patient Engagement Plan

Creating a strategy to implement a patient engagement plan is linked to the healthcare business (Lush, Rosner, Zant & Notte, 2016). Hospitals need to change, as the environment and expectations of service providers change. If changes are not made in a timely manner, the health care facility is perceived as "worse" - not meeting the patients' expectations, which in consequence can lead to a situation that it is no longer counted on the modern market. That is why the essence is to create a vision and implement a patient engagement plan at multiple levels including:

- **Organizational Level:**
    - Creating a strategy, developing a plan, stimulating action
    - Communicating to employees about changes that are being made, assigning responsibilities
    - Making conscious changes, controlling the implemented strategies at all levels
- **Team Level:** Employee involvement, employee relations with patients, establishing the boundaries of medical and patient responsibility, mutual communication, defining a model of doctor-patient -medical worker relationship
- **Individual Level:** Patient education, belief in the effectiveness of the idea of patient involvement, staff medical support for the patient

However, factors that impede patient engagement should be taken into account (Longtin, Sax, Leape, Shevidan, Donaldson, Pittet, 2010). These types of problems can occur at any stage. Most often, however, they concern the team or the patients themselves. The main reason is the lack of acceptance of the implemented idea or lack of willingness to participate in it. Table 1 illustrates the impediments leading to a lack of patient involvement.

Figure 1. Athenahealth Inc. 2014

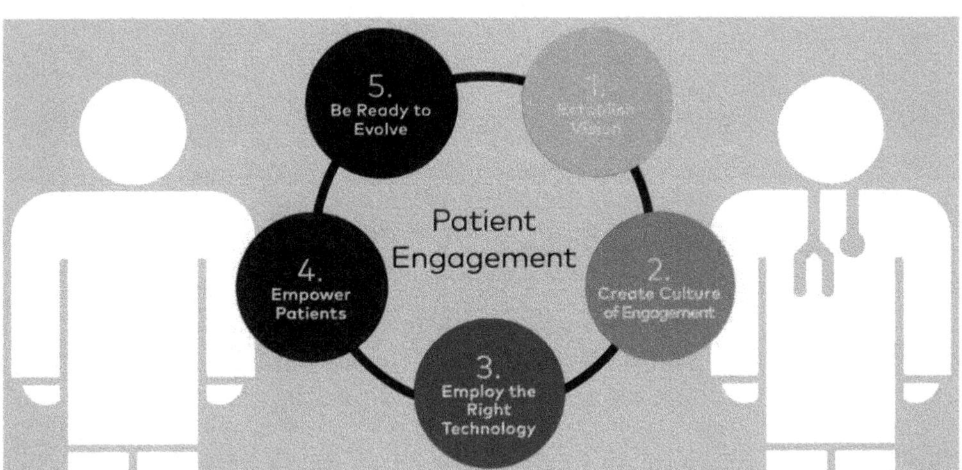

Table 1. Obstacles leading to lack of patient involvement: Team and patient perspective

Handicap	Medical Staff	Patient
Organization	Lack of acceptance	Lack of involvement
Team	Lack of time to educate the patient	Fear of responsibility
Individual	Work overload	Lack of information
	Ensuring own autonomy	Rejecting own role
	The need to stay in control	Problems with not being treated as an equal

Source: Author's own materials.

2. Creating a Culture of Commitment

Creating a culture of commitment aims to integrate the team, setting standards and value systems that will merge employees and patients in the healthcare facilities. Creating unified criteria that are designed to build good communication and mutual respect contributes to a culture of engagement. By doing so, negative emotions and conflicts in the organization are avoided (Harney, Madden, 2008). Figure 2 shows a model of engagement culture that the authors have developed for implementation in health care settings.

3. Active Cooperation

The fundament of active cooperation is communication, knowledge transfer and mutual education. It is also important to motivate the patient and convince him of the effectiveness of commitment. The compatibility of the patient's goals and priorities with the goals of the medical team contributes to the active cooperation of both groups in the health system (Reid, Bromiley, 2012).

However, sometimes it is difficult to build an active co-operation because of the asymmetric relationship. The search for the "golden measure" should begin with the answer to the question: Is it possible to meet one another's expectations?

Figure 2. A pyramid of the culture of engagement
Own materials.

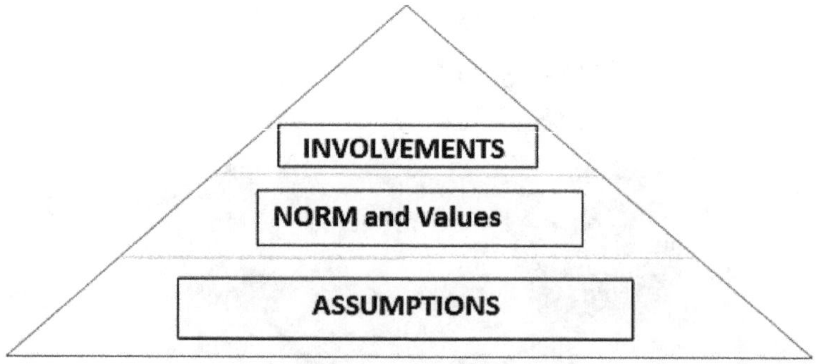

4. Changing Patient Expectations Requires Organizational Changes

Bowling, Rowe, Lambert et al. (2012) are increasingly being investigated and discussed as a factor in the selection of a medical facility by a patient. In scientific analysis, it is noted that both the survey of clients' expectations of medical institutions and their satisfaction with the medical service they are experiencing are valuable sources of information for the management of the medical institution (Kapala, Chudziński & Hyrcza, 2008). Correctly identifying the needs of your clients and then fulfilling them, contributes to a better assessment of the final medical service by the patient. This ensures a constant interest in patients for the health care institution and thus ensures that the healthcare provider is able to provide uninterrupted medical services with full use of the institution's human and material resources.

In the times of growing competition on the medical market, the patient's expectations are often the factor, that helps to choose the right medical facility (Bowling, Rowe, Lambert, Waddington, Mahtani, Kenten, Howe, Francis, 2012). It is noted in scientific analysis that both the survey of patients' expectations of medical institutions and their satisfaction with the medical services are valuable sources of information for the management of the medical institution (Kapala, Chudziński, Hyrcza, 2008).

5. Patient Involvement

This stage assumes the role of the patient. This is due to the key role he/she plays in the healing process when assessing the quality of health services from own perspective. In the past in many cultures the relationship between the patient and the medical staff was paternalistic, and the patient was a passive observer of the treatment process (McKinstry, 1992).

Modern medicine draws attention to the humanistic relationship model, which assumes that each patient has his or her own will and has the right to decide about their own health. The patient, as any other consumer, has the right to demand high quality services (Ezakiel, Linda, 1992). The patient taking part in the healing process benefits from his/her fundamental rights. Patient engagement helps in optimizing the healthcare system. WHO also emphasizes the need to promote patient involvement in the process of sustaining its well-being and enhancing the effectiveness of the health system (World Health Organization, 2007). Providing patients the opportunity to develop health awareness builds trust and promotes their rights. It will enable patients to act as an active partner in their healthcare. In practice this means the benefits of this approach for patients, healthcare professionals and healthcare systems.

- **Benefits for the Patient:**
    - Increase of health awareness
    - Increased sense of satisfaction
    - Sense of being needed
    - Increase of motivation
- **What Will the Engaged Patient Do in Practice?**
    - Look for health information
    - Comply with treatment plans
    - Verify own knowledge in consultation with a specialist
    - actively participates in the treatment process
    - Controls own health

- **Benefits for Healthcare Workers:**
  - Ability to deal with patients individually
  - Shared goals
  - Fewer patients' claims against doctors and medical staff
  - Impact on increasing awareness of rights and responsibilities of patients, coming from specific health behaviors and health decisions
  - Participation in decision-making process for patients' health and protection
- **Benefits for the Healthcare System:**
  - Improving the quality of treatment
  - Increase efficiency and efficiency by combining experience and expertise
  - Targeted use of health care resources according to real patient needs
  - Strengthening the links between health and other sectors, including education and social Support

6. The Will to Change the Organization

Being prepared to change should be seen as one of the key elements throughout the five-step strategy process. Without the will to change, the proper preparation, and the proper system for implementing patient engagement, the transformation will not be able to proceed correctly.

Patient Involvement in the Treatment of Chronic Diseases

The real challenge of our time is to promote medicine in a way, that treats the patient holistically rather than as a chosen disease unit. This is especially important in the context of the ever-growing number of people with chronic diseases, often classified as incurable. It raises the need for a new, individualized form of treatment that combines the achievements of western medicine and the complementary medicine with the understanding of psychosomatic causes. There are numerous discussions around the world about chronic and social diseases (Wagner, Weisz, 2014, Piddington, 2014, Rosenberg, 1998, Bjornotrop, 1998). Constant efforts are being made to find new ways to meet these challenge.

The main goal is to increase the involvement of citizens, patients and the healthcare sector in shaping and implementing health policies and raising public awareness in the fight against disease. Patient participation is crucial in the management of chronic diseases and is recommended as a way to improve patient safety. The World Health Organization (WHO) and the World Alliance for Patient Safety highlight the role that patients and their families can play in improving their health (World Alliance for Patient Safety). Many practitioners believe that engaging a patient in the treatment of a chronic disease is crucial to control the disease. This is because patients that are more focused on conditions and treatments are also more motivated to take care of themselves, and also monitor their own health so that treatment is more effective (Elisseen, 2016, Inzucchi, 2012; 2012).

Table 2 shows the involvement of patients with chronic diseases in the treatment process.

Although many medical practitioners see the benefits of patient engagement in the treatment process, there is also a large group of medical professionals not sharing this vision. One of the main reasons for this approach is the reluctance of medical staff to educate patients, to share knowledge and to abandon

Table 2. Involvement of patients with chronic diseases perceived by practitioners

• Patients with chronic diseases and greater experience with healthcare are more likely to participate in decision-making processes and participate more actively in the treatment process. • They are more likely to explore a comprehensive knowledge of their condition, monitor the effectiveness of treatment and the side effects of pharmacotherapy. • Many patients with chronic diseases require a full explanation of the diagnosis, proposed treatments and alternatives for deliberate and conscious choice. • They want to participate in healthcare to have an active impact on increasing the effectiveness of treatment

the traditional approach to the patient. Medical workers admit that they do not want to share the right to make decisions (Henderson, 2003). In practice they show resistance, which is mainly due to fear of loss of power, control and authority. Doctors use different methods to keep control. They limit the information and the possibility of discussion, which results in the patient's submission. Such behavior violates the patient's autonomy and rights. Medical staff justify this behavior with a line, that patients do not understand the medical language and they are therefore often forced to use categorical commands. This, however, arouses and upholds the feeling of disease-related uncertainty and thus reduces the involvement of patients in the treatment process. Paternalism in medicine and the authoritarian approach to the patient cause the fear to involve in own healing process and aversion to the treatment process itself (Weiss, 1985; Carter, 2015; Taylor, 2009; Hanson, 2008). Doctors and healthcare workers fears about the loss of authority is unjustified.

Integrated Healthcare Cooperation

With the aging of the population the number of people with chronic diseases increases (European Commission: DG Health & Consumers, 2015). WHO estimates that by 2030, two in three Americans will be struggling with chronic disease (Feinglass, 2002). According to McKinsey, chronic illness now accounts for 75 percent of global healthcare spending and is the leading cause of death and disability (Grant, 2010). However, the current healthcare system in many countries is not adapted to treat people with chronic diseases. There is no coordination and organized treatment for these individuals. Therefore, the modern way of providing healthcare needs changes. If the ways of providing healthcare remains unchanged, the treatment of chronic diseases will increase the cost of healthcare.

An integrated approach is required to avoid such consequences. Integrated healthcare is in fact the acceptance of the holistic perspective of human health as a result of many different factors. It is about emphasizing the role of cooperation, not only inside the healthcare sector itself but also involving active cooperation with the patient as a person responsible for his own health. A relational approach to patient care, understood as an integrated rather than segmented pathway of care delivery aims to improve the quality and effectiveness of healthcare. The relationship between efficiency and quality manifests itself strongly in integrated healthcare. Quality assurance increases the effectiveness of treatment giving better health outcomes for patients, and at the same time contributing to the cost of treatment. The increase of quality affect both service providers and the entire system (Peabody, Taguiwalo, Robalino, Frenk, 2006). This is mainly due to the reduction of duplicated research, the abandonment of unnecessary procedures, and the elimination of unnecessary resources.

Quality of Healthcare From a Patient Perspective

The opinion of patients is an extremely valuable source of information on the quality of healthcare services provided by healthcare institutions.

Healthcare institutions belong to organizations for which providing the highest quality of their services is a priority. Good quality improves health, trust, safety, and patient's life satisfaction (Institute of Medicine, 2001). Actions related to attracting and retaining the client, ensuring his or her trust and loyalty are most often seen in the dimension of organizations, whose main goal is to make a profit. However, for some time activities aimed at creating a good customer relationship to the organization are also made by non-profit entities, i.e. healthcare institutions. In healthcare institutions, as in other service companies, the external customer, which in this case is the patient, plays a key role. According to the World Health Organization, every person who uses medical services, regardless of whether they are healthy or sick, is a patient (Declaration on the Rights of Patients in Europe, 1994).

The high quality of services is achieved through understanding and fulfilling patient requirements. You cannot treat a client (patient) like a pet, he/she must be considered as the most important part of the organization structure, which should be above all activities of the organization. Adapting services to the needs and expectations of patients and designing conditions for hospitalization is key to achieving patient satisfaction with hospital treatment.

Meeting the expectations of patients requires, that healthcare executives pay attention to what the patient needs. The patient making a conscious decision to treat particularly points to: his / her own health needs, previous personal or family experiences related to hospital treatment, recommendation and opinion of friends, and the public image of the healthcare unit (hospital) on the medical services market (Figure 3). Figure 3 shows patient expectations that must be met in order for the quality of health services to reflect patient expectations.

Satisfying the Quality Expected by the Patient Compared to Patient Satisfaction With Hospital Treatment

Satisfaction of the patient with hospital care is a multidimensional concept. In the literature the subject is presented both from the perspective of a patient as well as from the perspective of the provider. It is an indicator of the quality of healthcare (Zandbelt, Smets, 2004). Evaluation of the patient's satisfaction is essential for continuous monitoring and improvement of the quality of health care (Sandoval, Brown, Sulivan, Green, 2006). However, patient's perception of the quality of hospital care may differ from the perception of physician (Rahmaqvist, 2001). The patient makes an assessment from his own point of view. If in his opinion all needs and expectations have been gratified then the patient will be fully satisfied with the hospital treatment. The patient's satisfaction level is influenced by a number of factors starting from admission to hospital, through medical care, nursing and communication during hospital treatment. In Poland the assessment of patients' satisfaction with the quality of received health services is a requirement imposed on healthcare institutions by hospital accreditation bodies.

Patients' satisfaction with medical care, including medical facilities, is important for payers, hospital directors, physicians and patients. Satisfaction refers to the experience that patients had with healthcare. It recognizes the role of the patient as a partner in protection of health and reflects the patient's right to

Figure 3. Patient expectations and patient satisfaction with received services
Own materials.

PATIENT EXPECTATIONS

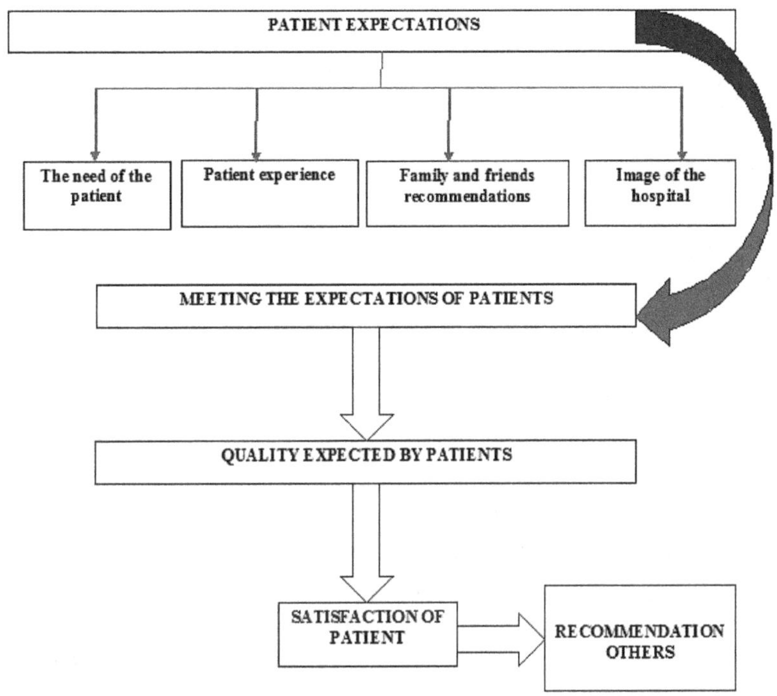

decide about the course of treatment (Platonova, Kennedy, Shewchuk, 2008). Behavior of a physician and good communication with the patient during treatment greatly increases the patient's satisfaction (Vogeus, 2016, Bescie, 2015). The quality of aspects in communication with a physician is particularly important, especially in closed therapy (Cunningham, 1991; Mishra, 2012; Degni, 2012). This idea relates not only to the global scale in public health, but also to the direct relationship of the physician to the patient in the hospital environment, who will decide whether or not the patient is satisfied with the medical consultation or hospitalization.

Considering the quality of medical services from the perspective of the patient there is no doubt that both medical and non-medical aspects must be taken into account which significantly influence the evaluation of the services received. This approach to quality issues is compatible with WHO recommendations, which identifies quality determinants, paying attention to the needs of the patient. The main determinants are:

1. Dignity of the patient
2. Availability of services
3. Patient's autonomy

4. Confidentiality
5. Access to mental support
6. Living conditions
7. Choice of medical services provider

In this sense, the quality of a medical service depends on the qualifications of the medical staff and the conditions under which the medical services are provided, as well as on the course of the procedures used and the atmosphere in which these procedures take place, and finally on recovery or health improvement after leaving the healthcare facility.

Ensuring Patient Safety: "Culture of Safety"

Pro-quality activities in healthcare institutions often face issues related to resistance or lack of awareness among medical staff about providing safety to the patient (Carayon, Wood, 2010).

The hierarchical organizational system in Polish healthcare facilities, strict organizational subordination, reluctance to share knowledge, internal conviction of infallibility of medical workers to their decisions and frequent ignoring of colleague's comments, restrict the organization's culture and thereby endangers the safety of patients. Failure to take precautionary actions to prevent risks causes that safety of the patient is only in theory.

Contemporary thinking about the functioning of a healthcare facility must take into account patient's safety. Healthcare institutions are specific facilities, often with an extended organizational structure such as hospitals. At one place they bring together sick people, caregivers and visitors, as well as direct and indirect care workers. Therefore, in order to seriously consider safety issues in health care, it is important to increase awareness of principles of patient's safe treatment and to build a "Culture of Safety" (Van, Nogueira, Gustafson, Wenda, Averch, Kim, 2016).

Building a secure organizational culture in medical settings involves several behaviors that contribute to achieving a high level of safety. The most important of these are:

- **Collective Prevention:** Its purpose is to make medical staff aware that any mistake should not be underestimated. Taking immediate action is to eliminate the cause of the error and reduce the likelihood of its occurrence in the future. It is important to draw conclusions from the mistakes and dangers and to take preventive action together.
- **Responsibility for Your Actions:** The essence is to treat the patient's safety as a superior value during the work performed. This principle can be fulfilled by:
    - Every time report to an internal team (person) of any errors, adverse events or activities that threaten the patient's safety,
    - Undertaking corrective or preventive actions to eliminate or minimize to an acceptable level any emerging threats affecting safety,
    - Maintaining vigilance while performing ongoing medical activities,
    - Speaking out loud about any issues that have or may have influence on the patient's safety,
    - Not accepting the behavior of personnel that may have or have been dangerous to the safety of the patient.

- **Exchange Observations and Comments Without Fear of Consequences:** Promoting such behaviors allows to create and maintain a security culture, which provides basis for implementing specific actions to minimize the occurrence of the risk and improving the quality and safety of patient care

What Forms the Culture of Security?

- The norms and values adopted in a given community,
- Human nature and interpersonal relationships,
- The organization's environment and the organization's relationships with the environment.

Ensuring a secure organizational culture in every medical institution is associated with taking action at the management level and with their proper enforcement at the operational level. This often requires making lots of efforts to ensure proper awareness, but also to implement it into daily action. Examples of mechanisms promoting a safe culture include:

- Strong and active involvement of top management in building safety awareness at the facility, for example by lack of tolerance for staff behavior that may endanger patients or promoting technological and IT solutions that reduce the risk of error;
- Linking e.g employee motivation system with activities increasing patient's safety and the level of involvement in identifying and eliminating hazards;
- Support by the management of cooperation between staff rather than competition through the creation of interdisciplinary and interdepartmental teams to exchange information on adverse events, mistakes or security measures implemented;
- Organizing systematic, mandatory training in patient's safety standards;
- Building effective communication between staff by implementing communication standards in various situations (natural and emergency) in the form of procedures, instructions or good practice;
- Creating policy and procedures to involve patients in the treatment process, providing them with information related to their state of health or treatment and specifying the time needed for questions and answers from the patient or his family.

Ensuring the right security culture requires creating an atmosphere of mutual cooperation and concern for patient's safety. Therefore, no medical facility can be indifferent to various types of information about hazards or errors furthermore should even provide the conditions for free exchange of information and monitoring of dangerous behavior among co-workers. By shaping a secure culture in the healthcare organization, it is important to remember that ensuring patient's safety is not just programs, plans, procedures or implemented management systems. They are only tools that help shape safety and quality. Safety begins with people most involved in the treatment process – doctors/physician, nurses, and technical support. High security awareness, interpersonal cooperation, lack of resistance or business impact before reporting errors or adverse events and drawing conclusions from any dangerous situation may make that the quality and safety will truly increase and the patient will feel safe. On Figure 4 shows why the safety of the patient should be investigated.

Figure 4. Why should we measure patient safety climate?
Adapted from Zohac 2014.

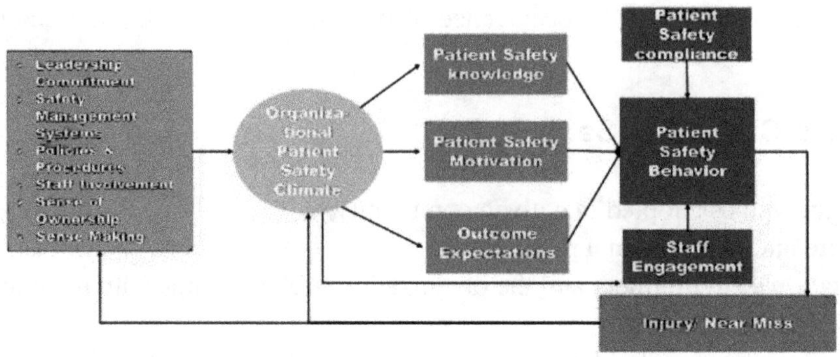

Improvement of Patient's Safety

The process of improving patient's safety requires the involvement of all stakeholders, as well as consistent commitment and continuous quality improvement. Changing the process requires involvement of the management to ensure adequate financial resources along with identifying their sources. Managers must facilitate and provide main stakeholders with the time needed to actively participate in changeing processes, provide administrative support and time to work on projects likewise emphasize that security is a priority for their organizations (Gerven, Deweer, Scott, Panella, Euwema, Sermeus, Vanhaecht, 2016). Success depends on motivated teams, involving everyone - from managers to employees with support of senior management. Table 3 shows examples of strategies to improve patient's safety in hospital.

Safety is the dimension of quality that is most valued by patients and their families. Security is not a value that automatically results from the functioning of a healthcare organization - it is a set value that has become a priority in more mature systems. National patient's safety programs are being developed and implemented. Creating such a policy is due to the fact that patients expect security and want to trust those who care for them. They also want to be informed about their health and confident that they are looked after by highly qualified staff.

Table 3. Examples of security improvement strategies

1. Involvement of all interested parties
2. Significant and strong support of management
3. Commitment and consistent implementation of commitments
4. Show commitment to improving patient's safety in writing form and in procedures performed
5. Appropriate financial resources
6. Time to actively participate in project implementation
7. Accept safety as an organization priority
8. Motivated team
9. Protocols adjusted to the needs of the patient
10. Education and training of the staff
11. Use quality improvement tools
12. Planned change of intervention
13. Upgrade your pre-planned activity while making changes to safety

Source: National Healthcare Quality Report, Agency for Healthcare Research and Quality. Rockville, MD 2006. http://www.ahrq.gov/qual/nhqr06/nhqr06.htm; Access: 3.02.2015. (National Healthcare Quality Report 2006).

Medical Errors and Patient's Safety Programs

Worldwide, health policy is being pursued to ensure patient's safety (Macdonalds, 2017, Andermann, 2013, Trenner, 2017). The necessity of these activities is related to the fact that only in the USA victims of medical malpractice are from 44 thousand up to 98 thousand a year. About 7 thousand patients die each year as a result of adverse events. According to WHO data, patient's safety is a global problem. Every year millions of patients suffer from many unnecessary and avoidable damages due to inadequate medical care. It is estimated that in developed countries about 5-10% of hospitalized patients are infected and 7.5% -10.4% patients staying in intensive care units show adverse drugs reactions. The main problem is that medical errors occur in hospitals around the world and can not be completely eliminated. Errors can only be reduced. According to a report by the Institute of Medicine: "To Err is Human" but it does not relieve responsibility and alertness to patient's safety and the implementation of the "Pimum non nocere" principle. As a result of the growing problem of patient's safety, programs have been developed to implement such a health policy.

There are many security programs in the USA. The Sentinel Events program, the Agency for Healthcare Research and Quality (AHRQ) initiative, the National Patient Safety Agency or the National Accreditation Program of the National Occupational Safety and Health Administration (JCAHO) are aimed at improving patient's safety and using proven and reliable measures of healthcare quality assessment (Finkelman, 2012; Dougherty, 2014; Catalano, 2006). Also in Europe created are national security programs: ANAES in France or NPSA in the UK (Panesar, Cleary, Sheikh, 2009). Council of Europe recommendations on patient's safety are included in Recommendation R (97) 17 on national quality in healthcare systems (US Join Commission, 1998). The procedures and processes for quality improvement are specified, determines the organization of the QA system in the Member States and the candidate countries, types conditions necessary for the introduction of the system and establishes the evaluation of the system.

Australia have a mature health system has: The Australian Council for Safety and Quality in Health Care, where the patient's safety program was introduced in 1997 (Second National Report on Patient Safety, 2002).

The Institut of Medicine report recommends a multi-faceted approach to improve patient safety (Sirota, 2000). It's down to:

1. Set priorities, develop tools and protocols to increase the knowledge base on safety.
2. Identify and learn from mistakes by creating a nationwide event reporting system.
3. Raising standards and expectations for improving safety through the work of supervisors, professional groups and patients.
4. Implement safety systems in healthcare facilities to ensure safety at the admission level for example to a hospital or healthcare facility.

Security should be a clear organizational goal. Implemented systems are designed to improve the reliability and safety of the patient care. Creating a secure care system requires data gathering, that determines information, as well as analysis, feedback and significant system remodeling where the problem has been identified. It is also necessary to build awareness and to understand the importance of safe health care, both in medical professionals and in patients; he involvement of the service recipients in the activity of improving the safety and quality of care, providing absolute confidentiality of anonymously provided data and information. High quality medical care is above all safe.

Involve the Patient in Improving Safety of the Treatment

World Alliance for Patient Safety seeks Patients for Patients Safety to provide patients with a significant role in improving care safety (World Alliance for Patient Safety, 2004). Patients affiliated in this movement are convinced that taking the patients and their families opinion into consideration is an essential part of changing the healthcare system to increase safety. Over the past ten years, patient safety has increasingly been recognized as a global issue. WHO initiative *Patient Safety,* facilitates development of policy and best practice on patient safety in all member states. The WHO has established patients as key entity in these activities. Although demonstrating the role of the patient in reducing the incidence of medical errors is difficult to prove, however, patient involvement is important to the success of the process of improving safety. One of the solution is to involve patients in improving the quality of health care through the development of educational programs, as well as interviewing other patients and their families about the safety of care.

Healthcare systems are becoming more and more complex, with the potential for adverse events and harm as a result of problems related to care and treatment or the functioning of the system. The patient receives healthcare from a variety of healthcare providers operating in different areas. The only people who are present throughout the diagnosis and treatment process are the patients and their families. They are a repository of extremely important knowledge. If they are involved in the whole process and have the potential to influence the safety of care, they can play a significant role in achieving positive outcomes in healthcare. Involvement of patients, and their families, who have suffered harm, can produce results in the form of organizational insights and conclusions. As a result they can be used in the future to improve the safety of care. Therefore it is important for the voice of the patients to be heard in the global healthcare arena. Figure 5 shows how to maintain patient safety and the quality of offered services.

Safe Clinical Practices

The main goal of implementing safe practices is to define uniform principles and ethical standards to ensure the protection and safety of participants (Keiffer, 2015). The guidelines have been developed with current good clinical practices in the European Union, Japan and the United States as well as in Australia, Canada and Scandinavian countries and the World Health Organization (WHO). Good practices relate to aspects such as:

Medical Reconciliation

The goal of the drug conciliation process is to ensure that accurate and consistent information about medications taken by the patients is provided when changing care. This process involves every patient and medical staff at all levels of healthcare.

Unwanted drug effects are one of the major causes of health breakdown and death in healthcare systems worldwide (Amoozegar, 2016, Institute of Medicine, 2006, Baker, 2004, National Audit Office, 2005). Many such cases occur due to improper or poor communication between the medical staff and between staff and patients and / or carers during transmission patient care, such as hospital admission, transfer

Figure 5. S.I. No. 171/2011 - Medical Council: Rules for the Maintenance of Professional Competence (No. 1)

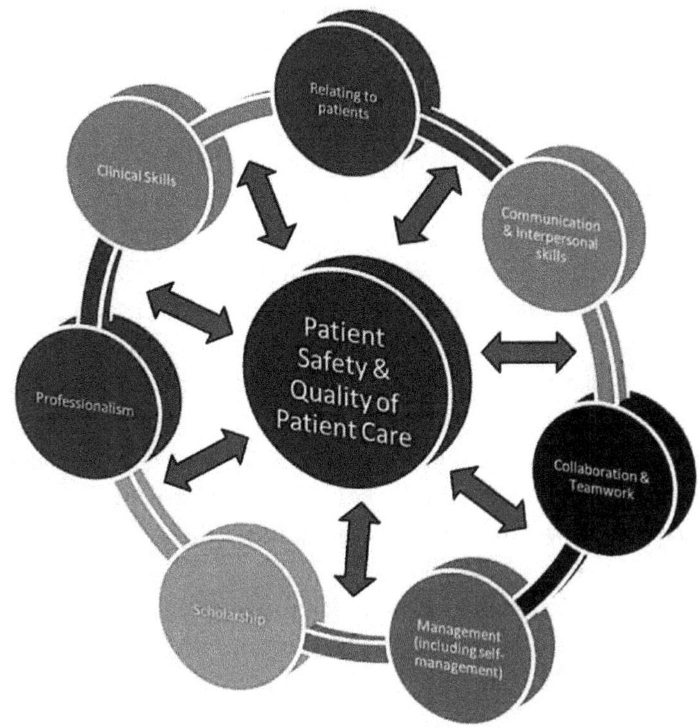

to another ward and discharge from hospital to home or long-term care facility. Misinformation about the medication taken may lead to discontinuation of the necessary treatment, resumption of a previously completed treatment, improper treatment or failure to diagnose a problem related to the medication. Most of these errors can be avoided by implementing drug conciliation, which goal is to increase the precision of collecting information about the medication being taken and useing this information when recommending drugs in the hospital and on discharge. Conciliation serves for better patients information and staff about changes in the pharmacotherapy plan (Dobranzil, Hammond, Holdsworth, 2002). Drug conciliation is a complex process that involves many areas of patient care. In hospitals in Poland the most often is lack of clearly defined process of conciliation or person responsible for its effective implementation. The lack of effective process of drug conciliation increases the risk of error and injury of the patient.

International cooperation has contributed to development of drug conciliation, which implementation requires introduction of systemic changes in existing procedures. Therefore, any organization (hospital) interested in implementation of proper pharmacotherapy should take into account all the elements of the strategy including:

1. **Management:** Support of the management and providing appropriate means to implement the conciliation process is necessary. Countries, where WHO High5s procedures are implemented, recognized that the leadership involved is a fundamental element. Essential leadership roles in the implementation of drug conciliation include:

   a. Ensuring that drug conciliation is a strategic priority, resulting in clearly defined expectations;
   b. Provide the necessary means and eliminate the obstacles.
2. **Action Strategies:** Rug conciliation concerns most patients at almost every stage of treatment. It represents a significant change in the way things are done and requires a strategy and a systemic approach to implement it.
3. **Context:** Local conditions have a significant impact on the success of the implementation process. There are valid external factors such as health policy, guidelines or accreditation requirements, as well as internal procedures governing patient care in hospitals. The success of the implementation can be determined by factors such as culture of the organization, structure of the hospital, the number of patients and other conditions for example liability for the introduction of conciliation and availability of resources. These factors should be taken into account at planning implementation strategy.
4. **Integration:** Effective and efficient implementation of drug conciliation requires integration with systems and functioning processes in the hospital. The drug reconciliation process should not be seen as an additional activity but as the innovative and the only appropriate solution in the planning of pharmacotherapy. In order to ensure effective implementation, hospitals should adopt a comprehensive perspective, which includes, among others:
   a. Numerous complementary strategies;
   b. Active engagement and effective communication in multidisciplinary teams;
   c. Adequate documentation, helpful in good communication and transferring information;
   d. Active involvement of the patient or his family.

Persons Involved in the Drug Conciliation Process

Medical Staff (Team of Doctors and Nurses)

The interdisciplinary team of medical staff in cooperation with patients and their families is responsible for the process of drug conciliation. The process of reconciling a list of drugs requires a team approach and the involvement of physicians, who order medicines, nurses, medical rescuers and pharmacists. Training is required for those involved in the process of conciliation. The tasks and responsibilities of the medical staff participating in the implementation of the conciliation will depend on local opportunities and conditions in particular hospitals.

Patient

Patients transferred between healthcare institutions are the only permanent element in the drug conciliation process. The action of reconciling a list of drugs works best with active involvement of patients and their families, as they can get up to date information about the medicines they receive (lists or information cards) (Forster, Clark, Menard, Dupuis, 2004). Patients should also engage in the remaining stages of drug conciliation, not only during information gathering. They should be kept informed about any changes and modifications to the treatment plan and the way drugs are taken. During discharge from the ward (to the home) and visits to clinics, during which pharmacotherapy is being modified, patients should receive clear written information and guidelines for updated treatment scheme. An assessment of the patient's understanding of the medication list provided to him, is a good way of confirming the correctness of the drug conciliation carried out at the time of discharge. Lack of full comprehension may indicate the need to improve this process.

Pharmacist

The role of a pharmacist who has been educated in an interdisciplinary chemistry and medicine is to provide patients with comprehensive and personalized help. By engaging a pharmacist in the patient care process, the patient's pharmacotherapy is monitored continuously, both in terms of efficacy and adverse events. The essence of this process is the pharmacist's responsibility to ensure that the medication used by the patient is as effective as possible, safest, most comfortable and in the most particular cases also the cheapest. This task requires great knowledge, discipline and proper organization of work.

On Figure 6 factors are shown to improve patient safety.

WHO Cochlear Operational Control Card

It aims to improve the safety of surgical procedures by participating in the World Health Organization (WHO) initiative "Safe surgery saves lives." It is part of the activities of the World Alliance for Patient Safety, aimed at reducing the number of complications and deaths of operated patients. By supporting the medical teams in reducing the incidence of such events, the WHO, following consultations with surgeons and anesthesiologists, anesthetics and operative nurses and patient representatives, has developed a Cochlear Operational Control Card, which can be used in any operating room around the world (World Alliance for Patient Safety, 2008).

Figure 6. Factors that improve patient safety

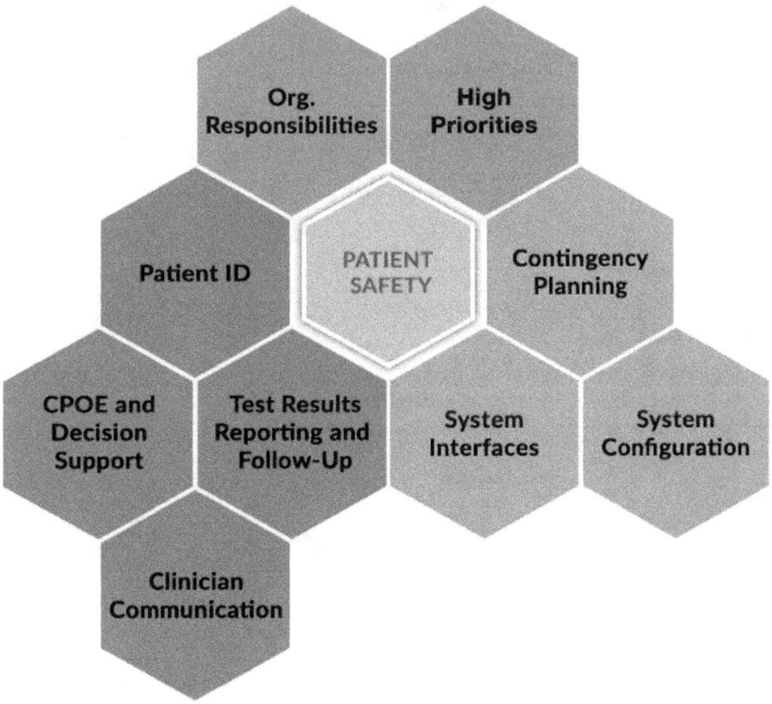

On Figure 7, a properly prepared card, documenting patient safety at the hospital.

Paediatric Early Warning Scores/System (PEWS)

The early warning system (PEWS) was developed to provide a repeatable assessment of the child's clinical condition during hospitalization (Gold, Mihalov, Cohen, 2014). Early identification of patients at risk of clinical deterioration and adapting adequate care to the disease is an integral part of high quality medical care to improve patient safety. The task of the PEWS system is not to replace a clinical assessment of a patient's condition. This is a tool to help you capture the moment of deterioration of a potentially stable patient. In addition, the introduction of such a system facilitates communication between medical personnel. The PEWS system also indicates patients at greater risk of transfer to intensive care units (Chaiyakulsil & Pandee, 2015).

SUMMARY

Involving the patient in the treatment process in close collaboration with the medical personnel is essential to improving patient's safety and the quality of service provided in healthcare settings. An atmosphere of mutual trust in which all members of the team can talk freely without mutual blame and punishment,

Figure 7. World Health Orgnization 2009: Surgical safety checklist

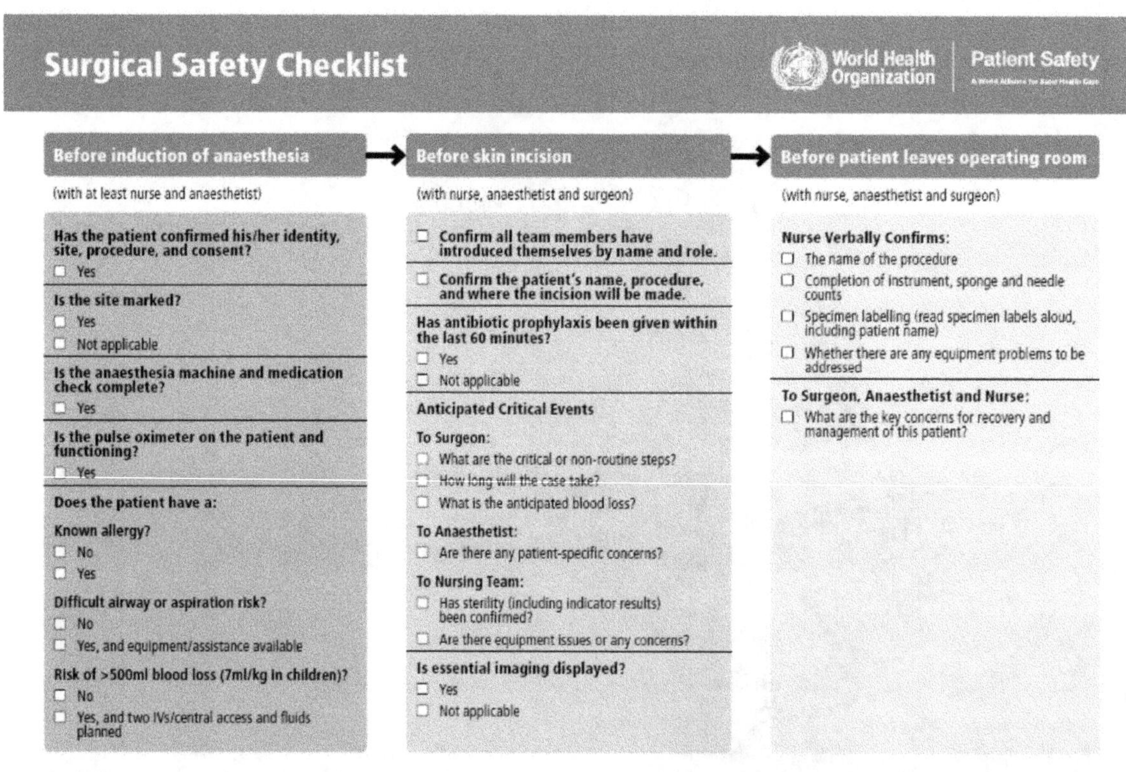

Surgical Safety Checklist

World Health Organization | Patient Safety

Before induction of anaesthesia (with at least nurse and anaesthetist)

Has the patient confirmed his/her identity, site, procedure, and consent?
- ☐ Yes

Is the site marked?
- ☐ Yes
- ☐ Not applicable

Is the anaesthesia machine and medication check complete?
- ☐ Yes

Is the pulse oximeter on the patient and functioning?
- ☐ Yes

Does the patient have a:

Known allergy?
- ☐ No
- ☐ Yes

Difficult airway or aspiration risk?
- ☐ No
- ☐ Yes, and equipment/assistance available

Risk of >500ml blood loss (7ml/kg in children)?
- ☐ No
- ☐ Yes, and two IVs/central access and fluids planned

Before skin incision (with nurse, anaesthetist and surgeon)

- ☐ **Confirm all team members have introduced themselves by name and role.**
- ☐ **Confirm the patient's name, procedure, and where the incision will be made.**

Has antibiotic prophylaxis been given within the last 60 minutes?
- ☐ Yes
- ☐ Not applicable

Anticipated Critical Events

To Surgeon:
- ☐ What are the critical or non-routine steps?
- ☐ How long will the case take?
- ☐ What is the anticipated blood loss?

To Anaesthetist:
- ☐ Are there any patient-specific concerns?

To Nursing Team:
- ☐ Has sterility (including indicator results) been confirmed?
- ☐ Are there equipment issues or any concerns?

Is essential imaging displayed?
- ☐ Yes
- ☐ Not applicable

Before patient leaves operating room (with nurse, anaesthetist and surgeon)

Nurse Verbally Confirms:
- ☐ The name of the procedure
- ☐ Completion of instrument, sponge and needle counts
- ☐ Specimen labelling (read specimen labels aloud, including patient name)
- ☐ Whether there are any equipment problems to be addressed

To Surgeon, Anaesthetist and Nurse:
- ☐ What are the key concerns for recovery and management of this patient?

This checklist is not intended to be comprehensive. Additions and modifications to fit local practice are encouraged. Revised 1 / 2009 © WHO, 2009 improves mutual relationships, patient's satisfaction with the services received and improves the quality of the services offered to the sick. Introducing simple mechanisms in daily work and educating patients on their role and involvement in the treatment process leads to significant improvement in patients' safety. It is necessary to develop awareness and understanding about how important safe healthcare is. Non-confrontational forms of communication and the use of patients' knowledge are conditioned by greater security and high quality of service. Such procedure brings benefits not only to the patient but also to the whole environment. The patient involved with the support of specialists is the foundation of a well-functioning healthcare system.

Existing in the society belief, that healthcare is in hands of physician, medical workers and healthcare units is evolving. The traditional paternalist model of medicine is changing slowly but towards a model in which patients and clinicians work together. The new look at healthcare draws attention to the fact that all parties involved, including patients and their families, are aware of their roles and responsibilities. In this context, there is opportunity to identify needs and to develop a quality of healthcare that will be satisfactory to all parties involved.

REFERENCES

Agency for Healthcare Research and Quality. (n.d.). National Healthcare Quality Report, Rockville. Retrieved 3.02.2015 from http://www.ahrq. gov/qual/nhqr06/nhqr06.htm

Amoozegar, J. B., Rupert, D. J., Sullivan, H. W., & O'Donoghue, A. C. (2017). Consumer confusion between prescription drug precautions and side effects. *Patient Education and Counseling.*

Dougherty, D., Mistry, K. B., LLanos, K., Lillie-Blanton, M., & Chesley, F. (2014, September–October). An AHRQ and CMS Perspective on the Pediatric Quality Measures Program. *Academic Pediatrics*, *14*(5 Suppl.), S17–S18. doi:10.1016/j.acap.2014.06.017 PMID:25169452

Anita, F. (2012). The Movement to Improve Care: The Institute of Medicine Quality Reports and Implications for the Advanced Practice Registered Nurse. *The Nursing Clinics of North America*, *47*(2), 251–260. doi:10.1016/j.cnur.2012.02.006 PMID:22579060

Anne, A., Wu, A. W., Angela, L., Peter, N., Kumar, A. N., Bates, D. W., & Itziar, L. (2013, December). Patient Safety Research Training and Education Expert Working Group of WHO Patient Safety. Case Studies of Patient Safety Research Classics to Build Research Capacity in Low- and Middle-Income Countries. *Joint Commission Journal on Quality and Patient Safety*, *39*(12), 553–560. doi:10.1016/S1553-7250(13)39071-0 PMID:24416946

Aujoulat, A., d'Hoore, W., & Deccache, A. (2007). Patient empowerment in theory and practice: Polysemy or cacophony? *Patient Education and Counseling*, *66*(1), 13–20. doi:10.1016/j.pec.2006.09.008 PMID:17084059

Baker, G. R., & Norton, P. G. (2004). The Canadian Adverse Events Study: The incidence of adverse eventsamong hospitalized patients in Canada. *Canadian Medical Association Journal*, *170*(11), 1678–1686. doi:10.1503/cmaj.1040498 PMID:15159366

Besciu, C. (2015). Patient Satisfaction in the Hospital's Emergency Units in Bucharest. *Procedia Economics and Finance*, *32*, 870–877. doi:10.1016/S2212-5671(15)01534-8

Bowling, A., Rowe, G., Lambert, N., Waddington, M., Mahtani, K. R., Kenten, C., & Francis, S. A. et al. (2012). The measurement of patients' expectations for health care: A review and psychometric testing of a measure of patients' expectations. *Health Technology Assessment*, *16*(30), 1–509. doi:10.3310/hta16300 PMID:22747798

Bravo, P., Edwards, A., Barr, P. J., Scholl, I., Elwyn, G., & McAllister, M. (2015). Conceptualising patient empowerment: A mixed methods study. *BMC Health Services Research*, *15*(1), 252. doi:10.1186/s12913-015-0907-z PMID:26126998

Bridges, J.F.P., Loukanova, S., & Carrera, P.M. (2017). Patient Empowerment in Health Care. Reference Module in Biomedical Sciences. In International Encyclopedia of Public Health (2nd ed., pp. 416-425).

Carter, S. M., Entwistle, V. A., & Littie, M. (2015, August). Relational conceptions of paternalism: A way to rebut nanny-state accusations and evaluate public health interventions. *Public Health*, *129*(8), 1021–1029. doi:10.1016/j.puhe.2015.03.007 PMID:25917003

Castro, E. M., Van Regenmortel, T., Vanhaecht, K., Sermeus, W., & Van Hecke, A. (2016). Patient empowerment, patient participation and patient-centeredness in hospital care. A concept analysis based on a literature review. *Patient Education and Counseling*, *99*(12), 1923–1939. doi:10.1016/j.pec.2016.07.026 PMID:27450481

Chaiyakulsil, C., & Pandee, U. (2015, August). Validation of pediatric early warning score in pediatric emergency department. *Pediatrics International*, *57*(4), 694–698. doi:10.1111/ped.12595 PMID:25639996

Cunningham, L. (1991). *The Quality Connection in Health Care: Integrating Patient Satisfaction and Risk Management*. San Francisco: Jossey-Bass Publishers.

Degni, F., Suominen, S., Essen, B., El, A. W., & Vehvilainen-Julkunen, K. (2012). Communication and cultural issues in providing reproductive health care to immigrant women: health care providers' experiences in meeting the needs of Somali women living in Finland. *Journal of Immigrant and Minority Health*, *14*(2), 330–343. doi:10.1007/s10903-011-9465-6 PMID:21465142

Den Brink-Muinen, V., Van Dulmen, S. M., De Haes, H. C., Visser, A. P., Schellevis, F. G., & Bensing, J. M. (2006). Has patients' involvement in the decision-making process changed over time? *Health Expectations*, *9*(4), 333–342.

Denis, C., & Robert, S. (2007). Taking Steps Toward Integration. *Health Affairs*, *26*, 69–71. PMID:17148492

Dobranzkil, S., Hammond, I., Khan, G., & Holdsworth, H. (2002). The nature of hospital prescribing errors. *Br. J. Clin. Govern.*, *7*(3), 187–193. doi:10.1108/14664100210438271

Economist Intelligence Unit. (2011). The future of healthcare in Europe [cited 2015 Mar 18]. Retrieved from http://www.janssen.pt/sites/default/files/The- Future-Of-Healthcare-In-Europe.pdf

Emanuel Ezakiel, J., & Emanuel Linda, L. (1992). Four models of the physician-patient relationship. *Journal of the American Medical Association*, *267*(16), 2221–2226. doi:10.1001/jama.1992.03480160079038 PMID:1556799

European Commission. (2015). DG Health & Consumers. European Core Health Indicators (ECHI). Self-reported chronic morbidity. Proportion of people aged 65+ reporting any long-standing chronic illness or longstanding health problem. Retrieved March 18, 2015 from http://ec.europa.eu/health/indicators/echi/list/

Feinglass, S. (2002). The Toll of Chronic Illness. *Health Affairs*, *21*(5), 297–298. doi:10.1377/hlthaff.21.5.297

Forster, A. J., Clark, H. D., Menard, A., Dupuis, N., & Chernish, R. et al.. (2004). Adverse events among medical patients after discharge from hospital. *Canadian Medical Association Journal*, *170*(3), 345–349. PMID:14757670

George, W. (2014). *Chronic disease in Twentieth Century. A history*. JHU Press.

Gold, D. L., Mihalov, L. K., & Cohen, D. M. (2014, November). Evaluating the Pediatric Early Warning Score (PEWS) system for admitted patients tn the pediatric emergency department. *Academic Emergency Medicine*, *21*(11), 1249–1256. doi:10.1111/acem.12514 PMID:25377402

Grant, J. (2010, January). What does it take to make integrated care work? *The McKinsey Quarterly*.

Hawley Sarah, T., & Morris Arden, M. (2017). Cultural challenges to engaging patients in shared decision making. *Patient Education and Counseling*, *100*(1), 18–24. doi:10.1016/j.pec.2016.07.008 PMID:27461943

Henderson, S. (2003). Power imbalance between nurses and patients: A potential inhibitor of partnership in care. *Journal of Clinical Nursing*, *12*(4), 501–508. doi:10.1046/j.1365-2702.2003.00757.x PMID:12790863

Peabody, J. W., Taguiwalo, M. M., Robalino, D. A., & Frenk, J. (2006). Improving the Quality of Care in Developing Countries. In Disease Control Priorities in Developing Countries (2nd ed.). New York: Oxford University Press.

Institute of Medicine. (2001). *Crossing the Quality Chasm*. Washington, DC: National Academy Press.

Inzucchi, S. E., Bergenstal, R. M., Buse, J. B., Diamant, M., Ferrannini, E., Nauck, M., & Matthews, D. R. et al. (2012). Management of hyperglycemia in type 2 diabetes: A patient-centered approach. *Diabetes Care*, *35*(6), 1364–1379. doi:10.2337/dc12-0413 PMID:22517736

Kaplan, S. H., Greenfield, S., Gandek, B., Rogers, W. H., & Ware, J. E. (1996). Characteristics of physicians with participatory decision-making styles. *Annals of Internal Medicine*, *124*(5), 497–504.

Kathleen, C. (2006, February). JCAHO'S National Patient Safety Goals 2006. *Journal of Perianesthesia Nursing*, *21*(1), 6–11. doi:10.1016/j.jopan.2005.11.005 PMID:16446238

Keiffer Melanie, R. (2015, June). Utilization of Clinical Practice Guidelines: Barriers and Facilitators. *The Nursing Clinics of North America*, *50*(2), 327–345. doi:10.1016/j.cnur.2015.03.007 PMID:25999074

Keith, T. (2009, February). Paternalism, participation and partnership- The evolution of patient centeredness in the consultation. *Patient Education and Counseling*, *74*(2), 150–155. doi:10.1016/j.pec.2008.08.017 PMID:18930624

Kravitz, R. L., Bell, R. A., Azari, R., Kelly-Reif, S., Krupat, E., & Thom, D. H. (2003). Direct observation of requests for clinical services in office practice: What do patients want and do they get it? *Archives of Internal Medicine*, *163*(14), 1673–1681. doi:10.1001/archinte.163.14.1673 PMID:12885682

Lush, M., Rosner, D., Zant, C., & Notte, S. (2016). Patient engagement strategies in a digital environment: Life sciences companies respond to changing patient expectations. *Delloite Review*, 18.

Makoul, G., & Clayman, M. (2006). An integrative model of shared decision making in medical encounters. *Patient Education and Counseling*, *60*(3), 301–312. doi:10.1016/j.pec.2005.06.010 PMID:16051459

Mary, H. (2008). *Building a Culture of Patient Safety*. Department of Health & Children.

McKinstry, B. (1992). Paternalism and the doctor-patient relationship in general practice. *The British Journal of General Practice*, *42*(361), 340–342. PMID:1457157

Mishra, P. H., & Gupta, S. (2012). Study of patient satisfaction in a surgical unit of a tertiary care teaching hospital. *Journal of Clinical Orthopaedics and Trauma*, *3*(1), 43–47. doi:10.1016/j.jcot.2012.04.002 PMID:25983455

National Audit Office. (2005). A safer place for patients: learning to improve patient safety. Retrieved from http://www.nao.org.uk/pn/05- 06/0506456.htm

Panesar Sukhmeet, S. (2009, July 1). Cleary Kevin, Sheikh Aziz. Reflections on the National Patient Safety Agency's database of medical errors. *Journal of the Royal Society of Medicine*, *102*(7), 256–258. doi:10.1258/jrsm.2009.090135 PMID:19605852

Pascale, C., & Wood, K. E. (2010). Patient Safety: The Role of Human Factors and Systems Engineering. *Studies in Health Technology and Informatics*, *153*, 23–46. PMID:20543237

Longtin, Y., Sax, H., Leape, L. L., Sheridan, S. E., Donaldson, L., & Pittet, D. (2010). Patient Participation: Current Knowledge and Applicability to Patient Safety. *Mayo Clinic Proceedings*, *85*(1), 53–62. doi:10.4065/mcp.2009.0248 PMID:20042562

Macdonald, A. L., & Sevdalis, N. (2017, March). Patient safety improvement interventions in children's surgery: A systematic review. *Journal of Pediatric Surgery*, *52*(3), 504–511. doi:10.1016/j.jpedsurg.2016.09.058 PMID:27717565

Per, B. (1998). Obesity: A chronic disease with alarming prevalence and consequences. *Journal of Internal Medicine*, *244*(4), 267–269. doi:10.1046/j.1365-2796.1998.00417.x PMID:9797490

Piddington R.A. (2014). Health and diseases. In *The Limits of Mankind* (pp. 32-56).

Piercy, N., & Morgan, N. A. (1994). The marketing planning process: Behavioral problems compared to analytical techniques in explaining marketing plan credibility. *Journal of Business Research*, *29*(3), 167–168. doi:10.1016/0148-2963(94)90001-9

Platonova, E. A., Kennedy, K. N., & Shewchuk, R. M. (2008). Understanding patient satisfaction, trust, and loyalty to primary care physicians. *Medical Care Research and Review*, *65*(6), 696–712. doi:10.1177/1077558708322863 PMID:18723450

Preventing medication errors. Institute of Medicine, 2006

Elissen, A., Hertroijs, D., Shaper, N., Vrijhoef, H., & Ruwaard, D. (2016). Profiling Patients' Healthcare Needs to Support Integrated, Person-Centered Models for Long-Term Disease Management (Profile): Research Design. *International Journal of Integrated Care*, *16*(2), 1. doi:10.5334/ijic.2208 PMID:27616957

Rahmqvist, M. (2001). Patient satisfaction in the relation to age, health status and background factors. A model for comparisons of care unit. *International Journal for Quality in Health Care*, *13*(5), 385–390. doi:10.1093/intqhc/13.5.385 PMID:11669566

Reid, J., & Bromiley, M. (2012). Clinical human factors: The need to speak up to improve patient safety. *Nursing Standard*, *26*(35), 35–40. doi:10.7748/ns2012.05.26.35.35.c9084 PMID:22708165

Riddle, M. C., & Karl, D. M. (2012). Individualizing targets and tactics for high-risk patients with type 2 diabetes. Practical lessons from ACCORD and other cardiovascular trials. *Diabetes Care*, *35*(10), 2100–2107. doi:10.2337/dc12-0650 PMID:22996182

Robin, H. (2008). Making sense of medical paternalism. *Medical Hypotheses*, *70*(5), 910–913. doi:10.1016/j.mehy.2007.09.002 PMID:17959323

Rogoziński, K. (2000). *Nowy marketing usług*. Poznań: Wydawnictwo Akademii Ekonomicznej.

Rosenberg, C., E. (1998). Patologies of Progress: The Idea of Civilization as Risk. *Medicine & Health*, *72*(4).

Roughead, E.E., & Semple, S. (2002). Second national report on patient safety: improving medication safety.

Sandoval, G. A., Brown, A. D., Sullivan, T., & Green, E. (2006). Factor that influence cancer patients; overall perception of the quality of care. *International Journal for Quality in Health Care*, *18*(4), 266–274. doi:10.1093/intqhc/mzl014 PMID:16809400

Sirota, R. L. (2000, November). The Institute of Medicine's report on medical error. Implications for pathology. *Archives of Pathology & Laboratory Medicine*, *124*(11), 1674–1678. PMID:11079023

Van, K. A., Nogueira, L., Gustafson, D., Tieu, W., Averch, T. D., & Kim, F. J. (2016, October). The Culture of Patient Safety Practice: Systematic Review. *Urology Practice*, 22.

Trenner M., Haller B., Storck M., Reutersberg B., Kallmayer M.A., Eckstein H.-H. Trends in Patient Safety of Intact Abdominal Aortic Aneurysm Repair: German Registry Data on 36,594 Procedures. *European Journal of Vascular and Endovascular Surgery, Available online 19 January 2017*

Tsao, K. J., & Browne, M.Tsao KuoJen. (2015, December). Browne Marybeth. Culture of safety: A Foundation for patient care. *Seminars in Pediatric Surgery*, *24*(6), 283–287. doi:10.1053/j.sempedsurg.2015.08.005 PMID:26653161

US Joint Commission. (1998). Patient safety incident Events: Approaches to error reduction and prevention. *Journal Quality Improvement*, *11*(6), 290–294.

Vahdat, S., Hamzehgardeshi, L., Hessam, S., & Hamzehgardeshi, Z. (2014). Patient Involvement in Health Care Decision Making: A Review. *Iranian Red Crescent Medical Journal*, *16*(1), e12454. doi:10.5812/ircmj.12454 PMID:24719703 van den Brink-Muinen A, van Dulmen SM, de Haes HC, Visser AP, Schellevis FG, Bensing

van den Brink-Muinen, A., van Dulmen, S. M., de Haes, H. C. J. M., Visser, A. P., Schellevis, F. G., & Bensing, J. M. (2006). Has patients' involvement in the decision-making process changed over time? *Health Expectations*, *9*(4), 333–342. doi:10.1111/j.1369-7625.2006.00413.x PMID:17083560

Van Gerven, E., Deweer, D., Scott, S. D., Panella, M., Euwema, M., Sermeus, W., & Vanhaecht, K. (2016, July). Personal, situational and organizational aspects that influence the impact of patient safety incidents: A qualitative study. *Revista de Calidad Asistencial*, *31*(Suppl. 2), 34–46. doi:10.1016/j.cali.2016.02.003 PMID:27106771

Vogus, T., & McClelland, L. (2016). When the customer is the patient: Lessons from healthcare research on patient satisfaction and service quality ratings. *Human Resource Management Review*, *26*(1), 37–49. doi:10.1016/j.hrmr.2015.09.005

Wagner Edward H. The role of patient care teams in chronic disease management. British Medical Journal 320.7234:569.

Weiss Gary, B. (1985). Paternalism modernized. *Journal of Medical Ethics*, *11*(4), 184–187. doi:10.1136/jme.11.4.184 PMID:4078856

WHO. (1994, March 28–30). A Declaration on the Promotion Rights of Patients in Europe, European Consultation on the Rights of Patients. Retrieved from http://www.who.int/genomics/public/eu_declaration1994.pdf?ua=1

(1996). WHO determinant with participatory decision-making styles. *Annals of Internal Medicine*, *124*(5), 497–504. doi:10.7326/0003-4819-124-5-199603010-00007 PMID:8602709

WHO. (n.d.). World Alliance for patient safety. Retrieved from http://www.who.int/patientsafety/worldalliance/alliance/en/

Wojciech, K., Sławomir, C., & Stefan, H. (n.d.). Oczekiwania pacjentów hospitalizowanych na oddziałach zabiegowych wobec personelu pielęgniarskiego. *Pielęgniarstwo Chirurgiczne i Angiologiczne*, *208*(1), 12-18.

World Alliance for Patient Safety. (2008). WHO surgical safety checklist and implementation manual.

World Alliance for Patient Safety. (2004, October 27). The Launch of the World Alliance for Patient Safety.

World Health Organisation. (2006). London Declaration: Patients for Patient Safety. Retrieved from http://www.who.int/patientsafety/patients_for_patient/London_ Declaration_EN.pdf

World Health Organization. (2007). Strengthening health systems to improve health outcomes.

Zandbelt, L. C., Smets, E., Oort, F. J., Godfried, M. H., & Haes, H. C. J. M. (2004). Satisfaction with the outpatient encounter. *Journal of General Internal Medicine*, *19*(11), 1088–1095. doi:10.1111/j.1525-1497.2004.30420.x PMID:15566437

Chapter 8
Building a Sense of Security in a Patient: A Psychological Perspective

Hanna Liberska
Kazimierz Wielki University, Poland

ABSTRACT

This chapter describes how biopsychosocial conditioning is a dynamic functional structure which included definitive aspects of health, somatics, social aspects, psychological parameters and spiritual health. The approach of the authors to include health and disease in terms of a system that governs the specific principles. The systems such as the human body and human psyche are open and relatively autonomous. Openness enables new factors, stimuli, information and experience to be introduced into the system, but also entails the risk of introducing harmful influences on health and psychosocial statuses. Autonomy and awareness of psychological structures are linked to the ability to control the biopsychosocial state. The conviction of exercising such control is a source of the sense of security.

INTRODUCTION

A lot of medical data indicate interrelationships between somatic and psychological health in the ontogenesis as well as with the context of life – past and present (Cierpiałkowska, Sęk, 2016, Liberska, 2016, Heszen & Sęk, 2017). Somatic health is the domain of physicians (doctors, physiotherapists, nurses), the psychological health – psychologists and psychiatrists. Nevertheless, numerous contemporary specialists in medicine and psychology claim that biopsychosocial approach seems worthwhile as it softens the competence borders with regards to the criterion of the effectiveness of treatment.

The biopsychosocial condition is dynamic and cannot be treated as a mean value or "simple resultant" of definitional aspects of health i.e. somatic, social, psychological and spiritual health (picture 1). The given aspects remain related with the life environment in the broad sense and human development. Therefore, at this point health and illness ought to be understood in terms of a system based on the rules of wholeness, equipotential, equifinality and mutual causality (von Bertalanffy, 1952; Laviolet, 1981; Janicka & Liberska, 2014).

DOI: 10.4018/978-1-5225-3946-9.ch008

This paper remains within the current of integrated approach to health and illness.

The human organism and its psyche are open and relatively autonomous systems. Openness allows new factors, stimuli, information, and experiences to enter the system, but also entails the risk of entering into the system factors harmful for health and biological and psychosocial functioning. Autonomy and awareness of psychological structures are linked to the ability to control the biopsychosocial state. The conviction of exercising such a control is the source of the sense of security.

According to the principle of wholeness, a system is an integral whole/ construction so it is much more than a sum of all elements making it. According to the principle of circularity each action or change in one element / subsystem causes a change in another element / subsystem with which it is in mutual relation. Changes in a system take place according to the feedback mechanism. Consequently, as follows from the principle of causality, everything that happens in the system has its causes and induces certain effects in the system. According to the principle of equipotentiality, different effects in the structure and functioning of the system can have the same causes. The system of any living organism (each living biological structure: human organism, animals, plants) is an integral part of a greater system (e.g. system of a family, hospital, society, etc.).

The health is influenced by genetic and socializing factors which include i.e. relations in a family, educational system or in the work environment, the condition of the natural environment, socio-economical system, especially the organization and quality of the health system as well as individual's own activity.

The Sense of Security and the Need for Security

The sense of security is the effect of a subjective impression of an individual concerning the fulfillment of their need for security. What is the need for security? It is one of the most rudimental human needs revealed from the very first moments of existence.

According to the theory of human motivation created by Maslow (1970), human needs create a hierarchical structure. The basis of the structure is formed by needs of dominant or compulsory character. They are fulfilled in the first place as remaining in the state of unfulfilled compulsory needs may threaten one's biological/physical existence. The needs, which are located higher in the hierarchy are fulfilled later as their immediate fulfilment is not necessary for keeping a subject alive.

In this respect, in a situation when a couple of needs on various levels of the hierarchy remain unfulfilled, including the need for security, the activity of a subject is focused on searching for signals indicating the possibility of fulfilling the needs from the category of dominant/compulsory. Providing that the primary needs are fulfilled, conditions arouse to develop new, higher-rank needs. Their fulfillment allows for creating needs of even higher rank in the hierarchy (in the pyramid of needs) (picture 2).

The needs located on the lower levels of the "pyramid of needs" showed in the picture 2, are aroused by signals or impression of deficiency which trigger out the so-called motivation of deficiency (Drat-Ruszczak, 2000). Its mechanism may be compared to the mechanism of negative feedback (conf. Lewicki, 1978). The needs located on the higher levels of the pyramid are connected with the motivation of growth as they are aroused by aspirations and expectations which stem from psychological structures rather than directly from the biological structures or physiological processes. The mechanism of the motivation of growth may be compared with the mechanism of positive feedback.

The needs set the direction and aim of activity, the strength of the realization undertakings and their dynamics. They regulate human current behaviour and their development in all dimensions. It is worthwhile that the source of needs is the body and the psychological structures shaped in the course of

Figure 1. The relationships between health aspects and their determinants in the biopsychosocial health and disease model
Liberska, 2016, p. 9.

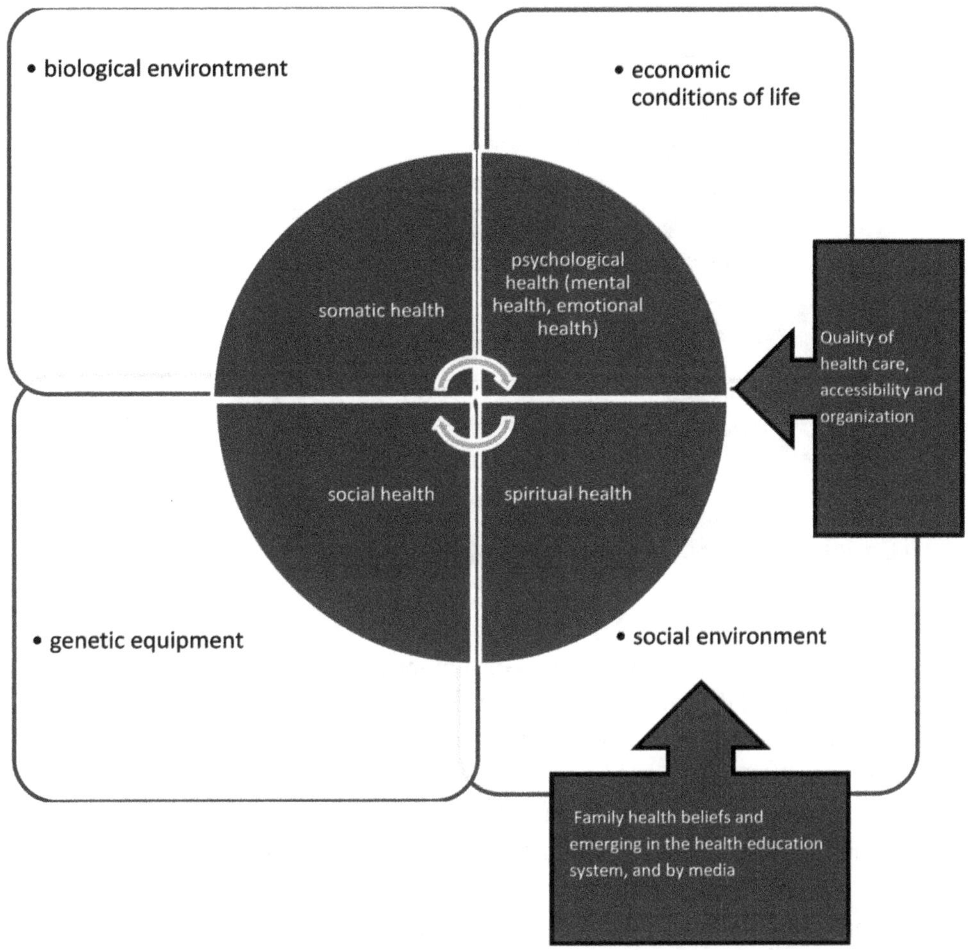

socialization as well as individual's own activity which, on the one hand, is the necessary condition for fulfilling the needs, on the other hand – is a factor of their development in the ontogenesis.

When the fulfillment of needs is difficult or impossible, an individual develops abnormalities and distortions of functioning on the biological and/or psychological level which are indicators of internal instability or homeostasis distortion. The may be the effect of the interaction of a subject (their properties, personality traits, hierarchy of needs et al.) and the environmental impacts (natural and/or social). Seeing no possibility of fulfilling certain needs in the environment, an individual may attempt to change the environment (e.g. changing job or workplace, changing partner, changing doctor etc.) or modify their hierarchy of needs.

Prolonged inability to fulfil primary needs (i.e.: deprivation of needs) may not only result in disorganization of physiological processes but also damage the biological structure of the body.

The need for security sets the border between physiological needs and higher-rank needs. Therefore, blocking the possibility of its fulfillment may lead to losing interest in higher-rank needs or even limit

Figure 2. Pyramid of needs according to A. Maslow
Own elaboration.

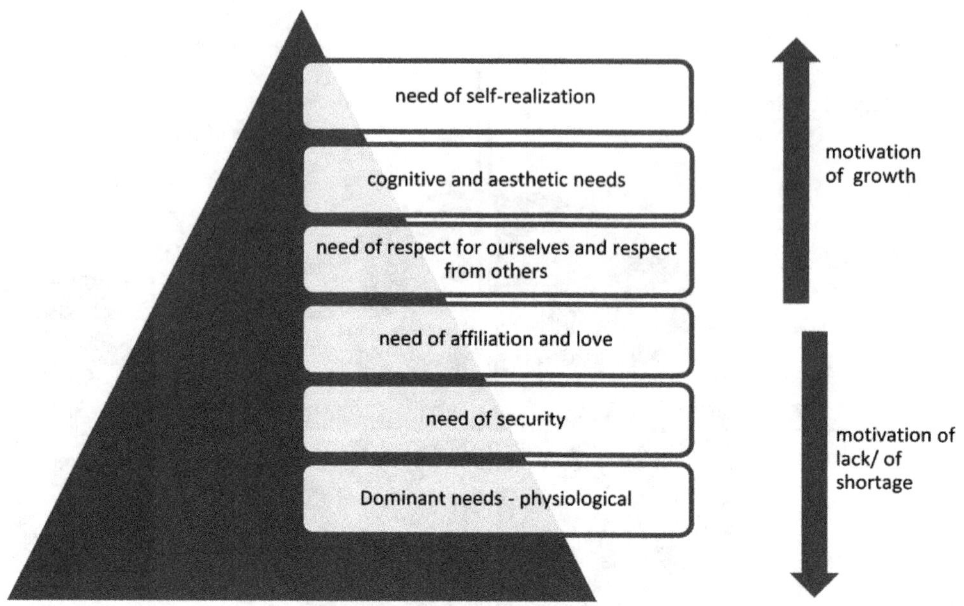

the proper, i.e. concordant with bodily parameters or requirements, fulfillment of physiological needs. It may lead to various biological dysfunctions. Its occurrence suggests that primary needs are unfulfilled, which leads to the deterioration of somatic health and decreases the interest in fulfilling needs from higher levels of the pyramid. This, in turn, may decrease the psychological condition of a subject in the shorter or longer run. The life energy and activity of a subject are limited, drastically at times, which may increase the symptoms of somatic illness and distort the psychosocial functioning. The abovementioned conditions of "double threat" to health within the biopsychosocial model (Liberska, 2016) suggest that it is worthwhile to provide a subject with both specialist medical and psychological care.

DISCUSSION

This article discusses the basic concepts of patient's safety and security. The importance of both factors for the hospital treatment process is presented. The consequences of failing to meet the need for patient security and the biopsychosocial state of the patient have been observed. Also, the opportunities related to the possibility of building a sense of security in a specialist care system are considered; this sense is important to convince the patient to exercise control over the treatment in hospital and beyond his hospital life. The approach to disease was emphasized as a manifestation of the dynamic imbalance in the body and its relationship with the environment. For this reason, it is considered a crisis event. In the remainder of this section, attention will be paid to the activation of the spiral of disturbances in the biopsychosocial functioning of the patient. The effects of internal imbalances on the quality of psychosocial functioning and intensification of disorganization of psychological structures are discussed. As a consequence of these negative changes, the subject may lose the sense of control over his or her life and the sense of security. The problem of personal resources (included sense of security) is analysed, which are important for the effectiveness of coping with illness and treatment. Then a discussion follows on the specialist support of the sense of security - treated as a kind of broadly defined social support and assistance available to a client-patient in a difficult situation - such as a situation of patient at a hospital. . The spheres, stages and categories of social support to the patient's sense of security as well as factors relevant to the supporting persons are also discussed. One way to improve the patient's sense of well-being and to improve his or her sense of health control is to change the lifestyle, i.e. rhythmic repetitive activities and habits. These are very effective methods that can bring long-term health improvement or stop the disease process. This is a very effective way of changing the pace of life and organization of life, which can bring long-term health improvements or stop the disease process.

The Meaning of the Sense of Security in Patients

The need for security is especially visible in the situation when life or health is threatened, i.e. illness, the necessity to undergo medical procedures (operations), hospital isolation etc. It is also revealed in different situations connected with, e.g., losing job, losing home, war, accidents and catastrophe casualties, being a victim of direct and indirect, physical, verbal or displaced aggression (Obuchowski, 2000, Farnicka, Liberska & Niewiedział, 2016). Identifying the signals threatening the sense of security may trigger out defensive activities or activities aimed at preventing its deterioration or loss. In the case of illness symptoms, their perception may be distorted (defensive mechanism) or blocked before they "enter" the cognitive structures of a subject. Although it may result in sustaining the sense of security, it does not permanently stop the illness, hence displays a rather short-term character. Another method of protecting the patients' sense of security (providing that the person has entrusted themselves with the specialist care) is submitting to the power of a competent person who runs or belongs to a medical team. This means that the patient trusts the specialist providing care and believes that the person holds proper skills and is reliable which sustains patients' conviction that they control their own lives and, therefore, sustains or amplifies their sense of security.

The subject develops the sense of security when their needs for predictability of events concerning themselves and their environment are fulfilled. It is based on the conviction about the relative stability of personal situation and the situation of the closest people, i.e. family situation, economic situation, professional status, health condition etc. It is reinforced by the recurrence of experiences, both positive and negative, providing that the subject has the impression that they coped with the threats and difficulties. The recurrence enables to get one's life in order and facilitates finding the meaning of life. The sense of comprehensibility and predictability of events, the conviction that an individual has the resources which enable them to cope with various challenges account for the sense of coherence which is an important factor in health protection (Antonovsky, 1987, Eriksson & Lindstöm, 2005, Heszen & Sęk, 2017, Cierpiałkowska & Sęk, 2016).

The Possibilities of Developing the Sense of Security in the System of Specialist Care

The conviction about the effectiveness of functioning gives the subject the sense of control over the events and their own life. The patients with such a positive attitude towards themselves and the world who has been convinced about the legitimacy of a certain therapy develops boosted sense of security.

It contributes to the engagement of their psychological resources in the cooperation with the medical team and may lead to increased effectiveness of treatment and further reinforce the patient's sense of security. This starts a chain of positive reinforcements between personal resources of the patient and therapeutic procedures as well as recommendations concerning the lifestyle after leaving the hospital.

Numerous studies indicate that even short-term impacts may be significant for our well-being. Positive mood facilitates greater optimism and creates positive attitude towards various objects, events or even health. Negative impacts, on the contrary, bring about more pessimistic attitude, increase criticism towards oneself and others. In the person who undergoes diagnostic procedures, medical procedures or therapy it may be revealed as negative behaviour toward the medical team, the method of treatment, recommendations or prognoses about the healing process. If the negative impacts last for a longer period or frequently reoccur, they may result in creating negative perception about the health condition and chances of recovery or may enhance the symptoms (Salovey & Birnbaum, 1989; Forgas & Moylan, 2002; Forgas, 2006, 2012). The biopsychosocial mechanism of these impacts is complex. It is presumed that the affective states may have a direct influence on the immune system and susceptibility to illness. The effects of this influence depend on the reaction of a subject to their emotions – whether they are revealed or contained (Labott and Martin, 1990; Labott et al., 2010).

The traits of the subject (here: patient), such as optimism, intensity of the experienced emotions, the level of anxiety or the effectiveness of regulating emotions (Salovey et al., 2001; Snyder, 1994), as well as psychical resistance or resilience (Ogińska-Bulik, Juczyński, 2012; Oleś, 2015) or coping difficulties, flexibility in coping stress (Basińska, 2016) influence their ideas on health and treatment and determine their possible changes in the course of treatment. It is presumed that they serve as mediators between the health/illness condition and the effectiveness of therapy (conf. Salovey et al., 2001; Forgas, 2010). The reference literature in this field indicates the significance of determining the "strengths" of a patient as factors contributing to quicker recovery after illness (Ryff & Spencer, 2002). Research into the neurobiological mechanisms of these impacts has been of interest to specialist all over the world (Heller, 2013). The majority of studies are interdisciplinary research taking into account the importance of sociodemographic factors (age, gender, race, social status, education, family structure, etc.) and psychological factors (psychological well-being, self-esteem, resilience, openness of cognitive structures, the need for taking risk, the emotional climate of a family etc.) as well as their relationship with biological factors for the functioning of the biological structure (including neurohormone regulation, inflammatory process and others .) (Boylan & Ryff, 2013). The studies are aimed at determining the mechanism embracing the sense of well-being and all aspects of the sense of security which may have health protective functions (Friedman & Ryff, 2012).

However, the analysis of the views of prominent psychologists indicates that the relatively strong sense of security is not the only factor facilitating patients' healing process and treatment. (conf. Maslow, 1970; Obuchowski, 2000). They can also be facilitated by a low sense of security. A patient who lacks the sense of security is focused on searching for signals which may instill such a sense. These signals may be provided by the doctor taking care of them (or collaborating psychologist). In such a case, the sense of security is "attached" to the doctor or another member of the medical team providing care for the patient. The patient starts to treat their doctor as the authority. According to the psychoanalytical approach they may perceive the doctor as a symbol of "the father" – i.e. a person who provides security to the child on the condition that the child is obedient (Freud, 1995). It has certain consequences for the functioning of the patient and the effectiveness of the therapy. Such an attitude on the one hand leads to the submission of a patient to doctor's orders, but, on the other hand, discharges the patient from the responsibility for the health condition and the recovery process. Moreover, it may increase the doctor's sense of responsibility which may become additional psychical load. Such behaviour is observed among patients with tumours especially when the prognosis for inhibiting the illness is negative (Compas, Beckjord & Agocha, 2006). A patient who is convinced about their inability to control the situation or influence their health condition has a limited access to the potential personal resources. As a consequence, the sense of coherence is decreased and the sense of helplessness strengthens. In such biopsychosocial conditions it is difficult to restore the patent's sense of security. However, a particular resource which contributes to patient's coping with a difficult situation seems to be the availability of avoidant or emotional stress coping styles (Endler, Parker, 1994, Basińska, 2016).

The stress coping style of a subject is formed by characteristic strategies or ways of coping (Heszen, Sęk, 2016). They reveal interindividual diversity. According to some researchers, the coping style depends on the situation and personal traits. Others claim that it is a rather stable disposition (conf. Lazarus, Folkman, 1984; Lazarus, 1986; Endler, Parker, 1994).

Endler and Parker differentiate three styles, i.e.: task-oriented, emotional and avoidant. The emotional style (anger, sense of guilt et al.) may result in decreasing the negative emotional tension of a patient remaining in a difficult situation – despite the lack of their engagement in the recovery process. The avoidant style (focused on refraining) allows for relieving of constant thinking about the difficult situation which the patient currently happens to be in (every illness is a difficult situation). It may be manifested as refraining from taking medicines, disobeying orders of the medical team, engaging in making contacts with other patients or their visitors, surfing the Internet etc. Such activities allow the subject to forget about the particular problem (illness) for a period of time. They give an ostensible sense of security engaging the patient in activities and undertakings connected with fulfilling needs from higher levels of the hierarchy. Focusing or directing attention to other issues indirectly connected with the illness such as: drawing up a will, confession, farewell letters, paying the last bills etc. may give the patient a feeling of being able to control the situation and their lives which allows impermanent sense of security. A change in the index of the experienced emotions (using the energy of negative emotions to arouse positive emotions) may indicate that the patient has managed to modify the stress coping style into a more effective, task-oriented one. However, at the same time, the tasks are modified from the initial overcoming illness to dealing with various "last" things. Coping with these tasks becomes a certain support for the patient (auto-support).

One of the methods of restoring patients' sense of security is including them in a network of support. It may be both institutional or extra-institutional.

The activation or aid in developing the task-oriented coping style proves similarly significant for the effectiveness of medical procedures in patients with lowered sense of security for whom the prognoses are positive. The signals of improving somatic health are related to primary needs as indicators or their fulfillment. It focuses the patients' interest on higher-rank needs, especially on the need which is next in the hierarchical order – the need for security. The restoration of the sense of security is a gradual process and, similarly to the patients whose prognoses are negative, it is connected with convincing the patients that they have personal influence on the situation and have regained control of their lives and health. As a consequence the patients are ready to take responsibility for the recovery process and take active part in the therapy.

Psychological Crises and the Sense of Security and Personal Resources of a Patient

An illness is an example of a destabilization or/and deterioration of the dynamic balance between the body and its relationships with the environment. Therefore, it is treated as a crisis event.

Crisis is defined as a psychological state which differs from other states as it constitutes a certain unity: (a) it has its beginning – unbalance, (b) its course – spreading of internal balance distortions and distortions of the balance in the relationships of a subject and environment, i.e. psychosocial dimension and (c) its final moment – regaining psychological balance, usually on a different level than before the crisis (conf. Płużek, 1997, Kuleta & Trzópek, 2003). Therefore, the notion of a psychological crisis is based on the subjective experiences and appraisals of a patient. Its core is a disorganization of the psychosocial functioning manifested in the transformations of the structure of needs, aims, values, interests, stress coping styles, world view (etc.) which coexist with a negative emotional tension and are also revealed on the level of physiological functions. The character of the changes is frequently drastic. As a consequence, the patient's life is limited to the level of biological activity (sleep, arousal, feeding, excreting, thermoregulation etc.). In case of the somatic illness symptoms – the balance is distorted also on the very basic level and its restoration frequently requires external help. Being on the primary level, such distortion spreads throughout other areas of human activity (psychological and social).

Crisis perceived by a person who experiences it, whether it was sudden and unexpected or brought about by long-lasting damaging stimuli or developmental processes, is a state or process over which the person has no control, is unable to predict future course of events nor modify them (Sędek, 1991). In contributes to the sense of helplessness in a person experiencing crisis and threatens their sense of security which conditions the realization of the majority of their needs (belonging, love, cognitive, aesthetic, self-realization). Leaving the psychological crisis may be treated as an effect of assimilation, accommodation and balancing processes occurring in the structures of the mind which led to their transformations and obtaining a higher level of internal balance and the balance between a subject and environment. It means, that regaining psychological balance by a patient requires contacts with external world and is connected with social relationships. It confirms the significance of social support as a particular resource of a patient necessary for the recover process according to the biopsychosocial approach to health and illness.

Roberts (2005) has proposed a similar definition of crisis: an acute disruption of psychological homeostasis in which one's usual coping mechanisms fail and there exists evidence of distress and functional impairment. The subjective reaction to a stressful life experience that compromises the individual's stability and ability to cope or function. The main cause of a crisis is an intensely stressful, traumatic, or hazardous event, but two other conditions are also necessary: (1) the individual's perception of the event as the cause of considerable upset and/or disruption; and (2) the individual's inability to resolve the disruption by previously used coping mechanisms. Crisis has two aspects: a) it is a process and b) it is also a state of an individual – relatively stable in shorter or longer time period (see: Roberts, 2005). It often has five components: a hazardous or traumatic event, a vulnerable or unbalanced state, a precipitating factor, an active crisis state based on the person's perception, and the resolution of the crisis.

L.M. Brammer (1985) defines crisis as a state of disorganization connected with the frustration of important needs and life aims or a strong distortion of the developmental cycle. It reveals the unreliability of the methods of coping with stressors. As a result, a person happens to be in a shock and experiences anxiety, distress, which is related to the threat to the need for security – the primary psychological need in the pyramid of needs by Maslow (figure 2).

The crisis is a mark of appearing barrier in the realization of important life aims including those concerning health, which, according to the patient, he is unable to overcome using the available methods of coping with difficulties (cf. Caplan, 1964). This leads to a decrease in the sense of controlling one's health and life as well as threatens the sense of security. The crisis, in such respect, leads to a disorganization of the psychological and behavioural structures. The direct effect of these changes is a temporary breakdown in the ability of psychological self-regulation which may be transferred onto the physiological level and increase or extend the scope of the symptoms of the illness.

If a patient makes strong relationships with other patients in the hospital, regardless of concentrating on the information about their own illness (which is understandable), he/she is able to sustain the sense of security.

The crisis, even if it does not have normative or developmental character, may initiate positive changes in the functioning of a patient determined as post-traumatic improvement (Ogińska-Bulik, 2013, 2016) and enlarge his psychological resources (Nowaczyk & Cierpiałkowska, 2016).

The Patients' Sense of Security and the Sense of Helplessness

Illness, as mentioned earlier, is an indicator and the effect of the distortion of homeostasis and the information about an illness distorts human psychological balance and results in distortions of social relationships. Therefore, a subject starts to experience the loss of balance in all dimensions of existence: biological, psychological, social and spiritual. It is a clearly uncomfortable state which loads the psychic and frequently results in increase in the perception of illness symptoms. A spiral of distortions in biopsychosocial functioning is being triggered out. The loss of internal balance distorts psychosocial functioning which, in turn, strengthens the processes of disorganization of psychological structures. At a certain point of these negative changes, a subject may lose –as mentioned before – the sense of control over oneself and their life. The appraisal of a situation as not subordinate to one's personal control forms the patient's conviction about the lack of relationship between their activities and occurring events. If such a situation of having no or limited control over the course of events and life lasts for a longer period of time or frequently reoccurs, a subject may develop the sense of psychological helplessness (Seligman & Maier, 1967). Patients find themselves in a situation perceived as limiting autonomous decisions and limiting the scope of activity. The appraisal of such a situation as necessary form the perspective of their somatic health does not modify – at least in certain patients – the sense of limited decisiveness or autonomy. The described chain of transformations in the appraisal of one's personal situation accounts for the mechanism of shaping the sense of helplessness. Its consequence is the deterioration or loss of the sense of security. Due to the interrelationship between all the areas of functioning – according to the biopsychosocial model of health and illness – the reduction of the sense of security may have a negative influence on the somatic condition and the effectiveness of the procedures carried out by the medical team.

The sense of psychological helplessness includes three areas of human functioning: cognitive, emotional-motivational, activity. The changes occurring in the cognitive areas lead to the conviction about the ineffectiveness of personal activities in the new situation. In case of a person staying in a hospital – the new situation is the hospital situation. Changes regarding motivational processes involve the decrease in motivation to undertake any activities. It is transferred onto the behavioural sphere and is revealed as an inhibition of activities, distraction leading to an increased number of mistakes during performing activities (e.g. following doctors' orders). In extreme cases patients may refrain from undertaking any activities including self-maintenance despite no real reasons for it and contrary to the general state of the patient. The patients may even lose interest in their health and treatment. The emotional deficits which account for the image of psychological helplessness manifest themselves in the patients' sense of threat, helplessness, anxiety, apathy, lack of hope for the improvement of health and regaining autonomy. In some patients, depressive symptoms may occur.

The sense of the learned helplessness leads to various behavioural distortions from passiveness to demoralization. It results in the occurrence of depressive symptoms, influences the course of somatic and psychic illnesses and may even lead to death (Peterson, Maier, Seligman, 1996).

It is worthwhile that these mechanisms are the same in children, adolescents and adults, somatically healthy as well as suffering from various somatic and psychical illnesses, however the triggering situations may differ. Such a situation may be a visit in hospital as a patient or a member of a patient's family. Also remaining in the same hospital room as another patient whose condition is not improving or deteriorating, finally the death of another patient may all become a stimulus initiating the mechanism of developing the sense of helplessness. The observation of a patient who is experiencing the sense of helplessness and lack of security may trigger out the process of modelling similar behaviour in other patients. In such cases one may talk about "infecting" with helplessness. On the one hand, the occurrence of the sense of having no control over their lives and the course of events concerning them is an uncomfortable situation, especially for patients who used to have a strong felling of internal control, and may lead to losing the sense of security. On the other hand, however, low sense of security in some patients may serve a protective role separating them from absorbing further negative information about health or blocking activities which could limit the effectiveness of the therapy (e.g. seeking other forms of treatment or a "wonderful medicine" etc.). There is another positive effect of the sense of helplessness developed due to being in hospital or another closed medical institution. It may be the particular function; the sense of helplessness has for the protection of a good image of a person. Refraining from activity, losing motivation to take care of one's health and the lack of interest in the recovery process gives ground for loading the medical team with full responsibility for the effect of the treatment. This allows for protecting self-esteem and good personal image. A patient who participates in the recovery process, taking partial responsibility for the treatment which does not bring the expected results – may cause not only physical loses (somatic state) but also psychological damages as it may arouse patient's sense of guilt for the ineffectiveness of the therapy. Further consequence would be a decrease in self-esteem and containing negative emotions. At this point the problem of the relationship between self-esteem and the sense of security arouses, however, its analysis is not directly connected with the topic of the paper. Nevertheless, it is noteworthy, that according to the concept of self-serving bias (Snyder, Stephan & Rosenfield, 1976), low self-esteem does not have to be connected with the lack of the sense of security. Occasionally, lowered self-appraisal (temporary or permanent), connected with learned—acquired in hospital—psychological helplessness may protect the self-esteem of a patient. A person of a high self-appraisal in a situation limiting their autonomy – as being in hospital is frequently perceived – will perceive lowered sense of security and a threat to their self-appraisal and self-esteem.

The sense of security will also be threatened in a person with low self-appraisal in a situation when they are persuaded to undertake moderately difficult tasks perceived as exceeding their realization abilities, e.g. maintaining a device, even of a simple structure and apparently easy operation such as insulin or derivatives injection pen or insulin mixes or stoma bags, etc.

In general, prolonged staying in hospital as a patient may lead to consolidation of psychological helplessness which may be negative from the perspective of autonomous life after leaving the hospital. If the patient has not regained full fitness, the consequences of consolidated sense of helplessness may negatively influence their sense of security and self-esteem as well as the perceived somatic health – even long after leaving the hospital. Restoring the sense of security and the conviction about one's agency may require specialist support.

The Sense of Security and Its Correlates

The sense of security involves a great deal of aspect of life and its temporal dimensions including aspirations and expectations about personal future. People of a higher sense of control over the events have a more positive attitude towards their future and stronger sense of well-being than people of lower sense of internal control (Liberska, 2004). Due to the relationship of the sense of control over one's life and the course of events and the sense of security the people who experience it ought to be characterised by a more positive attitude towards their future. As a consequence, they will have stronger motivation to undertake new activities in the long run. The small number of aims located in the future perspective is characteristic for people convicted about the lack of personal control over the events which makes them more susceptible to developing the sense of helplessness and threatens the sense of security. Occasionally, they trigger out a certain protective mechanism leading to creation of plans for distant future which are low in aims or the congestion of aims fall into the final stage of the plan. It means postponing the aims and tasks in time, yet their including in the plan gives the sense of security resulting from social comparisons. The subject is convinced that he or she is not considerably different from other at their age as they aspire to similar life aims. It provides a sense of belonging to a certain age cohort which, in turn, is the source of the conviction about the normativity of personal development (conf. Trempała, 2011) and fulfills the need for belonging located at one of the lower levels of the pyramid of needs. If a patient enters into strong positive relationship with other patients in the hospital, and focuses less attention to the information about their own illness, he or she gains the chance to maintain the sense of security.

However, perceiving future in negative terms increases the individual's fear of the change. In case of the patient hospitalization it may reveal itself as anxiety, even a fear of leaving the hospital. Therefore, a patient may attempt to persuade doctors that their health condition has not improved or may experience deterioration of health. The staying in hospital becomes the basis of their sense of security. Such patients form future plans of a specific construction: they are congested in two periods: close future and very distant future.

Patients of this group do not reveal great flexibility but fear of changes in their current status quo. After leaving the hospital they will probably experience difficulties in adapting to life in the external world and experience low sense of security. It loads the medical team with an additional task to prepare the patients for independent functioning after leaving the hospital, restoring their sense of security and the conviction about their agency. These factors are included in the personal resources conditioning the coping with difficulties.

Patient's Stress and Their Sense of Security

Stress, both from the perspective of physiological as well as psychological processes, may lead to disorganization of behaviour and deterioration of somatic health. However, stress also serves protective and adaptation functions. It prepares the body for undertaking struggle with the stressor or escaping from the battlefield where the stressor had occurred. Prolonged or recurrent physiological stress effects in negative changes in the human body due to its physiological "costs", inability to regain relative biological stability, homeostasis. Psychological stress is always accompanied by physiological stress. Therefore, psychological stress has a double impact on the behaviour and health of a person. In case of a person with somatic illness not only symptoms of physiological stress but also of psychological stress ought to be expected. The improvement of the somatic health does not necessarily involve the disappearance of the psychological stress. In case of psychosomatic illness, the relationships between psychological and physiological stress are very significant and medical and psychological research into this area have been carried out for a long period of time. Their results confirm the necessity of considering health and illness through the biopsychosocial model (Cierpiałkowska & Sęk, 2016).

The outlined relationship between the psychological and physiological stress (both aroused by stressors connected with social life and/or the functioning of a body as a biological organization) partially allows for understating the scope of threat to the sense of security perceived by patients raised in the introduction to this article.

The Sense of Patient's Sense of Security From the Perspective of Personal Resources

The concept of "personal resource" is understood in the reference literature as the complex of personality factors, cognitive, emotional-motivational structures and processes and attitudes which account for the psychological context of coping stress and difficulties. (Moos & Schaefer, 1993). Personal resources are regarded as relatively stable dispositional traits which decide about the selection of the cognitive appraisal processes and the effectiveness of the coping process. They include the sense of self-control over one's life and the course of events including events of stressful character, the sense of agency, positive adequate or slightly increased self-appraisal, high self-esteem, the sense of effectiveness, self-acceptance, optimism. The above-mentioned personal traits of an individual are important for coping with difficult and stressful situations. Apart from the personal resources understood as attributes of a subject, here: a patient, the resources also include social support received by the person. Part of this support may be connected with the first group of the resources (the traits of a subject) as they may be significant for receiving social support. In case of a patient who stays in a hospital especially significant seem those resources which concern maintaining, protection and regaining health. The authors own research indicated that for the active stress coping connected with illness and staying in hospital especially important proves to be the sense of control over the course of events, one's life and health as well as the sense of effectiveness in taking actions. For the emotional coping styles, which are self-esteem and effectiveness in taking action. For the coping style based on social support of utmost importance are the sense of effectiveness connected with either the conviction of the role of coincident in the course of events or the conviction of internal health control. Diagnosing the lack of the sense of control over health may suggest that the patient requires specialist support. Nevertheless, patients who display a strong conviction about having control over their health may also require specialist support. Up to this point it has not been possible to determine one particular factor of a decisive meaning for the support provided to a patient. However, the sense of personal effectiveness proves to be the primary condition for both relatively independent task-oriented or emotional coping styles as well as the relatively dependent coping style based on receiving social support. Still, a patient may not be qualified to a group requiring social support on the sheer basis of the conviction about controlling their own health.

The patients sense of personal effectiveness, its element of force as well as perseverance turned out to be the indicator of all three stress coping styles. The internal sense of controlling health and self-esteem are the predicates of the strategy of active stress coping and focusing on emotions. The external sense of controlling health – coincidence, indicates active stress coping style and seeking social support.

The obtained results indicated the particular role the sense of effectiveness has in the process of coping stress in children. This importance is also emphasized in the reference literature with regards to adults, especially by A. Bandura (1982) and A. Schwarzer (1999). The strong sense of self-effectiveness influences the choice, decision about undertaking a particular activity, the effort put into this activity, perseverance as well as the strength and quality of emotional reactions during the process of coping a problem. The sense of self-effectiveness also increase motivation. Particular importance is ascribed to the dimension of strength which is regarded as the most important aspect of the sense of effectiveness which determines the degree of certainty with which an individual appraises their possibilities of coping a problem. People of high sense of effectiveness tend to regard difficult situations as challenges and consequently strive to solve them. The stronger conviction about self-effectiveness the higher aims set by individuals and the stronger engagement in their realization even in the face of increasing failures (Schwarzer, 1997). Over last several years the expectations, including the sense of self-effectiveness, have been regarded as the key determinants of pro-health behaviour (Juczyński, 1998; Bishop, 2000). Another important variable which plays a significant role in the stress coping among children is the internal localization of the health control. It motivates the active coping style but also determinates concentration on emotions. A great deal of references analyses the more general construct of the perceived control also defined as the sense of personal control. People who believe in their ability to influence the stressful event tend to be able to cope with them and are more effective in struggling with them. The also reveal lower emotional tension and act more affectively (Bishop, 2000). The conviction about having personal control influences the coping process mainly through codetermination of the processes of the cognitive appraisal (Poprawa, 1996). It is said that people who located control internally are more prone to seek information about their problems, and their solutions. Children who are convinced that their health depends on themselves reveal a general tendency to perceive difficult situations as controllable which lead to their more effective coping.

Another variable which determines the stress coping styles among 11-12-year-olds is the sense of self-esteem measured through four separate factors regarding different areas of child's functioning. The predicate of active stress coping turned out to be the sense of self-esteem related to the functioning of a child at school, i.e. playing the role of a student as well as the functioning in the family which expressed the sense of understanding and acceptance by parents. On the other hand, the predicate of the emotional coping style was the self-esteem related to the child's functioning at school and among peers manifesting itself as being liked and accepted by peers. With regards to the third studied coping style i.e. seeking social support, the indicator is the personal sense of self-esteem related to general functioning of an individual, their trust in personal abilities and skills.

The importance of the sense of self-esteem as one of the personal resources is emphasized by numerous authors. The research carried out by M. F. Scheier and C. S. Carver (1987) proved that self-esteem and faith in one's abilities, positive expectations towards the results of personal activities enables people to maintain well-being in the face of stressful events. Carver et al. (1989) stated that individuals with high self-esteem, high level of optimism more often turn to active stress coping strategies. People characterised by having faith in their abilities undertake more activities to directly solve faced problems, are more focused on the efforts aimed at handling the problems and are more perseverant. They do not give in to failure as easily as pessimists.

The optimistic style of explaining, contrary to the sense of helplessness, is viewed by M. E. Seligman (1993) as being able to increase the resistance to stressful events. In case of children, higher self-esteem especially related to the functioning at school and in the family proved to be a good predicator of constructive coping with difficult situations.

Based on the obtained results, a conclusion may be drawn that increased sense of self-esteem may also improve stress coping strategies whereas shaping the sense of controlling one's health and increasing the sense of self-esteem related to the functioning of an individual at school and in the family may facilitate more frequent use of active coping strategies regarded as the most effective methods of coping stress.

It is noteworthy that the individual differences with regards to stress coping styles and personal resources are not the only factor which influence the process of coping stress. Differences resulting from every particular situation may not be omitted. In other words, the process of coping stress, as emphasized by House et al. (in: Rodin, Salovey, 1997) results from the interaction of individual and situational factors. It is also worthwhile to bear in mind that the process of coping stress (especially in a situation of long-lasting stress) may lead to depleting of personal and energetic resources of an individual.

Supporting Patients Through Changing Their Lifestyles

The lifestyle is understood as a complex of reactions, activities and undertakings which reoccur nearly every day and/or are of routine or habitual character. They attach a certain specific character to an individual's daily activity revealing itself as their own manner, distinctive from other people. In such perspective, lifestyle is a personal attribute. The lifestyle contains attitudes towards oneself and the environment, therefore, it includes knowledge, emotions and behaviour. Due to its routine character, lifestyle is difficult to be changed. Lifestyle may be the cause or one of the causes of some dysfunctions or illnesses, hence, it may be necessary to change it. Therefore, changing patient lifestyle may be an important part of the treatment. Such changes may be classified as developmental. The change may be triggered out on the behavioural level, i.e. shaping certain forms of activities (reactions, actions) and using them to replace the undesirable forms. The process of changing may be started by stimulating patient's reflection of their own lifestyle which may involve a cognitive analysis of a certain behaviour or attitude and allows for an inspect into the motives of certain behaviour as well as appraise its health effects. If the appraisal of the current lifestyle is negative, a space is created for providing the patient with knowledge about other forms of activity which are beneficial for their health and practicing such activities including effective stress coping strategies. Acquiring the awareness of the changes, their value and usefulness for the health of the patient enriches their personal resources, reinforces their sense of personal control over their health and life. In general, it contributes to the stronger engagement in the treatment. However, the change of lifestyle is not always quick. Frequently, the reinforcement of the changes requires a great deal of time: a couple of months or even years (Oleś, 2000). The changes may be of micro- and macro- character (Pietrasiński, 1990), however, regardless of the scale facilitate the development of an individual. The triggering of lifestyle changes is a process (Sniehotta, Schwarzer, Scholz & Schüz, 2005). Raif Schwarzer suggested a collective integrated model Health Action Process Approach (HAPA) (cf. Schwarzer & Luszczynska, 2015). It accentuates two components: a) spotting the threats to personal health by an individual and their self-appraisal and b) an analysis and appraisal of personal potential (resources and barriers) due to the specificity of the threats to health. It consists two main stages. The first stage involves arousing patient's motivation, i.e. making them formulate the intention. The second stage involves activating the will to introduce and implement the change. The perception of risk and the expected results (e.g. the recovery process, changing if the lifestyle) constitute the intention to build a plan of changes and its further realization which is adjusted to the stored personal resources and perceived personal barriers (cf. Wiedemann et al., 2011). Schwarzer draws special attention to the importance of self-effectiveness perceived by patients at various stages of changing pro-health behaviour (cf. Sutton, 2005). In case of people whose illness or staying in hospital decreased the sense of agency and self-efficacy, the initial procedures of the therapeutic team ought to be focused on increasing this feeling. The teams could attempt to shape relatively simple pro-health reaction – adequate to the health condition of the patient e.g. limiting the number of cups of coffee, 5-minute morning exercises adjusted to the abilities of the patient, eating fruit for lunch – or refraining from eating it etc. Being successful after a couple of days of such changes in activity may contribute to the patient's ability to control their own health. This leads to increasing of their sense of security as a result of the conviction of regaining control of their behaviour. It is worthwhile to emphasize that this is not an illusion but factual, gradual patent's regaining control over their own health and life.

According to the contemporary approach to the issues of health and illness a great deal of possibilities of improving the patient's condition may allow for determining the dynamic relationships between their psychic states (cognitive, emotional, motivational), behaviour and current somatic health. The understanding of the mechanisms engaged in the initiation and stabilization of beneficial behaviour patterns (including habits) is the starting point for creating psychological intervention programmes and promoting healthy lifestyle (Juczyński, 2001, 2009). Such programmes are valuable in the work of teams supporting the patients' struggles to improve health. Facilitating the process of changing lifestyle through professional impacts limits the risk of increasing emotional disorders in patients or deteriorating of their somatic health. The new behaviour shaped by the impacts and attempts of the supporting team of psychotherapists may account for a resource of a patient which may improve the effectiveness of the treatment provided by the medical team. All psychotherapeutic teams ought to be aware of the necessity to prepare the patient for possible occurrence of high risk situation concerning their health due to the recurrence of an illness (cf. Juczyński, 2014). It requires the ability to anticipate the situations facilitating the recurrence of an illness and sensitivity to the signals of such a threat. Providing patients with such competence allows them to sustain the sense of control of their health and the effectiveness of the undertaken pro-health actions (cf. Luszczynska, Mazurkiewicz, Ziegelmann & Schawrzer, 2007).

It is necessary to pay attention to the stress of taking on the role of a patient in a hospital, which due to the multitude of stressors seriously threatens the sense of security. Medical personnel are not always aware of this. According to the classification of stressful events, severe illness or injury occupy the sixth place in stress classification (Holmes, Rahe, 1967, Rahe, Mahan and Arthur, 1970). The patient's stay in hospital requires many changes in life. These changes concern the living conditions (29 places in the ranking of stress events), personal habits (30 places), sex (13 places), food (41 places), sleeping (39 places), social contacts (37 places) and contacts with family (40th place) and other spheres of life. The total number of points associated with these seven stressors is 190. According to the authors, there is a statistically significant relationship between the strength of the stressor and the probability of a serious illness. If the total strength of the stressors is 150 - 199 points, the probability of getting sick in 2 consecutive years is 37%. It follows that changes in the organization of life in relation to hospital stay pose a greater risk to the health of at least some patients (or their sense of well-being) than the illness that is the main cause of hospitalization.

The task of the team taking care of the patient is therefore to equip him with skills and methods to minimize the negative effects of stress resulting not only from medical treatment (eg surgery) but also from daily activities, schedule or organization of the day related to the rigors of hospital stay.

Some studies indicate that changes related to daily habits or problems (home cleaning, weight problems) - intensification of everyday difficulties - allow for a fairly accurate prediction of increase of stress, anxiety and depression, especially in women (Kanner et al., 1981; McLeod, 2010).

Support for the Sense of Security

The concept of social support still remains ambiguous (Schwarzer, 1988) despite the attempts which have been made over the last several years to specify its understanding and localization in the network of notions regarding health, illness, the quality of functioning and adaptation (Sęk & Cieślak, 2004). The research into the social support was initiated by the revelations of clinicists and social psychologists connected with self-aid groups (Caplan, 1961).

According to the Roberts (1985) model, effective patient support should include the following seven steps:

1. Planning and a thorough biopsychosocial and lethality/imminent danger assessment
2. Making psychological contact and rapidly establish the collaborative relationship
3. Identification of the major problems, including crisis precipitants
4. Encouragement of exploration of feelings and emotions
5. Generation and exploration of alternatives and new coping strategies
6. Restoration of functioning through implementation of an action plan
7. Planning follow-up and booster sessions

The realization of the above-mentioned seven steps requires the majority of patients to devote a great deal of time. Developing and reinforcing more efficient coping strategies as well as the control of their effects for the functioning of a patient, especially the sense of security does not infer the termination of supporting attempts. They are woven into the medical therapeutic process – its progress, inhibition periods, recurrence of symptoms their intensification and appearance of new symptoms. It may result in temporary decrease in the sense of security of patients and their conviction about being able to control their health and influence on the treatment. The attempts to stabilize the restoration of the sense of psychological security and physical condition ought to be harmonized with the changes in the symptoms observed among patients, their number, scope and intensification.

Therefore, the supportive procedures have a cyclic structure with recurrent laps of the mentioned impacts/steps. The supporting procedures undertaken by proactive professionals (cf. Caplan, Caplan & Erchul, 1994) – since a certain moment of the psychological crisis perceived by the patient – are the consequence of the changes in the cycle of overcoming psychological crisis. However, in order to block the laps of returning to the earlier stages of the crisis characterised by cumulated negative emotions and thoughts as well as destructive activities regarding health, introducing supportive activities and procedures which may anticipate the recurrence of these stages seems particularly worthwhile. This increases the patient chance to move on to the phase characterised by a greater stabilization and balance between the positive and negative emotions, thoughts as well as destructive and constructive activities.

The teams of proactive professionals are motivated to employ the currently available possibilities to achieve positive and permanent changes in the functioning of a person and its environment. Such activities are concordant with the ecological approach ("ecological field") propagated in the model of Caplanian mental health consultation (Caplan, Caplan & Erchul, 1994, p. 3). A great deal of patients require an incorporation of various social subsystems, including family and work subsystems, into the supportive system. Such a complex and extended structure of the supportive system increases the chances of stabilizing the imbalance between the impacts of all subsystems which the patient participates in. The mentioned imbalance may be one of the causes of distorted homeostasis and appearing illness symptoms in the patient.

These influences aim at: primarily – identification of the sources and lowering the intensity and time of the biopsychosocial stressors and the related tension which loads the patient; secondarily – hints and practical instructions concerning the strategies of coping with stressors – anticipated and/or expected in the ecological context; eventually – at mobilization of the system of social support in the broad sense, especially in situations of increased risk of occurring of stressors, health and life threats after leaving the specialist institution.

The task of the supporting people is to create situations facilitating the restoration or increasing self-esteem and problem-solving skills, also protect the patient from increased stress by providing intellectual and behavioural support and emotional support. As a result, the personal resources of the patient are enriched which contributes to their competence of independent coping with difficult situations. This restores patient's sense of self-efficacy and becomes the source of recovering – increasing the sense of security. In this respect the patient is able to increase their sense of well-being, capacity to play, work, study and love (Caplan, 1986). Therefore, the patient's attention is moved from the basis of the pyramid of needs to its higher levels including the need for self-realization.

In general meaning, social support is the assistance provided to a subject in difficult situation (Sarason, 1982, Sęk & Cieślak, 2004) by persons of significance and/or persons being the subjects' reference group. According to the structural approach to the idea of support, the source of support is a social structure defined as a social network whose activity and influence extends to the persons making it (por. Pommersbach, 1988, Sęk & Cieśla, 2004, Christakis, Fowler, 2011). In the functional approach to social support, the significance and types of interpersonal interactions in a difficult situation are considered, e.g. during the stay in a hospital as a patient. Developed interaction includes all types of support, informational, emotional, behavioral (instrumental) and material.

The studies show the differences in the effectiveness of the three types of support. Some researchers have indicated that informational support is related to higher level of self-care, instrumental support is related to lower level of self-care, and emotional support is important only for social functioning of the patient (Wilski & Sienkiewicz-Wilowska, 2014). However, emotional support is a very important source of potential patient resources for coping with stress and low positive mood (Wrześniewski & Włodarczyk, 2004).

The aim of social support is generation of conditions conducive to mobilization of the patent's strength and activization of the patient's developmental potential (Kowalik, 2007). The supporting activities provide the means for extension of the patients' personal resources needed for coping with the difficulties/problems or restrictions related to the health condition. Sometimes the supporting activities are factors moderating the relations between the sense of wellbeing and the level of stress or the effectiveness of coping with problems and the level of stress, depression and anxiety (Hwang, Moser & Dracup, 2014).

The Areas, Stages, and Categories of Social Support and Sense of Security

The supportive activities include cognitive, emotional and behavioural as well as material functioning of the person who is the recipient of support. We suggest to differentiate three categories of support with regards to the scope:

- The support of personal resources of the subject/patient – psychological, behavioural and habitual restructuring,
- Supporting the relationship of the subject/patient with the environment: changes in the patient – other people system,
- External support available for the subject/patient: social occasional and social systemic (institutional, material) (Figure 3)

Emotional support involves showing positive emotions towards the patient that reflect the positive attitude of the supporting person (source of support or communication sender) towards the person supported (support recipient or communication receiver). The positive emotions perceived by the patient, shown by the group of specialists taking care of the patient, lead to increased trust and improvement in the patient physical and mental state. The positive emotions increase the patient's sensitivity to signals of health improvement or hindering of the illness. They also increase the positive attitude of the patient towards the doctors and nurses and towards a given institution (surgery, hospital, sanatorium, etc.) and

Figure 3. Categories of support
Source: Self-created.

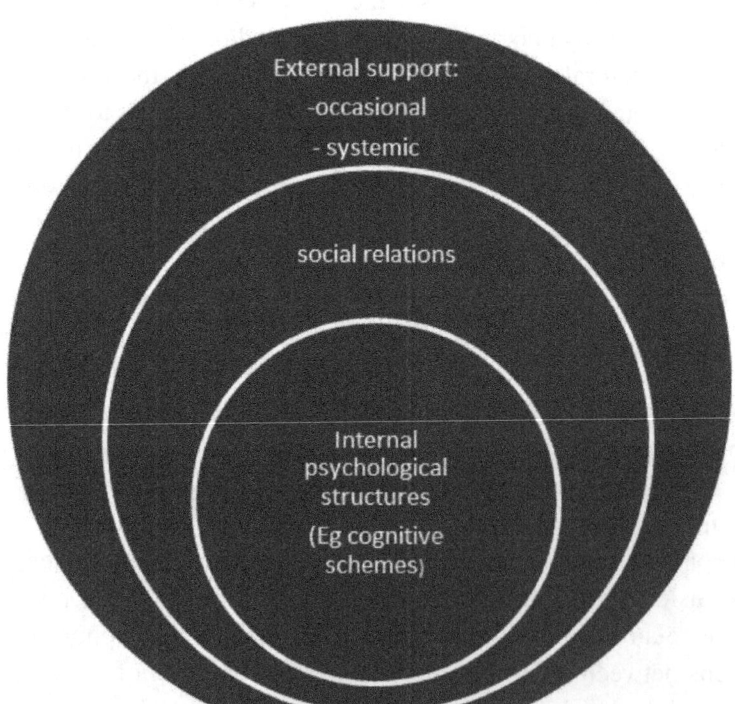

builds positive expectations of further therapy. It leads to increasing sense of security during the treatment at a given therapeutic institution. Emotional support is particularly effective towards the elderly. Such a support can be the basis for development of trust and attachment to a given member of the pertinent medical group or institution. The patient may not want to leave the hospital or other therapeutic institution and may try to prolong his/her stay at it. The informational support involves giving reliable information on the state of health, treatment planned, effects of the hitherto treatment and methods of coping with health problems, the principles of use of the rehabilitation devices, etc. Thanks to the information the patient better understands his/ her situation, meaning of the therapeutic procedures and reasons for further treatment. The changes that the patient observes are not a source of fear as they are expected. In this way the patient learns that he/ she has control over his/her health and feels relatively safe and secure. At the same time the trust to the medical team increases as the patients perceives it as competent. The informational support also includes the information on the effectiveness of actions taken by the patient, which permits a possible modification of behavior, adaptation to the standard, to instruction or to a specific situation (e.g. reading of the glucometer indications and appropriate modification of the next meal or the diet for the next day). Instrumental support is the assistance in everyday activities or in the use of rehabilitation devices the patient has to use because of the health status. Physical exercise, repetition of certain movements or activities aimed at improvement of certain actions, performed initially under intense control of the supporting person, permits development of necessary skills needed to cope with everyday tasks and limitations related to the current health condition. The instrumental support satisfies the patient's sense of security as instills in him/her the conviction of the ability to cope with certain problems. It also is a source of information on the patient's limitations.

The material support involves providing the patient with the appropriate equipment needed for rehabilitation or/ and for being relatively self-sufficient (e.g. prosthesis, wheelchair, ostomy pouch, nappies, etc.), at least in the first period after leaving the hospital or other health care institution, sometimes providing special orthopedic shoes or orthosis. It may happen that the patient has no financial means and then the instrumental support involves assistance in finding appropriate institutions, organizations, foundations that would help in this area and checking if the patient has applied to such institutions or organizations prior to leaving a hospital or other health care institution.

The informational and instrumental support also aims at preparing the patient for the use of further means of support, after he/she gets back home. The patient should be provided with the phone numbers and addresses of institutions and organizations or persons experienced in helping persons of the same health problems of the same life circumstances.

At first, it is important to identify the nature of the patient's health problem and next – to prepare a list of short-term goals and tasks, in cooperation with patient. The main goal of these intervention activities is helping the patient to develop the adaptive coping skills (Roberts & Ottens, 2005). But the success of the changes is limited by the level of sense of security in patient's perception.

The decision on the necessary forms of support in a given health care institution and their continuation after leaving this institution depends on the patient's condition, health prognosis and life situation. For many patients it is justified or necessary to provide a complex system of support including the family, neighbors, self-support groups, care institutions, charity organizations, foundations, etc.

The effectiveness of support depends on the specific health condition, the patient's sex and age. Social support is a process dependent on the following factors:

- Genotype of the patient
- Physical condition
- Intellectual level
- Emotional state
- Quality of family environment
- Quality of wider social environment (for children and the youth also educational environment)
- Quality of care and assistance in special needs
- Conditions of living environment (village, town, availability of special care centers, etc.).

A certain limitation of the effectiveness of special supporting activities are the stereotypes functioning in the social consciousness and concerning persons with relatively permanent impairments who are perceived as worse, less effective and condemned to life of poor quality. This stereotype restricts the patient's sense of security after leaving the hospital and blocks the realization of higher order needs.

In this paper we have proposed the use of the term 'support' to describe a wide range of special activities aimed at assisting the patient, covering rehabilitation procedures, correcting, compensating or supporting certain limited functions or structures of the organism, biological and psychological as well as applying to social environment outside the hospital or other health care institution. It should be emphasized that for many patients the support has individual character, so is adapted to the needs of individual patients and their particular life situations. In further stages the support may have group character as may be provided to a group of persons experiencing the same or similar problems in coping with life tasks following from their bio-psychosocial condition. The support is applied not only to those with somatic diseases but also to the persons suffering from problems with psychological or social functioning, actually very often problems appear in all spheres of functioning.

Finally, it should be mentioned that the aim of supporting activities addressed to the patient is solution of certain specific problems or at least control of a psychological crisis related to the health condition in order to regain the sense of security which is necessary for health condition improvement. The process of healing is understood in a broad sense as coming back to relatively self-sufficient and satisfying state of the patient, leading to the sense of wellbeing so in agreement with the ideals of positive psychology (Seligman at al., 2005). The patient is offered a chance of improving his/ her functioning in different areas of life, can regain or increase the sense of self-esteem and get convinced that he/she is not excluded from the hitherto social environment, although sometimes a change in life style is required.

A very important aspect of social support is its adaptation to the readiness of the support acceptance by the receiver. The patient may be not interested in active participation in the opportunities offered or may be disappointed by the first attempts which do not give satisfactory effects. Such situations require patience and understanding from the support-givers.

DIRECTIONS FOR FURTHER RESEARCH

Significant improvement in the patient's sense of security in hospital may change his attitude towards himself: to the body, psyche and social relations. The attitude of care for health and sense of security in full form consists of three elements: cognitive, emotional and behavioral.

Patient's Selfcare and the Sense of Security

Psychological literature provides many articles contributing to the discussion of the patient co-responsibility for his/her health (por. Kowalik, 2007). It is believed that patients should participate as partners in working out strategies for coping with problems after leaving the hospital or other health care institution. The necessary condition that should be satisfied prior to taking the decision on the patient's engagement in the process of healing, rehabilitation and adaptation to out-of-hospital environment, is acceptance of the patient's own limitations, difference or impairment. Often also the acceptance of oneself as a disabled person is required, including the acceptance of special needs, barriers in functioning or the need to find a new space for development.

The supporting group, taking care of the patient during his/her stay at the hospital or other health care institution should teach the patient to be responsible for his/her own health and convince him/her of the sense of health promoting behavior (cf. Pledger, 2003). The long-term goal is to develop the patient's selfcare which includes the conviction of the necessity of accepting responsibility for healing and quality of further life. In health psychology, the selfcare (or taking care of yourself) is a necessary regulatory function of control of behavior, consciousness, responsibility and self-awareness of the individual (see: Kowalik, 2007). It is the approach to oneself in which one accepts responsibility of one's life and which is manifested particularly in the face of adversity. This approach leads the individual towards taking up measures allowing changing the life situation to more desirable (Szmaus-Jackowska, 2011).

The results of the study indicate that such attitudes, which have been established in children and adolescents in the course of systematic education as well as intermittent interactions (for example, by media), are stronger and lead to the responsibility for somatic and psychological health. It is also manifested as the respect for health, greater interest in the condition of one's own health, but also greater concern for health than in adults. (Levenson, Morrow, Pfefferbaum, 1984). Many researchers point out that risky behaviors taken by young people lead to poor health (physical and psychosocial) which confirms the need for pro-health education in kindergartens and schools as well as cultural centers and sports clubs involving children and adolescents (James at al., 2017; Nelson, Patience & MacDonald, 1999).

A patient who is convinced that a team of care professionals treats him or her as a subject - respects his will, confers his or her autonomy in hospital-related matters and decision about the process of treatment. It is expressed in the readiness to subordinate to medical procedures, even if it imposes certain restrictions and requires realization of specific tasks (for example, the handling of medical equipment, self-education, some relatively simple activities such as self-injection, dietary change, daily gymnastics and others. Studies on psychosocial competencies of personel in hospitals have been conducted (also recently in Poland) but we note the lack of systematic analyzes of patients' expectations (Redo, Bielawska-Batorowicz, 2014). An important challenge for researchers is to study patients' views on relationships with medical personnel/staff and patients' expectations related to their need of security in hospitals. The ability to resolve conflicts with patients and their families by medical team members requires continuous improvement and effective training programs for patient-physician communications (Chrzan-Dętkoś & Pietkiewicz, 2015).

However, changing lifestyle, old habits, sometimes even family traditions (e.g. holidays on survival camps, high-altitude climbing, high-fat dinners and snacks, or passive holidays in front of TVs and others), as indicated above – are the source of many stressors. Even the eustres that is the result of effective treatment may not be able to overcome the dystres of changing the lifestyle and building the attitude including greater responsibility for health.

CONCLUSION

1. Health problems threaten the sense of physical and psychosocial security. Many people find it difficult or impossible to meet the needs of higher order (cognitive, aesthetic and the need on the top of the pyramid - the need for self-fulfillment).
2. Loss of sense of security can reduce the effectiveness of treatment because of lower involvement of the patient, who feels that he/she has lost control of his or her health and limited autonomy. This increases the stress experienced by him in the hospital. This is also the reason for further lowering of the sense of security. In the absence of satisfactory progress in treatment, a spiral of dissatisfaction is also associated with failing to meet the growing range of patient needs, not just those of higher levels. Prolonged treatment of patients experiencing the lack of control over their lives in connection with hospital stay may impair their well-being and the effects of medical treatment.
3. Specialist support to the patient should be tailored to his or her biopsychosomatic state, including spirituality, and to provide necessary information, emotional, biological and material support. It is not limited to recognizing the current state of somatic health, psychological needs, and social and economic circumstances of a patient, but is planned in the perspective of future needs - after leaving the hospital in a way that manages daily tasks and further develops his potential. This potential may be partially mitigated by the disease, but specialized effects, including services provided, are intended to provide new resources or to mobilize untapped potential.
4. Changes in the lifestyles in most patients are justified and necessary, but to the extent appropriate for the current state and further negotiations. It should be stressed that although it is necessary, it is a stressful task for a patient whose implementation may be difficult. The patient may even oppose this task (passively or actively), because at some point in their life they may find it too costly to be personally involved - and this may be due to the possible attenuation of psychological resistance following illness. When planning psychological therapy, the psychological characteristics of the patient should be taken into account, for example, temperament, emotional sensitivity, and so on. Some psychological traits have the status of moderators of psychophysiological costs of stress state (for example, temperament) (Strelau, 2000). Thus, tactics, patience, consequences and respect for the patient's personal dignity are expected (inter alia, to refrain from doing something that might threaten his or her sense of security).
5. Positive attitudes towards self-care for own health are not only important for individual development, but for the economic situation and organization of the health care system. However, this requires investment in development of health education for children and adolescents in the school system and lifelong education directed at everyone, not only children but also adults, of all ages.

REFERENCES

Antonovsky, A. (1987). *Unraveling The Mystery of Health. How People Manage Stress and Stay Well.* San Francisco: Jossey-Bass Publishers.

Basińska, M. (Ed.) (2016). Elastyczne radzenie sobie ze stresem w zdrowiu i chorobie [Coping flexibility with stress in health and in disease]. Bydgoszcz: Wydawnictwo Uniwersytetu Kazimierza Wielkiego.

Boylan, J. M., & Ryff, C. D. (2013). Varieties of anger and the inverse link between education and inflammation: Toward an integrated framework. *Psychosomatic Medicine, 75*(6), 566–574. doi:10.1097/PSY.0b013e31829683bd PMID:23766379

Brammer, L. M. (1985). *The helping relationship: process and skills.* Englewood Cliffs, N.J.: Prentice-Hall.

Caplan, G. (1961). *An approach to community mental health.* New York: Behavioral Publication.

Caplan, G. (1964). *Principles of preventive psychiatry.* New York: Basic Books.

Caplan, G. (1986). Caplan, G. (1986). Recent development in crisis intervention and in the promotion of support services. In M. Kessler & S. E. Goldston (Eds.), *A decade of progress in primary prevention* (pp. 235–260). Hanover, NH: University Press of New England.

Caplan, G., Caplan, R. B., & Erchul, W. P. (1994). Caplanian Mental Health Consultation: Historical Background and Current Status. *Consulting Psychology Journal: Practice and Research.* https://msrc.fsu.edu/system/files/Caplan%20G%20et%20al%201994%20Caplanian%20mental%20health%20consultation-20historical%20background%20and%20current%20status.pdf

Christakis, N. A., & Fowler, J. H. (2011). *W sieci. Jak sieci społeczne kształtują nasze życie* [On the Web. How social networks shape our lives]. Sopot: Smak Słowa.

Chrzan-Dętkoś, M., & Pietkiewicz, A. (2015). How can we cooperate better? The determinants of conflict solving competence in Polish pediatric nurses' relations with parents of hospitalized children. *Health Psychology Review, 3*(4), 345–351. doi:10.5114/hpr.2015.51906

Cierpiałkowska, L., & Sęk, H. (red.) (2016). Psychologia kliniczna [Clinical psychology] Warszawa: Wydawnictwo Naukowe PWN.

Compas, B. E., Beckjord, E., Agocha, B., Sherman, M. L., Langrock, A., Grossman, C. I., & Luecken, L. et al. (2006). Measurement of coping and stress responses in women with breast cancer. *Psycho-Oncology, 15*(12), 1038–1054. doi:10.1002/pon.999 PMID:17009343

Drat-Ruszczak, K. (2000). Teorie osobowości – podejście psychodynamiczne I humanistyczne. [Theories of personality - psychodynamic and humanistic approach] In J. Strelau (Ed.), *Psychologia* [Psychology. Academic manual] (Vol. 1, pp. 601–652). Gdańsk: Gdańskie Wydawnictwo Psycholgiczne.

Eriksson, M., & Lindstöm, B. (2005). Validity of Antonovsky's sense of coherence scale: A systematic review. *Journal of Epidemiology and Community Health, 59*(6), 460–466. doi:10.1136/jech.2003.018085 PMID:15911640

Farnicka, M., Liberska, H., & Niewiedział, D. (2016). *Psychologia agresji* [Psychology of aggression]. Warszawa: Wydawnictwo Naukowe PWN.

Forgas, J. P. (Ed.). (2006). *Affect in Social Cognition and Behavior.* New York: Psychology Press.

Forgas, J. P. (2012). Belief and affect: On the mental pre-cursors of health-related cognition and behaviour. *Journal of Health Psychology, 18*(1), 3–9. doi:10.1177/1359105312448869 PMID:22850972

Forgas, J. P., & Moylan, S. J. (2002). Affective influences on self-perception and self-disclosure. In J. P. Forgas & K. D. Williams (Eds.), *The social self: Individual, interpersonal and intergroup perspectives* (pp. 73–96). New York: Psychology Press.

Freud, S. (1995). Wykłady ze wstępu do psychoanalizy. Nowy cykl [Lectures from the introduction to psychoanalysis. New cycle]. Warszawa: KR.

Friedman, E. M., & Ryff, C. D. (2012). Living well with medical co-morbidities: A biopsychosocial perspective. *The Journals of Gerontology. Series B, Psychological Sciences and Social Sciences*, *67*(5), 535–544. doi:10.1093/geronb/gbr152 PMID:22377799

Gallant, M. P. (2003). The influence of social support on chronic illness self-management: A review and directions for research. *Health Education & Behavior*, *30*(2), 170–195. doi:10.1177/1090198102251030 PMID:12693522

Heller, A. S., van Reekum, C. M., Schaefer, S. M., Lapate, R. C., Radler, B. T., Ryff, C. D., & Davidson, R. J. (2013). Sustained ventral striatal activity predicts eudaimonic well-being and cortisol output. *Psychological Science*, *24*(11), 2192–2000. doi:10.1177/0956797613490744 PMID:24058063

Heszen, I., & Sęk, H. (2017). Psychologia zdrowia [Health psychology]. *Intervention (Amstelveen, Netherlands)*, *5*(4), 329–339. doi:10.1093/brief-treatment/mhi030

Hobfoll, S., Nadler, A., & Leiberman, J. (1986). Satisfaction with social support during crisis: Intimacy and self-esteem as critical determinants. *Journal of Personality and Social Psychology*, *51*(2), 296–304. doi:10.1037/0022-3514.51.2.296 PMID:3746613

Holmes, T. H., & Rahe, R. H. (1967). The social readjustment rating scale. *Journal of Psychosomatic Research*, *11*(2), 213–218. doi:10.1016/0022-3999(67)90010-4 PMID:6059863

Hwang, B., Moser, D. K., & Dracup, K. (2014). Knowledge Is Insufficient for Self-Care Among Heart Failure Patients With Psychological Distress. *Health Psychology*, *33*(7), 588–596. doi:10.1037/a0033419 PMID:23815766

James, S., Reddy, S. P., Ellahebokus, A., Sewpaul, R., & Naidoo, P. (2017). The association between adolescent risk behaviours and feelings of sadness or hopelessness: A cross-sectional survey of South African secondary school learners. *Psychology Health and Medicine*, *22*(7), 778–789. Published online14Mar2017. doi:10.1080/13548506.2017.1300669 PMID:28290218

Janicka, I., & Liberska, H. (red.) (2014). Psychologia rodziny [Psychology of family]. Warszawa: Wydawnictwo Naukowe PWN.

Juczyński Z. (2001). Spostrzegana kontrola a strategie radzenia sobie z przewlekłym bólem [Perceived control and coping strategies for chronic pain]. *Sztuka Leczenia*, *7*(2), 9-16.

Juczyński, Z. (2009). *Narzędzia pomiaru w promocji i psychologii zdrowia (wydanie drugie)* [Measurement tools in promotion and health psychology (2nd ed.)]. Warszawa: Pracownia Testów Psychologicznych PTP.

Juczyński, Z. (2014). Pomiar wsparcia społecznego – polska adaptacja Skali Znaczenia Innych [Measurement of social support - Polish adaptation of the Scale of Meaning of Others]. In E. Zasępa & T. Gałkowski (Eds.), Oblicza psychologii klinicznej. Pamięci Profesora Janusza Kostrzewskiego [Faces of clinical psychology. The memory of Professor Janusz Kostrzewski] (pp. 437–461). Warszawa: PWN.

Kanner, A. D., Coyne, J. C., Schaefer, C., & Lazarus, R. S. (1981). Comparison of two modes of stress measurement: Daily hassles and uplifts versus major life events. *Journal of Behavioral Medicine*, *4*(1), 1–39. doi:10.1007/BF00844845 PMID:7288876

Knoll, N., & Schwarzer, R. (2004). "Prawdziwych przyjaciół" Wsparcie społeczne, stres, choroba i śmierć ["Real friends" Social suport, stress, ilness and death.] In H. Sęk & R. Cieślak (Eds.), Wsparcie społeczne, stres i zdrowie [Social Support, Stress, Health] (pp. 29-48).Warszawa: Wydawnictwo Naukowe PWN.

Kowalik, S. (2007). *Psychologia rehabilitacji* [Psychology of Rehabilitation]. Warszawa: Wydawnictwa Akademickie i Profesjonalne.

Kuleta, M., & Trzópek, J. (2003). Zmiana stylu życia jako efekt przezwyciężenia kryzysu – szansa czy konieczność? [Change of lifestyle as a result of overcoming the crisis - chance or necessity?] In D. Kubacka-Jasiecka, & K. Mudyń (Eds.), Kryzys, interwencja i pomoc psychologiczna. Nowe ujęcia i możliwości [Crisis, intervention and psychological help. New shots and opportunities] (pp. 121- 144). Toruń: Wydawnictwo: Adam Marszałek.

Labott, S. M., Ahleman, B. A., Wolever, M. E., & Martin, R. B. (2010). The Physiological and Psychological Effects of the Expression and Inhibition of Emotion. *Journal of Behavioral Medicine*, 16(4), 182–189. PMID:2271804

Labott, S. M., & Martin, R. B. (1990). Emotional coping, age, and physical disorder. *Behavioral Medicine (Washington, D.C.)*, *16*(2), 53–61. doi:10.1080/08964289.1990.9934592 PMID:2364177

Laviolette, P. (1981). *A system view of man*. Boulder, CO: Westview Press.

Lazarus, R. S. (1986). Paradygmat stresu i radzenia sobie [Paradigm of stress and doping]. *Nowiny Psychologiczne*, *3*, 2–39.

Lazarus, R. S., & Folkman, S. (1984). *Stress, appraisal, and coping*. Berlin, Heidelberg, New York: Springer.

Levenson, P. M., Morrow, J. R. Jr, & Pfefferbaum, B. J. (1984). Attitudes toward health and illness. A comparison of adolescent, physician, teacher, and school nurse views. *Journal of Adolescent Health Care*, *5*(4), 254–260. doi:10.1016/S0197-0070(84)80127-8 PMID:6490480

Lewicki, A. (1978). Niektóre problemy teorii zachowania [Some problems of the theory of behavior]. In A. Lewicki (Ed.), Psychologia kliniczna [Clinical psychology] (pp. 21 – 43). Warszawa: PWN.

Liberska, H. (2004). *Perspektywy temporalne młodzieży. Wybrane uwarunkowania* [Temporar perspectives of adolescents. Selected determinants]. Poznań: Wydawnictwo Naukowe UAM.

Liberska, H. (2017). *Attachment and stress in adolescents during treatment in hospital* . Paper sent to the editor.

Liberska, H., & Boniecka, K. (2016). Introduction: biopsychosocial approach to transplantation. In H. Liberska & K. Boniecka (Eds.), *Selected psychosocial and medical problems of transplantation* (pp. 9–18). Warszawa: Difin.

Luszczynska, A., Mazurkiewicz, M., Ziegelmann, J. P., & Schwarzer, R. (2007). Recovery self-efficacy and intention as predictors of running or jogging behavior: A cross-lagged panel analysis over a two-year period. *Psychology of Sport and Exercise*, *8*(2), 247–260. doi:10.1016/j.psychsport.2006.03.010

Maslow, A. (1970). *Motivation and personality*. New York: Harper & Row.

McLeod, S. A. (2010). *SRRS - Stress of Life Events*. Retrieved from www.simplypsychology.org/SRRS.html

Moos, R. H., & Schaefer, J. A. (1993). Coping Resources and Process: Current Concepts and Measures. In L. Goldberger & S. Breznits (Eds.), Handbook of Stress. Theoretical and Clinical Aspects (pp. 234–257). New York: The Free Press.

Nelson, B. V., Patience, T. H., & MacDonald, D. C. (1999). Adolescent Risk Behavior and the Influence of Parents and Education. *Journal of the American Board of Family Medicine*, *12*(6), 436–443. doi:10.3122/jabfm.12.6.436 PMID:10612361

Nowaczyk, N., & Cierpiałkowska, L. (2016). Psychological profiles of patients with multiple sclerosis based on Hobfoll's conservation of resources theory. *Health Psychology Review*, *4*(4), 332–339. doi:10.5114/hpr.2016.59990

Obuchowski, K. (2000). *Galaktyka potrzeb. Psychologia dążeń ludzkich*. Poznań: Zysk i S-ka.

Ogińska-Bulik, N. (2013). The role of social support in people struggling with cancer. *Health Psychology Review*, *1*(1), 1–8. PMID:25793484

Ogińska-Bulik, N. (2016). The role of rumination in the occurrence of positive effects of experienced traumatic events. *Health Psychology Review*, *4*(4), 321–331.

Ogińska-Bulik, N., & Juczyński, Z. (2012). Resiliency as determinant of the positive and negative consequences of an experienced traumatic situation. *Polskie Forum Psychologiczne*, *2*(17), 395–410.

Oleś, M. (2015). Resilience and quality of life in chronically ill youth. *Health Psychology Review*, *3*(3), 220–236. doi:10.5114/hpr.2015.53246

Oleś, P. (2000). *Psychologia przełomu połowy życia* [Psychology of the mid-life breakthrough]. Lublin: Towarzystwo Naukowe KUL.

Parker, J. D. A., & Endler, N. S. (1994). Assessment of multidimensional coping: Task, emotion and avoidance strategies. *Psychological Assessment*, *6*(1), 50–60. doi:10.1037/1040-3590.6.1.50

Peterson, C., Maier, S. F., & Seligman, M. E. P. (1996). *Learned Helplessness. A Theory for the Age of Personal Control*. Oxford: Oxford University Press.

Pietrasiński, Z. (1990). *Rozwój człowieka dorosłego* [Development of an adult]. Warszawa: WP.

Pledger, C. (2003). Discourse on disability and rehabilitation issues: Opportunities for psychology. *The American Psychologist*, *58*(4), 279–284. doi:10.1037/0003-066X.58.4.279 PMID:12866393

Płużek, Z. (1997). Kryzysy psychologiczne i rodzaje kryzysów osobowościowych, [Psychological crises and types of personality crises]. In D. Kubacka-Jasiecka, & A. Lipowska–Teutsch (Eds.), Oblicza kryzysu psychologicznego i pracy interwencyjnej [Faces of the psychological crisis and intervention] (pp. 31-43). Kraków: Wyd. ALL.

Pommersbach, J. (1988). Wsparcie społeczne a choroba [Social support and illness]. *Przegląd Psychologiczny*, *31*(2), 503–525.

Rahe, R. H., Mahan, J. L. Jr, & Arthur, R. J. (1970). Prediction of near-future health change from subjects' preceding life changes. *Journal of Psychosomatic Research*, *14*(4), 401–406. doi:10.1016/0022-3999(70)90008-5 PMID:5495261

Redo, K., & Bielawska-Batorowicz, E. (2014). Expectations towards medical personnel – a study with infertility clinic patients. *Health Psychology Review*, *2*(3), 218–226. doi:10.5114/hpr.2014.45197

Roberts, A. R. (2005). Bridging the past and present to the future of crisis intervention and crisis management. In A. R. Roberts (Ed.), *Crisis intervention handbook: Assessment, treatment, and research* (3rd ed., pp. 3–34). New York: Oxford University Press.

Roberts, A. R., & Ottens, A. I. (2005). The Seven-Stage Crisis Intervention Model: A Road Map to Goal Attainment, Problem Solving, and Crisis Resolution. *Brief Treatment and Crisis Intervention*, *5*(4), 329–339. doi:10.1093/brief-treatment/mhi030

Ryff, C. D. (2014). Psychological well-being revisited: Advances in the science and practice of eudaimonia. *Psychotherapy and Psychosomatics*, *83*(1), 10–28. doi:10.1159/000353263 PMID:24281296

Ryff, C. D., & Spencer, B. (2002). Ironies of the human condition: well-being and health on the way to mortlity. In L. G. Aspinwal & U. M. Staudinger (Eds.), *A psychology of human strengths: Fundamental questions and future directions for a positive psychology* (pp. 271–287). Washington, D.C.: American Psychological Association.

Salovey, P., & Birnbaum, D. (1989). Influence of mood on health-relevant cognitions. *Journal of Personality and Social Psychology*, *57*(3), 539–551. doi:10.1037/0022-3514.57.3.539 PMID:2778638

Salovey, P., Detweiler, J. B., Steward, W. T., & Bedell, B. T. (2001). Affect and health-relevant cognition. In J. Forgas (Ed.), *Handbook of Affect and Social Cognition* (pp. 344–370). Mahwah, NJ: Lawrence Erlbaum and Associates.

Sarason, I. G., & Sarason, B. R. (1982). Concomitants of social support: Attitudes, personality characteristics, and life experiences. *Journal of Personality*, *50*(3), 331–344. doi:10.1111/j.1467-6494.1982.tb00754.x PMID:7143186

Schwarzer, R., & Luszczynska, A. (2015). Health Action Process Approach. In M. Conner & P. Norman (Eds.), *Predicting health behaviours* (3rd ed., pp. 252–278). Maidenhead, UK: McGraw Hill Open University Press.

Sędek, G. (1991). Jak ludzie radzą sobie z sytuacjami, na które nie ma rady? [How do people deal with situations that are not solved?]. In M. Kofta & T. Szustrowa (Eds.), Złudzenia, które pozwalają żyć [Illusions that allow you to live] (pp. 226-248). Warszawa: Wydawnictwo Naukowe PWN.

Sęk, H., & Cieślak, R. (2004). Wsparcie społeczne - sposoby definiowania, rodzaje i źródła wsparcia, wybrane koncepcje teoretyczne [Social Support - Ways to Defining, Types and Sources of Support, Selected Theoretical Concepts]. In H. Sęk & R. Cieślak (Eds.), Wsparcie społeczne, stres i zdrowie [Social Support, Stress, Health] (pp. 11-28).Warszawa: Wydawnictwo Naukowe PWN.

Seligman, M. E. P. (1975). *Helplessness: on depression, development, and death.* San Franciso: Freeman.

Seligman, M. E. P., & Maier, S. (1967). Failure to escape traumatic shock. *Journal of Experimental Psychology, 74*(1), 1–9. doi:10.1037/h0024514 PMID:6032570

Seligman, M. E. P., Steen, T. A., Park, N., & Peterson, C. (2005). Positive Psychology Progress: Empirical Validation of Interventions. *The American Psychologist, 60*(5), 410–421. doi:10.1037/0003-066X.60.5.410 PMID:16045394

Sniehotta, F. F., Schwarzer, R., Scholz, U., & Schüz, B. (2005). Action planning and coping planning for long-term lifestyle change: Theory and assessment. *European Journal of Social Psychology, 35*(4), 565–576. doi:10.1002/ejsp.258

Snyder, C. R. (1994). *The Psychology of Hope: You Can Get There from Here.* New York: The Free Press.

Snyder, M., Stephan, W., & Rosenfield, D. (1976). Egotism and attribution. *Journal of Personality and Social Psychology, 33*(4), 435–441. doi:10.1037/0022-3514.33.4.435 PMID:1271219

Strelau, J. (2000). Temperament. [Temperament] In J. Strelau (Ed.), *Psychologia. Podręcznik akademicki* [Psychology. Academic manual] (Vol. 1, pp. 683–719). Gdańsk: Gdańskie Wydawnictwo Psycholgiczne.

Sutton, S. (2005). Stage models of health behaviour. In M. Conner & P. Norman (Eds.), *Predicting health behaviour: Research and practice with social cognition models* (2nd ed., pp. 223–275). Maidenhead, England: Open University Press.

Szmaus-Jackowska, A. (2011). *Troska o siebie osób w starszym wieku* [Caring for oneself in old age]. Bydgoszcz: Wydawnictwo Uniwersytetu Kazimierza Wielkiego.

Trempała, J. (Ed.) (2011). Psychologia rozwoju człowieka [Psychology of human development]. Warszawa: Wydawnictwo Naukowe PWN.

von Bertalanffy, K.L. (1952). Problems of Life: An Evaluation of Modern Biological and Scientific Thought. New York: Harper.

Wiedemann, A. U., Lippke, S., Reuter, T., Ziegelmann, J. P., & Schwarzer, R. (2011). How planning facilitates behaviour change: Additive and interactive effects of a randomized controlled trial. *European Journal of Social Psychology*, *41*(1), 42–51. doi:10.1002/ejsp.724

Wilski, M., & Sienkiewicz-Wilowska, J. A. (2014). Social support as regulator of self-care attitude in persons with myocardial infraction. *Polish Psychological Bulletin*, *45*(4), 521–532. doi:10.2478/ppb-2014-0062

Wrześniewski, K., & Włodarczyk, D. (2004). Rola wsparcia społecznego w leczeniu i rehabilitacji osób po zawale serca. [Role of Social Support in Treatment and Rehabilitation of Persons After Heart Failure] In H. Sęk & R. Cieślak (Eds.), *Wsparcie społeczne, stres i zdrowie* [Social Support, Stress, Health]. (pp. 170–189). Warszawa: Wydawnictwo Naukowe PWN.

Zayas, V., & Hazan, C. (Eds.). (2015). *Bases of Adult Attachment: Linking Brain, Mind and Behavior*. New York: Springer. doi:10.1007/978-1-4614-9622-9

Chapter 9
Social Capital and Subjective Quality of Life

Monika Mularska-Kucharek
University of Lodz, Poland

ABSTRACT

This chapter describes how in recent decades, the concepts of social capital and quality of life have attracted the interest of both theoreticians and creators of social life. Both on the micro-, meso- and macrosocial levels, social capital has been viewed as one of the key elements of human well-being. Its positive influence on social well-being has been underlined by academics, practitioners of social life. In this chapter, the authors evaluate the relationship between social capital and the mental well-being of individuals. Through empirical analysis, the results of a representative research conducted among residents of one of the biggest Polish cities were examined. This concludes that social capital and social interaction are essential to the health of the individual.

INTRODUCTION

Questions about good life and happiness are by nature existential, pervasive and rhetorical. Nevertheless, they are significant enough to follow people throughout their lives. This issue takes on a particular importance in our times. Apart from research into quality of life and attempts at creating an adequate methodology, a number of efforts are underway to discover the mechanisms which determine a good life. Scholars and practitioners alike search for determiners which may improve the well-being of individuals and communities. Among the mechanisms which shape quality of life are also socio-cultural factors. One of the ever more significant ones is social capital, defined as a network of relationships between individuals and groups, shared norms and values, and trust. "These networks constitute a resource or asset – hence the term capital – that can be valuable in a range of situations." (Mclean and Page, 2005, p. 5).

The aim of this paper is to assess the relationships between social capital and subjective quality of life. The obtained data will be explored to verify the hypothesis that social capital is related to the mental well-being of individuals.

DOI: 10.4018/978-1-5225-3946-9.ch009

THEORETICAL BACKGROUND

The term "social capital" is ubiquitous in contemporary sociology. Its appeal rests, in part, on its capacity to stir in sociologists a renewed sense of the significance for collective action of social relations (Messner et al., 2004, p. 882).

Social capital is viewed as a set of resources created during the process of interaction which individuals have at their disposal in a given social situation (Halpern, 2005). Like any other type of capital, this value brings certain profits. If present, social capital may facilitate the production of individual and communal goods (Paxton, 2002). In Coleman's words (1990, p. 304), „social capital facilitates the achievement of goals that could not be achieved in its absence or could be achieved only at a higher cost".

Social capital brings social, political and economic benefits. Its use is commonly explored from the point of view of a community and rarely in its individual aspect. This adds particular interest to the analysis of social capital as an individual resource, which according to numerous authors (Coleman, 1990, 1994; Burt, 2000; Baker, 2000;) contributes to personal and professional success.

Moreover, the existence of social capital explains why some people get along in life better than others, despite seeming equally talented (Coleman, 1990). These differences manifest as a higher income, wider influence or better quality of life. According to Burt (2005), connection to other people makes some achieve their goals better and more efficiently than others. The resource of trust and social networks plays a significant role in the active participation of individuals in many dimensions of social life. Nevertheless, its main importance is for the economic aspect. "Social relations and non-market interactions of actors influence their behaviours toward one another on the market. Individuals choose behavioural strategies taking into account their own benefits and the probable behaviours of others. … This includes mutual trust, assessment of the propensity to cooperate and the willingness to maintain mutual contact in the short and long run" (Bartkowski, 2007, p. 56).

Social capital also influences the subjective dimension of quality of life. Individual dimensions of social capital – networks, trust, norms of cooperation – have a positive influence on the mental well-being of individuals. It is believed that there is a association between sociability and life satisfaction (Diener, 1984). In other words, people's life satisfaction is determined by the relationships they enter. Some studies conclude that it depends on having a spouse (Argyle, 1987). It turns out that married people are among the happiest ones, followed by people living as married, then widowed, divorced and separated (Helliwell, 2002). Even Aristotle said that a happy man is the one who has many friends (Aristotle, *Rhetoric*). Family support, both mental and financial, is an important aspect of the relations between social capital and quality of life (Giza-Poleszczuk, 2000). It is commonly believed that interpersonal relationships – social capital – are one of the most valuable things in life because they give more joy and happiness than material goods and satisfaction derived from one's own achievements. As Czapiński (2007) states, social networks played a crucial role among the adaptive resources after the changes which took place in Poland after 1989. A wide group of friends and strong social ties proved a rescue in this difficult situation. Single people were in a much worse mental condition than married ones.

The goal of this paper – to evaluate the relations between social capital and mental well-being of individuals – is not an easy task, not only due to the complexity of both concepts, but also due to the direction of this relation (meaning, does social capital impact quality of life, or is it the other way round). The literature of the subject favours heavily the first approach.

Berger-Schmitt (2000, p. 15) indicate that at the empirical level, positive associations between social capital and quality of life have been observed. The results of several studies point towards favourable effects of various aspects of social capital on … well-being. Scheffert et al. (2008) prove that people who are socially connected are happier and healthier. Connected people are more likely to be aware of the medical help they need, and they seek it out. They are also more likely to monitor their use of health resources (for example, to keep a doctor's appointment). Noghani et al. (2009) indicate that social capital has a greater role in explanation of quality of life relative to income and education. Income is the most important factor for explanation of the objective quality of life and social capital is the most important factor for explanation of subjective quality of life. Abdul-Hakim et al. (2010) indicate that the result of their study suggests that social capital plays a role in improving quality of life. Ounagh and Ounagh (2011) conducted a comparative research about social capital and quality of life in Delhi and Tehran. The results of multiple regressions in this study indicated that in both societies there is a significant relationship between social capital and quality of life. In addition, the study found that there is significant difference in impact of social capital on quality of life in Delhi. Bjornskov (2003) suggests a few possible explanations in regard to the relationship between social capital and quality of life (life satisfaction). Firstly, social capital could lead to higher economic growth rates, which in turn, may create optimism for the future. The optimism about the future then may lead to higher life satisfaction. Secondly social capital could help countries to cope with external shocks successfully. The ability to cope successfully with external shocks will help promote stability in the economy. This in turn may reduce economic uncertainty, and hence raise the level of life satisfaction. Finally, social capital inherently is good in itself. Having social interaction and knowing many friends could lead directly to the feeling of good about oneself and may raise the individual or societal level of life satisfaction. Karimzadeh et al. (2013) gave following arguments that social capital is regarded as an important determinant of quality of life. They indicate a positive relation between quality of life and all dimensions of social capital (view towards locality, locality solidarity, social trust, social communication and social participation) which means higher social capital will lead to higher quality of life in India.

METHODS

The empirical material consists of the results of quantitative studies performed in 2010 among 497 adult residents of Lodz, one of the largest Polish cities. The sample is representative. The research was conducted using the PAPI method, i.e. paper and pencil interview. However, the territorial limits of the study do not allow for a wider generalisation of the results, which gives them a utilitarian character. The results were compared to numerous studies by Polish (Czapiński, 2007; Theiss, 2007; Działek, 2011) and international researchers (Baker, 2000; Mellor et al., 1999; Putnam, 2000; Woolcock, 2001; Leung et al., 2010), both confirming their findings and supplementing them with new paths for research. Hence, it may be assumed that the findings on social capital and quality of life as well as their mutual relations, diagnosed in the researched community, are not an isolated phenomenon but rather a sign of more general patterns. The results presented here may therefore form an inspiration for further research on these phenomena, so significant for the development of societies.

The examined phenomena are by nature qualitative, not quantitative, which makes detailing the rules of measurement adopted in this paper even more important.

The vast number of approaches to social capital makes the concept difficult to operationalise for research purposes. Nevertheless, an overview of the basic theories of social capital shows that components of social capital exist as parts of three attributes of social life. Most authors list contact networks, norms and values, as well as various types of trust as the main elements of social capital (Putnam, 1995; Inglehart, 1997; Woolcock, 1998; Paxton, 1999; Theiss, 2007; Starosta and Frykowski, 2008), and such an approach was adopted in this paper. In the process of operationalising this concept, the following constitutive dimensions of social capitals were adopted:

- Social trust level, examined in the following dimensions: a vertical one (toward various institutions), and two horizontal ones – private (toward familiar people) and generalised (toward the majority of people)
- The density and range of maintained networks of social interactions,
- Level of shared social norms related to cooperation, the common good, democracy and the subjectivity of individuals in a given society or social group.

If one assumes that social capital consists of three basic components: networks, norms and trust, then the potential of social capital may be presented as a sum of the indicative values of the elements listed above (which was done for the purposes of this study).

When it comes to quality of life, the project analyses its two dimensions, subjective and objective. This paper discusses only subjective quality of life.

The analysed variables (social trust, quality of life) were treated as multidimensional concepts, which led to creating a synthetic scale for each of the three items. In both cases, original solutions were used, which adapted and expanded internationally recognised research tools.

Social capital was measured based on the methodology of the World Bank, namely Social Capital Integrated Questionnaire (Grootaert and van Bastelaer, 2002; Grootaert et al., 2003). The questions were divided into groups pertaining to the individual elements of social capital, including organisations and social networks, trust in the local environment and the existing models of cooperation. General and partial indicators of social capital were constructed, including indicators of vertical, horizontal and general trust, social norms approval indicator and social network indicator.

Social capital consists of the elements mentioned above, i.e. networks, norms and trust; on the individual level social capital resources are determined by the level of the features believed to be its constitutive elements, and the configuration of these elements determines the type of the capital. Therefore the study assumed that the total value of social capital is determined by the sum total of the discussed elements. Source questions were measured using a seven-point Likert scale. Due to the fact that the indicators of the analysed components of social capital consist of varying numbers of items, all partial variables included in the components mentioned above were transformed into variables with discrete values from the –1 to +1 interval. This ensured a full comparability of the selected subscales, which made it possible to maintain equal weights for all the subscales when determining the general indicator of social capital. Social capital level (in general) assumes values from -3 to +3. The higher the value, the higher the social capital of the individual.

When assessing quality of life, the authors assumed, as cited in Borys and Rogala (2008), that a complete view of quality of life can only be obtained by examining both its objective and subjective dimension. The assessment of subjective quality of life was based on the methodology of the European Social Survey, which refers to Campbell's (1976) proposal, used for almost 20 years in Poland (including periodic studies of the Public Opinion Research Centre (CBOS), TNS OBOP, the Social Diagnosis, and Polish General Survey on Quality of Life – Ostasiewicz 2004). The empirical indicators of subjective quality of life were questions about general life satisfaction and satisfaction with specific areas of life (immediate family relationships, financial situation of the respondent's family, relationships with acquaintances (a group of friends), current family income, possibility to meet nutritional needs, health, life achievements, situation in the country, living conditions, standard of the available goods and services, perspectives for the future, sexual life, education, free time activities, job, children, marriage, safety in one's place of residence, health care facilities near place of residence, participation in culture, political elites of the country). The source questions (diagnostic variables) were measured using a seven-point Likert scale. Subjective quality of life, similarly to social capital, was considered a multidimensional concept. Therefore a synthetic indicator of subjective quality of life was created by adding the values of the partial variables listed above. This variable took on values from the 27–146 interval, where higher values indicated a higher subjective quality of life.

The most important data pertaining to the constructed scales and as a result to the synthetic indicators are presented in Table 1.

A descriptive analysis was performed on the sample, and the results were expressed as means (M), standard deviations (SDs), frequencies and percentages. Cronbach's α values were calculated to evaluate the validity and reliability of social capital scale (SC) and quality of life scale (QoL). Factor analysis was used to evaluate the "coherence" of social capital scale. The significance of differences among populations was evaluated using a one-way analysis of variance. Association between qualitative variables was measured using a chi-square test of independence. The strength of the association between the variables was measured using the Cramer's V coefficient. The study assumed a standard level of significance ($\alpha = 0.05$). The calculations were performed in SPSS 21.0.

RESULTS

The first part of this analysis consisted of examining the association between social capital level and subjective quality of life. The analyse of independence indicated that only selected indicators of subjective quality of life are statistically related to social capital. Firstly, it was concluded that social capital statistically significantly determines life satisfaction ($\chi^2 = 14.532$; p = 0.006**), with a higher level of social capital meaning a better assessment of one's own life. The data show that people with rich resources

Table 1. Main features of the social capital and quality of life scales constructed

Indicator		Variation Interval	Cronbach's α Coefficient	M	SD
Social capital	Total	-3 ÷ 3	0.723	0.20	1.25
	Social trust (T)	-3 ÷ 3	0.836	0.40	1.22
	Acceptance of social norms (R)	-4 ÷ 4	0.733	2.88	1.78
	Social networks (N)	-7 ÷ 7	0.701	2.95	2.28
Subjective quality of life (SQoL)		27 ÷ 146	0.856	97.77	18.46

Source: Own work.

of social capital feel much more satisfied with their lives that people with a low level of this potential. It must be added that people with a high social capital level did not give a negative evaluation of their lives. In fact, over 90% of respondents evaluated their lives positively. Therefore, it may be concluded that a wide network of social contacts, displaying trust in interpersonal relations and sharing pro-social norms positively influences one's life satisfaction. Psychologists claim that the quality of interpersonal relationships is vital for happiness (Csiksztenmihalyi, 1990). "Developed social networks lead to happiness, growth, satisfaction and a meaningful life" (Baker, 2000, 16). However, trust and openness to other people also impact life satisfaction (Seligman, 1995). Trust is a good predictor of social relations stability. Life satisfaction also depends significantly on the last component of social capital, that is social norms. Their existence provides individuals with a sense of security and psychical comfort. Functioning within an existing axionormative system is undoubtedly crucial for life satisfaction.

Furthermore, the analyses pointed to a statistically significant association between social capital and satisfaction with one's education ($\chi^2 = 22.128$; $p < 0.0001$***). The research shows that most people satisfied with their education have a high social capital level (73.6%). Among this group, people dissatisfied with their education constitute only 5.6%, whereas in the group of respondents with a low social capital level, as much as 20% express dissatisfaction. The obtained data corroborate the theoretical and empirical conclusions pertaining to the association between social capital and education. According to Baker (2000), the fact that people can communicate with one another is a sign of the social relations included in human education. The ability to read and write is mainly a function of learning opportunities created by other people. Through social relationships, individuals achieve successive levels of education, thereby investing in human capital, which is a significant element of success. Such personal investments are made possible due to social contacts, as it is social capital that facilitates the creation of human capital (Baker, 2000, 7). Coleman (1988) also believes in the importance of social networks for educational achievements. In his publication about the role of social capital in the creation of human capital, he discusses the importance of micro-social ties for individuals' learning achievements. He maintains that familial social capital is crucial for the intellectual development of children. It determines their educational aspirations and their individual attitudes to education. Family relationships, parents' interest in school and their participation in school life create a so-called bridge in the intergenerational transfer of resources. Therefore, Coleman (1988, 109–115) underlines the importance of locational stability, as it facilitates the creation of social ties between students' parents and teachers, as well as between students and teachers or other members of the community.

The relation between social capital and satisfaction with the perspectives for the future is another statistically significant association ($\chi^2 = 14.410$; $p = 0.021$**). The analyses showed that a high level of social capital is conducive to positive expectations for the future. It can be explained by the fact that the perspectives for the future depend on the individual components of social capital. Trust plays a great role here, as it is omnipresent in everyday life and contributes greatly to one's functioning in the complex social reality. People with a high social trust level are open to others, initiate social contacts eagerly, show initiative and complete planned goals. Besides, as Sztompka (2007, 45) says, "to face the future in an active and constructive way, we must show trust". The modern world requires trust because it becomes a resource which allows individuals to cope with an ever-changing environment. However, plans for the future are also shaped by the social networks at one's disposal. Family, close and distant friends may form a potential source of support for individuals, the more so when the future is possibly associated with uncertainty, changes and risk. In such situations social support, which is a consequence of belonging to a social network, is often needed and has an enormous importance in the everyday battle with stress (Sęk, 2001), including the stress related to one's future. Finally, individuals' attitudes to the future depend on the axionormative system, the norms and values shared by the members of social groups which provide the framework to their functioning. The axionormative system determines human behaviour and forms the criteria of what to do and how to act in interpersonal relations. Therefore, the approval of social norms gives psychological comfort.

The analyses conducted confirmed also the relations between social capital and financial sphere. It turned out that this individual resource is significantly correlated with the satisfaction with one's family's financial situation ($\chi^2 = 27.101$; $p < 0.0001$*** and with the satisfaction with one's income ($\chi^2 = 21.435$; $p < 0.0001$***). The association has the following character: the higher the social capital level, the better the respondents' satisfaction with their family's financial situation and their own income. It turns out that most people satisfied with the analysed sphere of life are among the one with a high level of the examined phenomenon, and the group with low levels of this potential has the lowest number of people satisfied with the discussed sphere.

The impact of social capital on economic capital was documented in numerous studies. Baker (2000) claims that people with a rich social capital are better paid and are promoted faster. He maintains that social capital is connected to many benefits. If individuals have social capital, they can use it e.g. when looking for a job. Besides, those better equipped in social capital will more frequently find work through unofficial channels. Finally, as Boxman et al. (1991, 52–54) state, social capital has an independent influence on income.

Moreover, social capital determines in a statistically significant way the satisfaction with one's health ($\chi^2 = 14.182$; $p = 0.007$**). The obtained data show that most people satisfied with this sphere of life have a high level of social capital. It should be noted that there is a significant difference between the high and the medium and low levels of social capital when it comes to the satisfaction with one's health. The association between the variables is as follows: the higher the social capital level, the higher the satisfaction with one's health. The influence on individual and public health is one of many benefits of social capital. The literature of the subject points to "three types of the association between social capital and health, which are the results of: firstly, social support; secondly, socio-economic diversity; and finally, the impact of political economics" (Theiss, 2007). "The impact of social relations on health improvement was documented in a number of cases, from decreasing a risk of a serious illness to alleviating a common cold" (Baker, 2005, 16). It turns out that people with rich resources of social capital are in better mental and physical health. In turn, people with strong social networks get better the fastest (House et al., 1988). Other research indicates that couples where partners treat each other with respect suffer less frequently from contagious diseases. Unhappy marriage increases the risk of falling ill by 35% and shortens one's lifespan by 4 years (Gottman and Silver, 2000). On the other hand, Woolcock and Szreter (2004) claim that the impact of social capital on health is confined to highlighting the role of social support which it provides. The association between individual social capital and health is explained by drawing attention to the benefits of social contact networks, which may form a source of mental support and help for individuals.

To summarize, the analyses discussed here concern the association between social capital and elements of subjective quality of life. As mentioned before, not all indicators of this dimension of quality of life correlate statistically with the examined phenomenon. Nevertheless, it is worth noting that such a association was diagnosed in most aspects of life. Those which correlate the strongest with social capital were discussed at length.

Taking into account the synthetic subjective assessment of quality of life (SQoL), a statistically significant effect of the social capital variable for all three cases may be isolated. The analyses pointed at a statistically significant difference between people with a high and low social capital level. The graph of the averages showed that the highest satisfaction with life and its aspects might be observed in people with rich resources of social capital (M = 0.23; SD = 0.76), and the lowest in those whose level of social capital is low (M = -0.09; SD = 0.74). The obtained data therefore confirm the hypothesis concerning the impact of social capital on subjective quality of life.

DISCUSSION AND CONCLUSION

The importance of social capital for life satisfaction is mainly discussed in the context of social support which is understood as "objectively existent and available social networks whose distinguishing feature is the fact that through the existence of ties, contact and the sense of belonging they act as a help for people in difficult situations" (Sęk and Cieślak, 2004, 14–15). The expressed support may concern various aspects. Due to social relations, people may obtain, firstly, emotional support through the communication of supportive and calming emotions, which are signs of trust and a positive attitude to the person being supported; secondly, informative support, which includes the exchange and imparting of information and advice which foster a better understanding of one's situation, position in life and problems; furthermore, instrumental support through direct help in the form of loans, gifts and services; and finally, spiritual support, concerning the most difficult situations when the remaining forms of support are not conducive to a positive resolution of the situation (Kawula, 1997; Sęk and Cieślak, 2004). Social capital is connected with a positive attitude to life, active dealing with difficulties, satisfaction with life, striving to achieve important goals, joy of life, subjectivity etc. It has a significant influence on the mental well-being of individuals.

As Baker (2005) says, social capital is an indicator of happiness and determines one's lifespan. According to psychologists, the main motivation in life is participation: the expansion and development of connections to other people (as cited in: Baker, 2005; Miller and Stiver, 1997). Wide social networks give individuals a feeling of happiness and satisfaction. What is more, people with rich social networks live longer. "A number of studies show that social ties and relations may play a significant role in determining health status" (Berkman and Syme, 1979, 79). Admittedly, according to Baker (2005), not all the mechanisms are fully understood, but the association between social networks and longevity seems to be a result of both behavioural and biological changes. This thesis is confirmed by research which shows that a frequent participation in religious services reduces mortality, partly because of behavioural changes – a tendency to more frequent social contacts, improvement in health practices and remaining in marriage – but also because of the importance of religion in human life (Strawbridge et al., 1997). The research of Berkman and Syme (1979), who for ten years studied the relationship between social networks, lifestyle and health practices, offers similar conclusions. On the basis of the obtained results, she concluded that lonely people had a three times higher chance of death than people who sustained social ties. Moreover, studies documenting the relations between social ties and the length of life showed that it is the number of social ties that matters, not their type. It is important as far as social capital offers a certain protection to individuals (as cited in: Baker and Hallowell, 2001). It also plays the role of a personal resource which may be used in situations difficult for the individual in question, including a new social order and the need to adapt to a rapid and profound social change (Sztompka, 2002). It is confirmed by Czapiński (2007, 56), who writes, "A wide group of friends and strong social ties proved a rescue in the difficult years following the change. Single people were in a worse mental condition than married ones." Social capital integrates people, hence it is often compared to a "social glue", a substance which brings people together in a literal or indirect way (Bartkowski, 2007).

The exploration provided arguments for the thesis that social capital is significantly correlated to the assessment of quality of life. Taking into account the findings up to now, it may be concluded that social capital has a significant influence on the mental well-being of individuals. The results presented here are important for everyone who asks for a recipe for a successful life. No ready solution is included here, as it obviously does not exist, but the conclusions of the conducted research may be useful when looking for tips to achieve a high quality of life. As Czapiński (2004) claims, one of the most important, if not the single most important, correlate of happiness seem to be good social relationships.

REFERENCES

Abdul-Hakim, R., Ismail, R., & Abdul-Razak, N. A. (2010) The relationship between social capital and quality of life among rural households in Terengganu, Malaysia, *International Journal of Sustainable Development,* 1(5). Retrieved 20 May 2014 from http://www.ssrn.com/link/OIDA-Intl-Journal-Sustainable-Dev.html

Argyle, M. (1987). *The psychology of happiness*. London: Methuen.

Arystoteles. (2008) *Retoryka. Reotoryka dla Aleksanda. Poetyka.* Warsaw: PWN.

Baker, W. (2000). *Achieving Success Through Social Capital: Tapping the Hidden Resources in Your Personal and Business Networks*. Michigan: Jossey-Bass.

Bańka, A., & Derbis, R. (1994). *Psychologiczne i pedagogiczne wymiary jakości życia (The Psychological and Pedagogical Dimensions of Life)*. Poznan: Gemini.

Bartkowski, J. (2007). *Kapitał społeczny i jego oddziaływanie na rozwój w ujęciu socjologicznym (Social Capital and Its Impact on Developemnt: A Sociological Perspective*). In M. Herbst (Ed.), *Kapitał ludzki i kapitał społeczny a rozwój regionalny (Human and Social Capital versus Regional Development).* Warsaw: SCHOLAR.

Berger-Schmitt, R. (2000) Social Cohesion as an Aspect of the Quality of Societies: Concept and Measurement (Working Paper 14). EU Reporting. Mannheim: ZUMA.

Berkman, L. F., & Syme, S. L. (1979). Social Networks, Host Resistance, and Mortality: A Nine-year Follow-up Study of Almeda County Residents. *American Journal of Epidemiology, 109*(2), 186–204. doi:10.1093/oxfordjournals.aje.a112674 PMID:425958

Bjornskov, C. (2003). The happy few: Cross country evidence on social capital and life satisfaction. *Kyklos, 56*(1), 3–16. doi:10.1111/1467-6435.00207

Boxman, E., De Graaf, P., & Flap, H. (1991). The impact of social and human capital on the income attainment of Dutch managers. *Social Networks, 13*(1), 51–73. doi:10.1016/0378-8733(91)90013-J

Burt, R. S. (2005). *Brokerage & closure. An introduction to social capital*. New York, Oxford: Oxford University Press.

Burt, S. R. (1997). A note on social capital and network content. *Social Networks*, *19*(4), 355–373. doi:10.1016/S0378-8733(97)00003-8

Campbell, A., Converse, P., & Rodgers, W. (1976). *The Quality of American Life: Perceptions, Evaluations, and Satisfactions*. New York: Russel Sage Foundation.

Coleman, J. (1988). Social Capital in the Creation of Human Capital. *American Journal of Sociology*, *94*, 95–120. doi:10.1086/228943

Coleman, J. (1990). *The Foundations of Social Theory*. Cambridge: Harvard University Press.

Csikszentmihalyi, M. (1990). *Flow: The Psychology of Optimal Experience*. New York: Harper Collins.

Czapiński, J. (2004). *Ekonomiczne przesłanki i efekty dobrostanu psychicznego* (*Economic determinants and effects of mental well-being*). In T. Tyszka (Ed.), *Psychologia ekonomiczna (Economic psychology)* (pp. 192–242). Gdansk: GWP.

Czapiński, J. (2007). Indywidualna jakość życia (Individual Quality of Life). In J. Czapiński, & T. Panek (Eds.), Diagnoza społeczna [Social Diagnosis]. Warsaw: VizjaPress@IT.

Diener, E. (1984). Subjective Well-being. *Psychological Bulletin*, *95*(3), 542–575. doi:10.1037/0033-2909.95.3.542 PMID:6399758

Działek, J. (2011). *Kapitał społeczny jako czynnik rozwoju gospodarczego w skali regionalnej i lokalnej w Polsce (Social capital as the determinant of economic growth in Poland in regional and local perspective)*. Krakow: Jagiellonian University Press.

Giza-Poleszczuk, A., Marody, M., & Rychard, A. (2000). *Strategie i system. Polacy w obliczu zmiany społecznej [Strategies and the System. Polish People against a Social Change]*. Warsaw: Institute of Philosophy and Sociology at the Polish Academy of Sciences.

Gottman, J. M., & Silver, N. (2000). *The Seven Principles for Making Marriage Work*. New York: Crown.

Granovetter, M. S. (1973). The Strength of Weak Ties. *American Journal of Sociology*, *78*(6), 1360–1380. doi:10.1086/225469

Grootaert, C., & Van Bastelaer, T. (2002). *Understanding and Measuring Social Capital. A Multidisciplinary Tool for Practicioners*. Washington, DC: The World Bank. doi:10.1596/0-8213-5068-4

Grootaert, C., *Narayan, D.,* Nyhan Jones, V. and Woolcock, M. (2003) *Integrated Questionnaire for the Measurement of Social Capital*. he World Bank.

Halpern, D. (2005). *Social capital*. Cambridge: Polity Press.

Helliwell, J. F. (2002). Social Capital, the Economy and Well-being. *The Review of Economic Performance and Social Progress*. In K. Banting, A. Sharpe, & F. St-Hilaire (Eds.), *The Review of Economic Performance and Social Progress* (pp. 43–60). Montreal, Ottawa: Institute for Research on Public Policy and Centre for the Study of Living Standards.

House, J. S., Landis, K. R., & Umberson, D. (1988). Social Relationship and Health. *Science*, *241*(4865), 540–545. doi:10.1126/science.3399889 PMID:3399889

Inglehart, R. (1997). *Modernization and Postmodernization. Cultural, Economic and Political Change in 43 Societies*. Princeton: Princeton University Press.

Karimzadeh, M. (2013). Impact of Social Capital on Quality of Life: Evidence from India. *International Journal of Economic Practices and Theories*, *3*(4), 264–270.

Kawula, S. (1997). Spirala życzliwości: od wsparcia do samodzielności (The Kindness Spiral: From Support to Self-Reliance). *Wsparcie Społeczne*, *1*, 13–21.

Leung, A., Kier, C., Fung, T., Fung, L., & Sproule, R. (2011). Searching for Happiness: The Importance of Social Capital. *Journal of Happiness Studies*, *12*(3), 443–462. doi:10.1007/s10902-010-9208-8

Mclean, J., & Page, M. (2005) Social Capital and Quality of Life. In *Proceedings of the 7th Australian Conference on Quality of Life*.

Mellor, D., Cummins, R., & Loquet, T. (2012). Life quality and wealth: a qualitative and quantitative comparison of affluent and poor people. *Journal of Social Research and Policy*, *3*(2), 7–18.

Messner, S., Baumer, E., & Rosenfeld, R. (2004). Dimensions of Social Capital and Rates of Criminal Homicide. *American Sociological Review*, *69*(6), 882–903. doi:10.1177/000312240406900607

Miller, J. B., & Stiver, I. P. (1997). *The Healing Connection: How Women form Relationships in Therapy and in Life*. Boston: Beacon Press.

Noghani, M., Asgharpour, A., Safa, S., & Kermani, M. (2009) *Quality of life and Social Capital in Mashhad City in Iran, Conference of health and society*. Retrieved 27 November 2012 from http://profdoc.um.ac.ir/paper-abstract-1021206.html

OECD. (2001). *The Well-Being of Nations: The Role of Human and Social Capital, Education and Skills*. Paris: OECD Centre for Educational Research and Innovation.

Ostasiewicz, W. (2004). *Ocena i analiza jakości życia*. Wroclaw: Wroclaw University of Economics Press.

Ounagh, N., & Ounagh, M. (2011). A Comparative Study of Social Capital and Quality Of Life in Delhi and Tehran. *Journal of Exclusion Studies*, *1*(1), 19–35. doi:10.5958/j.2231-4547.1.1.002

Paxton, P. (1999). Is Social Capital Declining in the United States? A Multiple Indicator Assessment. *American Journal of Sociology*, *105*(1), 88–127. doi:10.1086/210268

Paxton, P. (2002). Social Capital and Democracy: An Interdependent Relationship. *American Sociological Review*, *67*(2), 254–277. doi:10.2307/3088895

Putnam, R. D. (1995). *Demokracja w działaniu*. Krakow, Warsaw: Znak Press, Batory Foundation.

Putnam, R. D. (2000). *Bowling Alone: The Collapse and Survival of American Community*. New York: Touchstone. doi:10.1145/358916.361990

Scheffert, D. R., Hornvedt, J., & Chazdon, S. (2008). *Social Capital and Our Community*. Minnesota: University of Minnesota Press.

Sęk, H., & Cieślak, R. (2005). *Wsparcie społeczne, stres i zdrowie (Social Support, Stress and Health).* Warsaw: PWN.

Seligman, M. (1995). *Optymizmu można się nauczyć (Optimism Can Be Learned).* Poznan: Media Rodzina.

Starosta, P., & Frykowski, M. (2008). Typy kapitału społecznego i wzory partycypacji obywatelskiej w wiejskich gminach centralnej Polski (Types of social capital and models of the civic participation in the rural communities of central Polish). In M. S. Szczepański, K. Bierwiaczonek, & T. Nawrocki (Eds.), *Kapitały ludzkie i społeczne a konkurencyjność regionów [Human and social capitals vs. region's competitiveness].* Katowice: Silesian University Press.

Stone, W., & Hughes, J. (2002) Social Capital: Empirical Meaning and Measurement Validity (Research Paper 27). Australian Institute of Family Studies, Melbourne.

Strawbridge, W. J., Cohen, R. D., Shema, S. J., & Kaplan, G. A. (1997). Frequent attendance at religious services and mortality: A 28-year follow-up. *American Journal of Public Health, 87*(6), 957–961. doi:10.2105/AJPH.87.6.957 PMID:9224176

Szreter, S., & Woolcock, M. (2004). Health by association? Social capital, social theory, and the political economy of public health. *International Journal of Epidemiology, 33*(4), 650–667. doi:10.1093/ije/dyh013 PMID:15282219

Sztompka, P. (2002) Integracja europejska jako szansa kulturowa. O moralności, tożsamości, zaufaniu [European Integration as a Cultural Opportunity. On Morality, Identity and Trust]. Nauka, 2, 59–66.

Sztompka, P. (2007). *Zaufanie. Fundament społeczeństwa [Trust. The Cornerstone of Society].* Krakow: Znak Press.

Theiss, M. (2007). *Krewni – Znajomi – Obywatele. Kapitał społeczny a lokalna polityka społeczna [Relatives – Friends – Citizens. Social Capital and the Local Policy].* Torun: Adam Marszałek Press.

Woolcock, M. (2001). The Place of Social Capital in Understanding Social and Economic Outcomes. *Canadian Journal of Policy Research, 2*(1), 11–17.

Woolock, M. (1998). Social Capital and Economic Development: Toward and Theoretical Syntesis and Policy Framework. *Theory and Society, 27*(2), 151–208. doi:10.1023/A:1006884930135

Chapter 10
Patient Satisfaction

Nafisa Vaz
Goa Institute of Management, India

ABSTRACT

This chapter describes how there are three major stakeholders in a patient's hospitalization: the patient, the healthcare providers, and the hospital. Satisfaction with the care and hospital experience is important to the patient because evidence suggests satisfied patients are more likely to adhere to self-care instructions and have better clinical outcomes. Hospitals have aimed to provide care and service that is highly satisfying to patients because it is the right thing to do and because reputation affects volume and revenues which in turn impacts the fiscal bottom line. Unfortunately, not all patients enjoy equal levels of satisfaction in the health care system. To succeed amongst today's competition; healthcare organizations must be patient-centered and win the loyalty of their patients by providing an outstanding patient experience, then retaining these patients, increasing the number of patients through positive word of mouth and continually delivering greater value.

INTRODUCTION

The system of medicine has evolved over centuries. There are major developments that have taken place in the health systems in the last few years. You now have the establishment of corporate hospitals equipped with the latest facilities, the advent of third-party payers (insurance companies, governments, companies, etc.), increasing awareness among patients, freely available information through the internet, higher expectations in patient care, and the increasing litigations in the healthcare industry.

This has made the health care industry a very challenging service industry. What was once considered a noble profession is no longer thought as one. Patient satisfaction is an important component of evaluating care. Patient satisfaction describes how patients value and regard their care; it is a process as much as an attitude, so it must be, monitored continually, and frequently measured.

DOI: 10.4018/978-1-5225-3946-9.ch010

THE THEORETICAL FRAMEWORK

Patient as a Consumer

The last few years health systems have revamped the way of delivering care, patient have become the center of focus and new organizational models have been applied in order to provide patient-oriented services. Marketing experts are aware that consumers make their decision about utilization of services on the basis of their perception of the service rather than the reality and hence marketing and patient satisfaction have become of paramount importance as mouth-to-mouth publicity and personal referral is the most common and influential cause of using a particular health facility. Healthcare facility is very difficult to measure; hence, it is a challenge to a healthcare provider to influence a patient's perception of quality of care. A patient's satisfaction may not be totally influenced by the quality of physician available, but it reflects how the medical care has been delivered. To provide the highest level of satisfaction that is profitable to both the patient and the provider, management must control both the perception of expectation and the quality of delivery of the healthcare services. Knowledge of expectation and the factors affecting them, combined with knowledge of actual and perceived healthcare quality, provides the necessary information for designing and implementing programs to satisfy patients. With the advancement in technology and stiff competition, hospitals are always striving for improvement in their services. Patient expectations are constantly changing, so what satisfies a patient at one point in time may not satisfy him at some later date. As you improve your service levels on some patient satisfaction 'attributes,' you will change patient expectations on the remaining attributes.

Defining Patient Satisfaction

It is important to know what it is. Defining and understanding patient satisfaction will help to structure an evaluation process which will provide an organization with adequate measures of the variables that contribute to patient satisfaction. Most patients even if they are usually satisfied with the services, they may not be uniformly satisfied with all aspects of the care they receive. The management would need to be in a position to be constantly aware as to how much is enough to result in high patient satisfaction and to make them keep coming back. (Naidu, 2009).

Patient satisfaction is "a person's positive feeling of pleasure or disappointment resulting for comparing a product or services perceived performance or outcome in relation to his or her expectations" (Anand, Kaushal, & Gupta, 2012; Rashmi & Vijakumar, 2010).

A patient's experience is based on numerous encounters with various situations. The experience can begin with the various touchpoints, that could even mean getting to your website, then by physically visiting the facility, the admissions process, meeting with the doctors, nurses, lab technicians and support staff. This could also cover physical aspects such as the location of the patient rooms along with the care and concern they receive while in their room, the discharge process. There are many factors that could impact the perception of the care provided during an inpatient stay. It can also include the cleanliness of the environment, appearance of the facility, the ease of access to specific locations, the waiting time, the clarity of the communication by the physicians, the outcome from the care provided, the cost of the visit, the quality of the food and the list can go on.

Patient satisfaction is defined as "the extent of agreement between what a patient expects to receive from the healthcare experience and the perception of the level of care they actually receive".(Babu, 2012).

Patient satisfaction is related to the extent to which general healthcare and condition-specific needs are meet. Patient satisfaction is a multidimensional constructs that includes the degree of patient's positive feeling on satisfaction, quality of service, interpersonal behaviour, communication, financial aspects, time spent with physicians, nurses, administrative staff, pharmacy service, accessibility to health care service, convenience, availability of care and condition of facilities during their health care services (Vadhana, 2012).

Clients' satisfaction was defined as the result of matching one's expectation of healthcare services with actual experiences whether it is pleasant or disappointed in Advances in Service Marketing and Management.

Many articles about patients' satisfaction suggested the following significant relationship:

- Satisfaction is the result of perceiving service implementation against expectation.
- Willingness to buy or come back to receive the same services is the effect of satisfaction.
- Expecting and willingness to have services create alternatives for patients.
- The more the patients are pleased, the greater the level of satisfaction will be.

Findings from various articles suggested that most patients are very sensitive to what is going on with their health condition. They honestly insist on knowing exactly what the problems are, the ways treatment might be taken into account and the consequences that might happen. They still do even though it might frighten or disappoint them in anyway Sometimes, it is hard for the service providers to meet some patients' high expectation. Some researchers have found out that the characters of socio-demographic factors vary vastly according to the actual aspects (Heng, 2011). The nature of patients' expectation may be widely different and complicated. One cannot base on a set of standard rules to satisfy different groups of people and to expect that they will show a similar satisfaction level. Therefore, significant factors around them might become effective tools to predict what they really want.

People with a low standard of living tend to experience a low level of healthcare services when they have health problems. In addition, because they really have to work hard to survive, they might not be able to follow more schedules of treatments. In some case, their physicians do not treat them equally as the patients who have full coverage of insurance. This factor unavoidably might lead them to have a low level of satisfaction.

The concern about the relationship between age groups and level of satisfaction has also been studied. Some previous researchers have suggested that the older Respondents seem to give more scores to the service providers since they have been going through the social services all their lives. They are said to be more Understanding and accepting than younger respondents who usually have less Social and commercial experiences of the real world and seem to judge things very quickly.

Many reports have associated a low level of patients' satisfaction with low family income. They say that people's monthly incomes play important roles in purchasing power of goods and services. It also classifies the users' social status with a set of standard quality of services, which is usually highly expected by the user of healthcare services.

The Importance of Patient Satisfaction Evaluation

Why should Patient Satisfaction be a Top Priority? Improving the quality of patient care in hospitals is very necessary. Listening to your patients is the single most critical component of establishing a long-term relationship with your patients. From the patient's feedback, we can measure the patient satisfaction level and accordingly offers an insight into the healthcare provider's level of success.

The healthcare community has been assessing patients. Developments in the medical environment and the increase in competition have promoted the health care organizations to recognize the patients as valuable customers. In the last few years, health systems changed the way of thinking and delivering care, the patient has become the center of the overall care process and providing patient-centred services has become an important focus. (Sajid & Ali, n.d.)

Patient satisfaction is a very important measure and is a primary means of measuring the effectiveness of health care delivery. The competitive environment has forced health organizations to focus on patient satisfaction as a way to maintain market share and stay ahead in the market. If you are not aware of your strengths and weaknesses you cannot compete effectively. There are several studies that have shown that higher hospital-level patient satisfaction scores were associated with lower hospital inpatient mortality rates and negatively correlated with a hospital's 30-day readmission rates (Environment, n.d.).

The data gathered through patient satisfaction studies indicates the level of care delivered by staff and doctors and can serve as a tool in decision-making and performance appraisal. Patient satisfaction surveys can be tools for learning. They also serve as a means of holding doctors and other staff accountable. Doctors and other staff can be asked to prove that they have acceptable levels of patient satisfaction, which can be used as a performance indicator. Patient satisfaction data can also be used to document the quality of health care, to accrediting bodies nationally as well as internationally.

Patient satisfaction surveys are important as they have the capability to identify and resolve potential problems before they even break into major issues. They could also be used to assess and measure the benefits of any specific initiatives or projects in the service delivery. They can identify those faulty operations and processes that require better explanation to patients. Most importantly, they can increase patient loyalty amongst the patients by demonstrating that they care about their perceptions and are looking for ways in order to improve the experience. There are a number of challenges that small facilities, in particular, face with conducting patient satisfaction surveys.(Murante, 2010) For example, tighter budgets, lack of commitment from administration and lack of funding, small sample size, designing a statistically valid sampling process, obtaining acceptable response rates, reporting survey data, converting findings into information that can be utilised for quality improvement efforts and selecting a survey instrument that will produce valid and reliable results are also major challenges to consider.

Patient satisfaction has a significant and strong direct influence on loyalty and word-of-mouth communication, while loyalty and retention have a substantial influence on profitability. Research shows that there is a clear correlation between patient satisfaction and financial benefits to the organization.

Health Service's Nature and Value

Like quality in most services, healthcare quality is difficult to measure owing to inherent intangibility, heterogeneity, and inseparability features. Healthcare is dynamic – considerable customer changes have taken place and competition is increasing. Consequently, healthcare quality evaluations raise problems owing to service size, complexity, specialization, and expertise within healthcare organizations. Patients may be unable to assess medical service technical quality accurately; hence, functional quality is usually the primary determinant. Healthcare quality can be assessed by considering the opinions and perceptions of friends and family as these groups represent potential future patients and are major influencers of healthcare choices.(Messina, Scotti, Caney, & Zipp, 2009; Powell, 2004)

Contributing Factors for Patient Satisfaction

There has been a thorough review provided about the concept of Customer Experience Management and although research shows that a good patient experience could result in more satisfied customers, it is important to determine from the literature what factors are also considered to be contributing towards this goal.

The fulfillment of promises is an important factor in achieving patient satisfaction. This is very important since the reputation of a service provider is often measured or determined by its ability to meet its obligations and fulfill its promises. (Powell, 2004; Qu, Platonova, Kennedy, & Shewchuk, 2011)

The following determinants help ensure patient satisfaction:

- Attentiveness
- Helpfulness
- Responsiveness

Providing information to patients in the case of delays creates a positive attitude towards the organization's attentiveness and empathy towards the customer.

THE MEASUREMENT OF QUALITY

Steps Involved Are

- Specification of attributes to be measured
- Choice of an approach to measurement
- Choice of phenomenon to be measured
- Formulation of criteria and standards
- Obtaining information about care.

Patient satisfaction depends primarily on the outcome of care; since it is ultimate well-being that results from acceptable care. Satisfaction or dissatisfaction can also result from patient's judgment on certain aspects of care, calibrating the degree of their acceptability. Satisfaction also contributes to the success of future care (O'Brien & Shea, 2011).

Dimensions That Outline Patient Satisfaction

Various frameworks have been analyzed and some elements have been identified to determine patient satisfaction which are:

1. Accessibility
2. Doctor's care and communication
3. Ancillary staff's care and communication
4. Information provision
5. Pain control
6. Physical environment
7. Delivery of promised services
8. Customization of services

Components of Patients' Satisfaction

The main elements of satisfaction proposed by the researcher in the Khmer-Soviet friendship Autonomous Hospital comprise of convenience, courtesy, and quality of care.

Convenience

Convenience is defined as the comfort in approaching a set of standard quality of care such as chances of seeing wanted physicians, adequate waiting time, ease of meeting the required expectation and qualified services.

Users usually will come back to receive services from where they used to be satisfied. Researchers can use this characteristic to differentiate the quality of services provided. Furthermore, one main factor that should be considered for predicting the level of convenience is waiting time (Kunarantnapruek & Boonpadoong, 1989). In a study of patients' satisfaction in the Outpatient Department of Chulalongkorn Hospital by Sriratanabul and Pimpakovit, a significant factor led the majority of the respondents to feel uncomfortable with the services provided was long waiting time. 83% of the respondents showed positive feeling towards services provided by the department while disappointed with very long waiting time to receiving services.

Again, Likun mentioned waiting time services in a study of "Ways and Means to reduce the Waiting Time and Improve Patient Satisfaction" in 1996. He revealed that there was a significant relationship between waiting time to receive service and patients' satisfaction level. The majority of his respondents, 61% complained that waiting was not good for them.

Likewise, in a research in Ramathibodi Hospital, long waiting time was indicated as the significant factor for a low level of satisfaction. There is a report that the respondents who were highly educated showed a low level of satisfaction in the Registration section while similar effect also happened in the Pharmacy section (Ammo, Abu-shaheen, Kobrosly, & Al-tannir, 2014)

Quality of Care

Nowadays, hot issues like qualified health care service and patients' satisfaction are being crucially discussed throughout the world. Many different institutions have adopted a means to reflect on their service providing. Hi-tech, humanistic approach, educational backgrounds, communication, and means of transferring qualified service quality to the patients constitute the vitality of patients' satisfaction (Al-Bashir & Armstrong, 1991).

Efficacy, effectiveness, efficiency, optimality, acceptability, legitimacy, and equity are the seven main factors in assessing the services quality provided. Significant changes in healthcare service evaluating and enhancement is opening a new health care portrait for the service user. Formally accepted principles and apparatus to assessing and improving health care service users are dated to the American College of Surgeon's 1971, Hospital Standardization Program when it evolved into the Joint Commission on Accreditation of Healthcare Organization Accreditation Process (Williams & Calnan, 1991).

A new trend in combining quality assurance from other commercial industries with health care delivery strategies is the main indicator for quality of care. Generally accepted and hi-tech methods of health care services have led the industry to the contemporary way of qualified healthcare management.

The quality of hospital care was created by The American College of Surgeons as a fundamental formula in 1933 and gradually this principle in 1917 became its hospital standardization program. Furthermore, The Canadian Hospital Association with American College of Physicians, The American Hospital Association, and American Medical Association has established a Joint Commission on Accreditation of Hospital (JACHO) that originated the criteria based audit method. (Ammo et al., 2014).

An article regarding Resource Dependency was written by P. Garpenby from Sweden in 1999. It mainly indicated the relationship between the aspect of national-level clinical profession and patient satisfaction level. It also suggested that service quality advancement should be the main focus in order not to lose the public expectation. He also mentioned that the health care framework should be regarded as in other industries by characterizing its quality profession. An accepted set of qualified standards of care such as accessibility, availability, personnel's qualifications, and mutual understanding are not only the significant factors considered by the management level, but also by the users of the healthcare services who are normally called clients.

Courtesy

The last-mentioned element of patients' satisfaction is courtesy. Courtesy is usually defined by respect, attentiveness, and care shown by the clinical personnel.

Putting Patients First to Improve Patient Satisfaction- Patient Centricity

It is very important to put patients first because today we very well know that with the competition we have, our patients have choices for their care. If health systems want to improve the patient experience, they need to put the patients first and at the center of everything they do. The "soft stuff" counts to patients, and patients will continue to gauge their quality of care on their own proxy measures (like being treated respectfully) because that's what they understand. Hospital leaders may believe that patients are more concerned about issues like long wait times, but the data shows otherwise.

To really become transformational and succeed in the value-based care environment, hospitals need to understand their patients' needs. Even though we can't fix every little problem, we can zero in on the things that matter. The only way to know how to zero in what matters is by looking at the data.

Patient Delight

It is described as a positive emotional response as a result of surprisingly high levels of performance. Now one will wonder if this is even possible in the healthcare space. It is vital for a healthcare organization to build an emotional relationship with the patient and its relatives, as this would result in patient loyalty. Patient delight or approval does not just become a logical preference but instead will create an emotional attachment to the other party. It can, therefore, be considered as the ideal to strive for.

A delighted customer most likely makes use of the repeated and positive word-of-mouth referrals much more than a moderately satisfied customer.

Delight lasts as a long-term memory. The achievement of customer delight may result in a more stable loyalty and in line with what companies seek. It, therefore, gives another reason for companies to strive towards achieving a higher level of satisfaction, or customer delight. It can also be considered to be in line with the aims and objectives of a Customer experience management approach.

Patient Loyalty

This term patient loyalty is used in order to describe the attitude of repeat patients, those that offer good ratings, and testimonials. Some patients do a great service to the hospital by offering favorable word of mouth publicity regarding a product, thus adding more to the number of loyal customers. Patient Loyalty is a process, a program, or a group of programs geared that aim towards keeping a patient and their families happy so that they would provide more business in the future. In previous research, strong arguments were made to support the notion that satisfied patient will become loyal patients.

Patient loyalty can be enhanced by creating a perfect patient experience. These concepts seem to be interlinked and it is necessary to look into the concept of loyalty and how this interrelates with a profitable and lasting working relationship with customers.

Loyalty, over the past decade, has become a vital construct. The European Customer Satisfaction Index (ECSI) model was used as basis to try and clarify loyalty by using the constructs of trust and communication and identifying its effect on loyalty. (Ako-Nai, 2011; "SERVICE Quality and customer satisfaction," 1994)

Major changes in the healthcare space makes it more challenging for marketers to build a lasting patient loyalty. Organizations should be careful whilst doing this as superficial efforts may be more obvious to customers or patients and can actually lead to mistrust.

Although loyalty is a well-known and often-used term it cannot be easily defined, due to its nature of being an intangible and elusive concept. Loyalty is defined as the feeling a customer or in this case, a patient has about a brand and that it ultimately generates positive and measurable financial results. Another definition of loyalty is "When customers continue staying on with their service providers and make use of word-of-mouth to recommend it to their friends, and even influences their friend's decisions". Loyalty is a feeling of commitment towards the company's people, product or services. Having loyal customers or patients is an asset for organizations and should be a point of focus for budding organizations.

Loyal customers are individuals who remain, clients of their original service provider, even if a competitor proposes better offers. These clients basically cannot be deterred from the service to which they have built a bond. They are the most profitable ones and they are free marketing channels in terms of benefits received by companies from word-of –mouth. These customers are the most liked and they should be most treasured as in a healthcare organization, due to the sensitive nature of its service should work largely in promoting such a relationship. (Chase, 2000)

Good Customer Service

It is about meeting the needs of the patient as a customer. Patients have an inherent expectation as well as a fear due to their vulnerable nature. They need to be reassured through good service that they would be treated well, in a friendly, kind, and respectful manner. Answering their questions and being kept informed about their health status and treatment plan is also a feature of good patient service. If you deliver the service you promised, in the manner in which you promised, and help the customer or the patient overcome any difficulties or challenges they may have faced with the service, and the customer/patient is ultimately happy with the experience, that's good customer service.

Good patient service is about safeguarding that the patient is receiving the appropriate treatment they truly need and not do any unnecessary procedures.

Superior Patient Service

It's all about going the extra mile to please the Patient. For example, when a patient just delivered her baby, the medical team including the doctor joined in a small celebration. It was unexpected and the mother and the rest of the family looked delighted. A person who experiences a negative patient service is more likely to share it with others than someone who experiences a positive patient service. It is, therefore, important for healthcare organizations to go out of their way and strive for an exceptional patient service in order to avoid the negative image and response for that matter.

Designing a Service Excellence Strategy With Analytics

When your organization has its moment of truth, how will it measure up? Organizations whose business has service at its core and whose activities focus mainly on service design, management, and delivery are likely to find increasingly that, for survival, service is a matter of life or death. Analytics can help improve the experience of the patients by conducting a robust quantitative and qualitative study to see exactly what patients wanted. Data are collected at several points but not utilized to the fullest. Once data is collected, analytics should be used to dig deeper to gain valuable insights (Ako-Nai, 2011).

The patient satisfaction measurement can use either qualitative modalities or quantitative modalities.

In establishing patient satisfaction, some of the usual goals are to Measure patient satisfaction, Monitor changes in satisfaction, Measure performance on attributes that affect satisfaction and Monitor changes in performance.

Employee Engagement Strategies to Build a Patient First Culture

It is a generally heard phrase that employees are the organization's most valuable asset. This is particularly correct for well-trained and loyal staff coming directly in contact with patients. It is important that patients should receive customized treatment and that the systems should also be personalized in such a way that employees can transfer that principle. The employees of an organization are most vital to ensure that the business is successful in creating loyal customers.

This is referred to as organizational citizenship behavior (OCB) and can be defined as a global concept that includes all relevant positive behaviors of individuals which exist within an organization. Patient satisfaction is the responsibility of everybody in the organization; from the Manager to the cleaner. All staff members must always be reminded of how valuable patients are, so your staff knows how to treat clients in the appropriate and valued manner. (Environment, n.d.)

To make things smooth, an organization should focus on the barriers of patient satisfaction:

- Right Staffing to meet patient needs

The ability to right-staff is important to staff satisfaction and retention. Forward-thinking healthcare organizations are finding ways to harness analytics to gain a deeper understanding of patient needs and how to match the right staff with those patients to meet their needs.

- Reduce overtime costs

Overtime carries a price tag higher than the burden it puts on labor costs. Extensive overtime also has a negative impact on employee engagement and patient satisfaction. Working long hours can take a toll on employees. Studies have also shown that when nurses work long hours, patient satisfaction suffers. The impact carries through to both staff satisfaction and patient experience.

- Increase and improve patient engagement
- Improve patient outcomes
- Patients role in continuous quality Improvement
- Build patient loyalty.

With the ability to make data-driven staffing decisions, health systems reap the benefits of streamlined processes, better patient care, engaged staff and ultimately a far healthier bottom line. That allows caregivers to more efficiently and effectively provide outstanding care to their patients, and that's a huge satisfier for staff.

Hospitals have always been in the business of providing patient care. However, with the inception of Value-Based Purchasing, the measurement of successful patient care delivery has been redefined. The move from fee-for-service to pay-for-performance also means that reimbursements are tied to the quality of care that is delivered. Hospitals that provide a higher quality of care than their peers will receive reimbursement incentives, and hospitals that provide a lower quality of care will be penalized.

The quality of care is measured by two metrics: patient outcomes (70%) and patient satisfaction (30%). With patient satisfaction scores now having a direct impact on the bottom line, the measure and management of patient satisfaction have become a top priority at health systems across the country. In fact, more than half (54%) of healthcare executives say patient experience and satisfaction is one of their top three priorities, according to HealthLeaders Media's 2013 Industry Survey data (Experience, 2010).

Trust

Trust can be considered as one's confidence in organizations reliability, honesty and integrity and the belief that the organization always acts in one's best interest. Trust is a function of one's credibility. There can thus be no doubt that the presence of mutual trust is not only a vital prerequisite for the establishment of a lasting and beneficial relationship. This will also lead to a much higher customer or patient retention rate. There has been an increased awareness, of harm associated with healthcare errors. With this came an increased concern amongst policy makers, hospital administrators, and professionals about patient safety. Those who trust have an expectation that the trusted person/organization will behave with goodwill towards them and with competence in the domain in which he or she is trusted. Organization or doctor trust issues may lead patients to stop using a particular hospital's services owing to negative word-of-mouth. Basic principles outlined in healthcare studies include: Trusting patients are vigilant, and trust is not simply an inexplicit hope or thinking optimistically; healthcare service providers must keep a focus on zero errors in the course of their care and providing treatment. Some checking by the patient is appropriate even when there is trust particularly when honest mistakes are possible, which may be easily spotted and corrected. Patients may continue to trust even if harmed, particularly if the provider shows remorse, is apologetic and takes corrective action. Healthcare provider's trust in their patients may positively affect healthcare experience and outcomes.

Using Acuity-Based Staffing Models for Nurses and Nurse Communication

Acuity can be defined as the measurement of the intensity of nursing care required by a patient. An acuity-based staffing system regulates the number of nurses on a shift according to the patients' needs, and not according to raw patient numbers. Patients may range from needing minimal care on the day of their discharge to needing a dedicated nurse around the clock after a complication puts them in the ICU. In today's digital world, computers and specialized software can support nursing managers who are using an acuity-based staffing model. Acuity-based staffing systems can help a nurse manager determine the best core-staffing pattern for every shift, based on patient data.(Powell, 2004)

Nurse communication is a very important factor that is a part of nurse's service in outpatient department. The patient can consider the ability and experience of the nurse, suggestion of how to take care of oneself, clarification of diagnosis and care during their visit. Communication is fundamental and vital to all healthcare functions. Communication is a means of transmitting information and making oneself understand by another or others. Communication is the creation or exchange of thoughts, ideas, emotions, and understanding between nurses and patients. It is essential to building and maintaining relationships in the workplace. Although nurses spend most of their time communicating, meaningful communication does not necessarily occur in all exchanges. Communication can occur even through facial expression, eye contact, body posture and touching, as well as through speech. The successful communication demands an accordable cognitive effort and awareness of the patients of communication.

The nurse can play an important role in communicating with patients who seeking medical care services. Nurse communication is crucial role in all of the medical fields during their patient caring in health care center. Professional nursing practice requires the ability to appropriately and effectively communicate with patients. The quality of interpersonal communication is related to health outcomes, including quality of life and patient satisfaction.

Design of the Patient Experience: A new Perspective for Performance Evaluation Systems in Health Sector

This would initially involve the framing of an entire process which would need to be designed with the consumer. Firstly one would need to develop an understanding of the requirements needed to achieve the desired patient satisfaction. This would have to be achieved via patient interactions through various modes. Once this data is received, it is of utmost importance that one works on this data inorder to identify the flaws and good experiences faced by patients and accordingly maintaining satisfaction. This system should be followed by constant feedback to keep a tab that satisfaction levels are being maintained.

Mayo Clinic Model of Care

This model is defined by high quality, compassionate medical care delivered in an integrated medical institution. The Mayo clinic has a set of core elements that each employee imbibes into during the patient care and is instilled in the Mayo clinic environment. Patients report that the most significant difference between Mayo Clinic and other healthcare centers is that at Mayo Clinic everyone cares about them. Patients recognize Mayo Clinic as a place of trust where they are treated with dignity and compassion. Mayo clinic considers employees as their most valuable asset. The Mayo School of Health Related Sciences ensures a constant source of highly trained allied health professionals.

Cleveland Clinics Principle of "Patient First"

Putting patients first requires more than world-class clinical care – it requires care that addresses every aspect of a patient's encounter with Cleveland Clinic, including the patient's physical comfort, as well as his or her educational, emotional and spiritual needs. Cleveland Clinic's Office of Patient Experience has dedicated resources and programs that enhance the patient and family experience, while also improving clinical outcomes. There are several survey instruments and processes that have been designed to measure patient satisfaction at different touch points.

Patient Retention

The worst case scenario in any relationship is when a patient ends the relationship, without the service provider even being aware, due to an unpleasant service experience and then continues to spread a negative word-of-mouth message about their bad service experience to many other prospective customers or patients over a prolonged period of time. It is very difficult to reverse the effects of negative word of mouth, which has a rippling impact. No organization can assume that all the patients will be customers for life, especially in the changing healthcare scenario of today. Therefore patient should be a focus priority and related to the aims of establishing and maintaining satisfied and loyal patients. In today's competitive environment the ability to retain patients is a vital survival strategy. Many businesses are starting to focus more on retaining current patients than acquiring new ones.

There was a situation once where more than 50% of executives indicated in a study that they were satisfied with the service they received and they changed to another service provider soon afterward. This indicates that patient satisfaction measurements should not be treated casually and that patient retention strategies cannot be merely based on superficial observations. Dissatisfied patients will not necessarily complain, but may end the relationship without reporting their problem, this is something that one should always keep in the back of their minds. It is vital that organizations should create opportunities where dissatisfied patients can point out to problem area early, before the situation worsens. This helps in rectifying the situation to result in satisfaction of the patient, thus retaining them and ensuring that other patients are not lost due to the same problem.

Physician Role and Patient Behavior

It was found that patients in large multi-speciality organizations were more satisfied with physicians who fit an expected demographic norm. There is a clear relationship between medical care satisfaction and patient compliance; when patients are dissatisfied with medical advice they are less likely to cooperate. The research found that doctors' and other medical personnel's behavior were central determinants of patients' attitudes about a hospital as a whole. But the other touchpoints also have a lasting impact. (Heng, 2011)

Barriers to Patient Satisfaction

- **Poor Accountability:** Each employee should be held accountable to the patient to ensure patient satisfaction. They should not be encouraged in blame game, which will then result in a relaxed attitude.
- **Insufficient Systems:** The systems used in dealing with patients should be working optimally. Patients will get frustrated very quickly if the turn- around time is long. Hence if any issues then the same should be attended to quickly.
- **Communication of Patient Value:** That patient satisfaction is everyone's responsibility it should be instilled and constantly reinforced amongst all employees.
- **Lack of Incentive:** The suitable incentive should be given to staff for outstanding service to patients. If they are not motivated and happy, they may not go that extra mile for the patients. The organization should bring in means to ensure their staff is constantly motivated and are empowered to service the patients to the best of their abilities.
- **Lack of Understanding about Patient Needs:** Patient satisfaction data should be regularly analyzed. Only if this is done will the healthcare organization have an understanding of where lies the deficit in the providing of services and satisfaction of their patients and ultimately result in market success.
- **Failure to Deliver on Brand Promise:** Organizations should be very careful of what they promise to their customers, through their advertisements etc. It is through these modes of communication that an expectation is built and then it is the organization that has the onus to ensure the promises are met.

CONCLUSION

A hospital cannot go wrong if it has the right focus on the right aspects necessary for patient satisfaction. Every healthcare organization should constantly re-enforce their employees and management with the values they stand for, thus helping everyone to be on the same page. With the entire organization aligned to the same goals can help healthcare organizations to be successful in achieving patient satisfaction.

REFERENCES

Ako-Nai, E. A. (2011). *Effect of Customer Service on Customer Satisfaction, a Case Study of Fidelity Bank* (p. 85). Kumasi: Adum.

Ammo, M. A., Abu-shaheen, A. K., Kobrosly, S., & Al-tannir, M. A. (2014). Determinants of Patient Satisfaction at Tertiary Care Centers in Lebanon. *Open Journal of Nursing*, *4*(December), 939–946. doi:10.4236/ojn.2014.413100

Babu, T. S. and N. S. (2012). A STUDY ON PATIENT SATISFACTION IN HOSPITALS (A Study on Three Urban Hospitals in Guntur District, Andhra Pradesh) T. *International Journal of Management Research and Business Strategy*, *1*(1), 100–118.

Chase, A. (2000). Information to users. doi:10.16953/deusbed.74839

Environment, V. (n.d.). *The Rising Importance of Patient Satisfaction in a Value-Based Environment.*

P. Experience. (2010). Focus on the Patient Experience Save the Date.

Heng, C. C. (2011). Customer's satisfaction towards service quality of private hospitals in Kuching.

Messina, D. J., Scotti, D. J., Caney, R., & Zipp, G. P. (2009). The Relationship Between Patient Satisfaction and Inpatient Admissions Across Teaching and Nonteaching Hospitals. *Journal of Healthcare Management*, *54*(3), 177–190. Retrieved from http://search.ebscohost.com/login.aspx?direct=true&db=buh&AN=41033454&lang=de&site=ehost-live PMID:19554798

Murante, A. M. (2010). Patient satisfaction: a strategic tool for health services management. *Scuola Superiore Sant' Anna.*

Naidu, A. (2009). Factors affecting patient satisfaction and healthcare quality. *International Journal of Health Care Quality Assurance*, *22*(4), 366–381. doi:10.1108/09526860910964834 PMID:19725209

O'Brien, M., & Shea, J. (2011). Disparities in patient satisfaction among Hispanics: The role of language preference. *Journal of Immigrant and Minority Health*, *13*(2), 408–412. doi:10.1007/s10903-009-9275-2 PMID:19626440

Powell, L. (2004). Patient satisfaction surveys for critical access hospitals. *National Rural Health Resource Center*, *1*, 26–45.

Qu, H., Platonova, E., Kennedy, K. N., & Shewchuk, R. M. (2011). Primary care patient satisfaction segmentation. *International Journal of Health Care Quality Assurance*, *24*(7), 564–576. doi:10.1108/09526861111160599 PMID:22204089

Sajid, A., & Ali, H. (n.d.). Impact of Process Improvement on Patient Satisfaction in Public Health Care Facility in Pakistan.

Service quality and customer satisfaction. (1994). Customer based definitions for Quality: Value based definitions for Quality (Ch. 4, 109–133).

Vadhana, M. (2012). assessment of patient satisfaction in an outpatient department of an autonomous hospital in Phnom Penh, Cambodia [Thesis]. *Public Health Management*, (September).

Chapter 11
Formal Methods for Assessing Patient Satisfaction in a Patient–Doctor Relationship

Aleksandra Mreła
Kujawy and Pomorze University, Poland

Oleksandr Sokołov
Nicolaus Copernicus University, Poland

ABSTRACT

When patients visit a doctor, they not only expect to be cured, but also to feel that they are taken care of. The patients like to be treated like guests, sit in a nice place during waiting for a doctor and feel that they are taken care of seriously at the reception desk. All these factors are important for the patients but the relationship with doctors seems to be the most valid. When the patients can choose a clinic where they want to make an appointment with a doctor, the owners and managers of the clinics try to persuade people to choose their clinic. Hence more and more often managers of the clinics try to find out the opinion of the patients, so scientists carried out the research on this phenomenon and called it Patient Satisfaction. This chapter presents the application of fuzzy sets and fuzzy relations to gather and analyze the information from patients and compute their contentment. Using classical logic is less appropriate because the patients can only choose two values: they are satisfied or dissatisfied. Fuzzy logic let the patients choose more phrases for their opinions.

INTRODUCTION

When people visit a doctor, they expect that doctors will cure them immediately and if they understand that it is impossible they want a doctor to spend some time trying to get to know not only patient's pain but also, they expect that the doctor should take into account the circumstances of the disease. It is not so important when the sickness is not so serious but it is really significant if the treatment takes weeks, months and years.

DOI: 10.4018/978-1-5225-3946-9.ch011

On the other hand, doctors have quite a few patients every day and sometimes they do not have enough time to talk about something else than only symptoms of the illness. In Poland magazines and newspapers debate about it and for example according to rynekzdrowia.pl the National Health Fund does not specify the length of time that the family physician should spend with a patient (but requires that the visit with specialists should take about 15-20 minutes) (Rynekzdrowia.pl, 2009) and on the portal Gazeta prawna.pl B. Lisowska writes that family physicians would like to have it specified (Lisowska, 2015).

Nowadays people can use the Internet to write about their dissatisfaction with a too short visit as Joan Eisenstodt did after very short meeting with a specialist: "He looked up my nose, said it was inflamed, told me to see the nurse for a prescription and was gone" (Rabin 2014). One person wrote in an email to the portal tvp.info (Tvp.info, 2015) "I am sending a record of visits to a doctor's office in Gdańsk. … The family doctor takes 90 people in 7 hours. The average visit time is about 4.5 minutes, assuming that the doctor is working completely without the break for the toilet, etc."

Of course, the length of time spent on the visit with a doctor is not only one decisive factor of Patient Satisfaction but it is really important. Thus, we can ask ourselves what is Patient Satisfaction? According to Bhanu Prakash (Praksh, 2010) "Patient satisfaction is an important and commonly used indicator for measuring the quality in health care." By Radosław Plentara, Anna Knyszyńska and others (Plentara, 2015) the concept of Patient Satisfaction has started to be used in the context of health services only at the end of the 1990s but according to E. Kabengele Mpinga and P. Chastonay this concept "has a long history of controversy and debate" and started "in the fifties" (Kabangele, 2011).

Why carrying out the research on Patient Satisfaction is important? According to B. White "The truth about patient satisfaction surveys is that they can help you identify ways of improving your practice" (White, 1999). Thus, we should do it if we run a clinic or a medical office. Moreover, by R. Kravitz, "Measuring and reporting on patient satisfaction with health care has become a major industry" (Kravitz, 1998).

As the concept of Patient Satisfaction (PS) is not explicitly defined yet, it will be discussed within three main area of concern:

1. A_1 : Registration with a doctor in a clinic;
2. A_2 : Meeting a doctor;
3. A_3 : A clinic.

EXPERT SYSTEM

We will discuss the situation when we examine not many people: only 10 patients and 10 doctors. However, the statistical analysis is more reliable when the questionnaire is administered to more people, for example more than 100 hundred patients. According to doctors, the situation is different, we can ask only employed doctors.

Performing calculations, even if there are not many respondents takes some time, but in the case of many respondents or when we perform this study continuously it takes a lot of time, so it is better to design an information system. The system we propose is based on fuzzy relations and their composition.

In Encyclopedia Britannica we can find the definition of an information system, thus it is "an integrated set of components for collecting, storing, and processing data and for delivering information, knowledge, and digital products". The information system (IT) is consisted of software, hardware and telecommunications. Moreover, we can distinguish in the IT system: human resources and procedures, information technology, databases and data warehouses.

Among IT systems we can differentiate the expert system. Its definition was stated by Ketty Peeva and Yordan Kyosev as "...a computer-based system with artificial intellect that emulates the reasoning process of a human expert within a specific domain of knowledge." (Peeva, 2004). According to Shu-Hsien Liao, we should use the expert systems because "Expert Systems provide powerful and flexible means for obtaining solutions to a variety of problems that often cannot be dealt with by other, more traditional and orthodox methods. Thus, their use is proliferating to many sectors of our social and technological life, where their applications are proving to be critical in the process of decision support and problem solving" (Shu-Hsien, 2004). Nowadays there are designed more and more expert systems for solving many problems because as Masić, Ridanović and Pandza stated they "give explanation and advice to human experts when performing certain tasks" (Masić, 1995). Of course, there are also designed, examined and developed medical expert systems (Shortliffe, 1986) and (Shusaku, 1996).

Moreover, we can also differentiate decision support systems (DSS), which are designed to help people make a decision especially in the case when we have to solve a problem, we have to analyse a lot of data. The DSS contains Knowledge Base, Data Base, Inference Engine, Decision Support and User Interfaces (UI) (comp. Figure 1).

Knowledge Base is designed for storing knowledge which is gathered and collected by experts, one or a few people who understand the problem. In our case experts can be doctors, psychologists, nurses, managers and maybe patients. The experts must study fuzzy relations to the extent that they can build fuzzy relations with the help handed by designers of the system. The definitions of given fuzzy relations and composition of them must be coded, so the experts need some help from designers to describe the fuzzy relation in such a way they can be coded using the programming language. Because fuzzy logic imitates the way of human thinking, it is really useful to build Knowledge Base using fuzzy relations.

Figure 1. The structure of Decision Support System

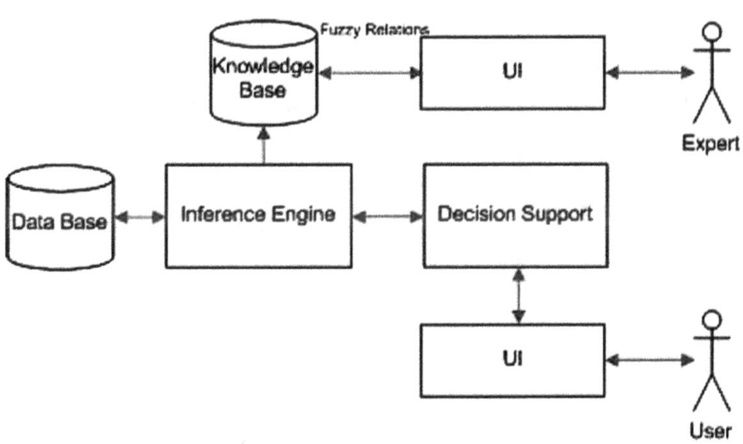

The next part of the expert system is Data Base, where a lot of data is stored. The Inference Engine is the main part of the system, imitates the human way of thinking (rules used by the Engine are given with the application of fuzzy logic) and produces solutions to drawing data from the Data Base and rules (fuzzy relations) from the Knowledge Base. The User can ask questions, describe problems and receive solutions with the use of the User Interfaces in order to connect with the expert system. The Decision Support explains to the User the reasons of given answers to the problem or more specific questions.

As mentioned above during designing the expert system, the experts should be employed. The role of the experts is giving knowledge about the health care system and/or the examined clinic. Thus, among them there can be doctors, nurses, registration nurses, managers and administration officers and of course patients.

Why Fuzzy Logic?

Communication in all areas of life is really important, so people have to formulate their thoughts in such a way that the others can understand them. Thus, they try to describe their ideas, opinions and suggestions as precise as they can. But our languages have a lot of imprecise words and phrases which we have studied to understand. For example, we can say that "I drove fast" and from the context we understand the meaning which is different in the case of a car in a city or on the highway. We do not usually say "I drove 70km/h on average" or more precise sentence "At the beginning from my home to the first turn I was driving 30km/h, then I could drive faster 52km/h till I met a slow car and I had to slow down to 46km/h".

The same situation is in medical treatment, people studied how to understand the vague phrases like for example "I coughed heavily yesterday evening". However, what does it really mean? To understand better we can ask more precise questions: "How long?", "All evening?", "Wet or dry?" and so on.

To help people communicate, philosophers and mathematicians have been trying to develop logic which is, according to the classical definition (Kotarbiński, 1985), "the study of the ways of clear and precise formulation of thoughts, rules of correct reasoning and justification of theorems". Moreover, according to Stanford Encyclopedia of Philosophy, "a *logic* consists of a formal or informal language together with a deductive system and/or a model-theoretic semantics".

According to T. Kotarbiński classical logic was considered as a two-level logical system and each sentence can be estimated to be true (logical value 1) or false (logical value 0) (Kotarbiński, 1985). Based on this logic, the mathematical concept of a set was developed. According to Encyclopedia of Mathematics, a set is "an aggregate, totality, collection of any objects whatever, called its elements, which have a common characteristic property. "A set is many, conceivable to us as one" (G. Cantor)".

Application of Fuzzy Relations

Let X be a universe and let $A \subset X$ be a set. Assume that $x, y \in X$ are two objects such that x belongs to set A and y does not. Thus we can say that the grade of membership of object x to set A is equal 1 and the grade of membership of y to set A is equal 0. For example, let A be a set of all people in some clinic with the fever. Then a person with the temperature 38°C belongs to this set (its grade of membership is equal 1) and a person with the temperature 36.6°C does not (its grade of membership is equal 0). Whenever we like to talk about sets with respect to classical logic, we will name them "crisp sets" in order to distinguish them from fuzzy sets.

Sometimes the classical logic and classical concept of sets are good enough to solve problems, but in the case of Patient Satisfaction we can get better results if we use fuzzy logic and fuzzy sets. Let us consider the following example. The director of a clinic had been considering the problem whether patients liked the registration office and had asked the registration manager to ask a sample of 10 patients. They decided to use the following rule of carrying out research: If the patients like the registration office, they will say "yes" and then the grade of membership is equal 1, if they do not, they will say "no" and the grade of membership is equal 0. Let us assume that they got 4 answers "yes" and 6 – "no". What does this answer mean? Did these 6 patients think that the registration system was completely wrong? Or maybe it was not perfect, so these people said "no" because there was not possibility of indicating this imperfectness.

Using fuzzy logic is more useful in the case of social science because we do not need to stick to answers "yes" or "no", we can have much more possibilities like for example "little", "very much" and so on. According to Stanford Encyclopedia of Philosophy, "fuzzy logic is intended to model logical reasoning with vague or imprecise statements … It refers to a family of many-valued logics and thus stipulates that the truth value (which, in this case amounts to a degree of truth) of a logically compound proposition, like "Carles is tall and Chris is rich", is determined by the truth value of its components."

Returning to our example patients can answer "not at all", "very little", "so so", "very much" and so on. To this value we can describe the grade of membership (a number belonging to interval [0,1]. For example, we can agree that the grade of membership of the phrase "not at all" is 0, the grade of membership "very little" is 0.2 and so forth. Using the fuzzy logic, we can give the respondents a wide variety of possible answers, not only "yes" or "no".

Patient Satisfaction (PS) is considered as a fuzzy set of patients with discrete membership function which values indicate the level of satisfaction of the patient. Let us recall the definition of a fuzzy set.

Let X be the universe. The type 1 fuzzy set A (Zadeh, 1965) is a set of all pairs $(x, \mu(x))$, where $x \in X$ and μ is a function which domain is X, and the set of values is interval $[0,1]$. Function μ defines the grade of membership of element x to set A.

For example, let

$$PS = \frac{0.8}{J.Kowalski} + \frac{0.6}{A.Nowak} + \frac{0}{P.Piotrowski} + \frac{1}{K.Krawczyk},$$

where the nominator shows the grade of membership of the object located in the denominator and the sign $+$ indicates the union of elements. This fuzzy set shows that J. Kowalski is satisfied on the level 0.8 or at 80%, A. Nowak is satisfied at the level 0.6 or at 60%, P. Piotrowski is deeply dissatisfied and K. Karwczyk is completely satisfied. These values give the director of the clinic some information about PS however in this case not too much because the levels of satisfaction are really dispersed. Of course, Patient Satisfaction cannot be examined on the sample of 4 people and moreover it is well known that researchers can get more real answers if patients are asked anonymously.

After defining fuzzy sets, we can describe their compositions. Let (A, μ_A) and (B, μ_B) be two fuzzy sets. T -norm of these two fuzzy sets is a fuzzy set (C, μ_C) which the membership function is defined as follows: $\mu_C(x) = \min\{\mu_A(x), \mu_B(x)\}$. S -conorm of these two fuzzy sets is a fuzzy set (D, μ_D) which the membership function is defined in the following way: $\mu_D(x) = \max\{\mu_A(x), \mu_B(x)\}$.

Let, for example,

$$A = \frac{0.8}{J.Kowalski} + \frac{0.6}{A.Nowak} + \frac{0}{P.Piotrowski} + \frac{1}{K.Krawczyk}$$

and

$$B = \frac{0.7}{J.Kowalski} + \frac{0.2}{A.Nowak} + \frac{0.3}{P.Piotrowski} + \frac{0.4}{K.Krawczyk}.$$

Then

$$C = \frac{\min\{0.8, 0.7\}}{J.Kowalski} + \frac{\min\{0.6, 0.2\}}{A.Nowak} + \frac{\min\{0, 0.3\}}{P.Piotrowski} + \frac{\min\{1, 0.4\}}{K.Krawczyk}$$
$$= \frac{0.7}{J.Kowalski} + \frac{0.2}{A.Nowak} + \frac{0}{P.Piotrowski} + \frac{0.4}{K.Krawczyk}$$

and

$$D = \frac{\max\{0.8, 0.7\}}{J.Kowalski} + \frac{\max\{0.6, 0.2\}}{A.Nowak} + \frac{\max\{0, 0.3\}}{P.Piotrowski} + \frac{\max\{1, 0.4\}}{K.Krawczyk}$$
$$= \frac{0.8}{J.Kowalski} + \frac{0.6}{A.Nowak} + \frac{0.3}{P.Piotrowski} + \frac{1}{K.Krawczyk}.$$

When we analyze the results of a survey, the situation is different, because we do not talk about objects, we discuss pairs of them. Hence, we do not discuss fuzzy sets, we talk about fuzzy relations. For example, let us assume that the questionnaire is consisted of two questions Q_1, Q_2 and it is administrated to two patients P_1 and P_2, then

$$R = \frac{0.2}{(P_1, Q_1)} + \frac{0.9}{(P_1, Q_2)} + \frac{0.4}{(P_2, Q_1)} + \frac{0.8}{(P_2, Q_2)}.$$

We understand that patient P_1 answering question Q_1 determined the level of agreement equal 0.2. Let X and Y be two universes and let $X \times Y$ be the Cartesian product of them, so $X \times Y = \{(x, y), x \in X, y \in Y\}$.

The fuzzy subset R of $X \times Y$ is called a fuzzy relation.

Similarly as in the case of fuzzy sets, we will define the composition of them, which is called $S - T$ composition. Let X, Y and Z be the universes and let $X \times Y, Y \times Z$ and $X \times Z$ be the Cartesian products of them. Let $(R_1, \mu_1) \subset X \times Y$ and $(R_2, \mu_2) \subset Y \times Z$ are fuzzy relations. Then using $S - T$ composition we get the fuzzy relation $(R3, \mu 3) \subset X \times Z$ which membership function can be defined in the following way:

$$\mu_3(x,z) = S_{y \in Y} T(\mu_1(x,y), \mu_2(y,z)) = \max_{y \in Y}\{\min\{\mu_1(x,y), \mu_2(y,z)\}\}.$$

We often write values of a fuzzy relation in the form of a table. Let R_1 be a fuzzy relation between areas of Patient Satisfaction and questions. Assume that there are 3 areas of PS $(A_1 - A_3)$ and questions (Q_1, Q_2). Let experts describe levels of importance of the questions to understand Patient Satisfaction in these areas as follows.

Let R_2 be a fuzzy relation between questions and patients and the values of this relation be put in Table 2.

Now using the $S - T$ composition (max-min composition) we will calculate values of relation R_3 between the areas of PS and patients. Thus

$$\begin{aligned} R_3(A_1,P_1) &= \max\left\{\min\left\{R_1(A_1,Q_1), R_2(Q_1,P_1)\right\}, \min\left\{R_1(A_1,Q_2), R_2(Q_2,P_1)\right\}\right\} \\ &= \max\{\min\{0.6, 0.2\}, \min\{0.8, 0.9\}\} = \max\{0.2, 0.8\} = 0.8. \end{aligned}$$

Table 1. Sample relation R_1 between areas of PS and questions

Areas of PS	Questions	
	Question Q_1	Question Q_2
Area A_1	0.6	0.8
Area A_2	0.7	0.6
Area A_3	0.4	0.7

Table 2. Sample relation R_2 between patients and questions

Questions	Patients	
	Patient P_1	Patient P_2
Question Q_1	0.2	0.4
Question Q_2	0.9	0.8

It means that Patient P_1 is satisfied in 80% of the services within area A_1. Applying the same method, the values of the fuzzy relation R_3 were calculated and put in Table 3.

Experts should also prepare fuzzy relation R_0 between areas of PS and Patient Satisfaction. Let us assume that experts prepared the table of the fuzzy relation between areas of PS and Patient Satisfaction which values are put to Table 4.

Applying $S-T$ composition (max - min composition) we can calculate values of the fuzzy set PS. Hence:

$$PS(P_1) = \max\{\min\{R_0(PS, A_1); \min\{R_3(A_1, P_1)\}; \min\{R_0(PS, A_2); \min\{R_3(A_2, P_1)\};$$
$$\min\{R_0(PS, A_3); \min\{R_3(A_3, P_1)\}\} = \max\{\min\{0.7; 0.8\}; \min\{0.8; 0.6\}; \min\{0.5; 0.7\}\}$$
$$= \max\{0.7; 0.6; 0.5\} = 0.7.$$

Similarly, we can calculate $PS(P_2)$ and put these values to Table 5.

Notice that in this case both patients are satisfied on the same level 0.7. Moreover, we can say that they are well-satisfied.

Table 3. Sample relation R_3 between areas of PS and patients

Areas of PS	**Patients**	
	Patient P_1	**Patient P_2**
Area A_1	0.8	0.8
Area A_2	0.6	0.6
Area A_3	0.7	0.7

Table 4. Sample fuzzy relation R_0 between patient satisfaction and areas of PS

Areas of PS	**Area A_1**	**Area A_2**	**Area A_3**
Patient Satisfaction	0.7	0.8	0.5

Table 5. Sample fuzzy set Patient Satisfaction (PS)

Patients	**Patient P_1**	**Patient P_2**
Patient Satisfaction	0.7	0.7

We would like to recall one more concept of fuzzy sets, namely α-cuts of a fuzzy set $A = (X, \mu_A)$ (Piegat, 1999). Let α be an arbitrary number belonging to interval [0,1]. Then α-cut of fuzzy set A is a crisp set A_α defined in the following way:

$$A_\alpha = \left\{x \in X, \mu_A(x) > \alpha\right\}.$$

Returning to our example, let $\alpha_1 = 0.6$ and $\alpha_2 = 0.7$. Then

$$PS_{0.6} = \{x \in X, \mu_{PS}(x) > 0.6\} = \{P_1, P_2\} \text{ and } PS_{0.7} = \{x \in X, \mu_{PS}(x) > 0.7\} = \Theta,$$

where the symbol Θ denotes the empty set (the set with no elements).

Patients' Survey

At the beginning of the research we have to find, as usually, experts who know the world of clinics and hospitals, understand rules and methods of medical treatment and know problems of patients, doctors and administration of clinics. Of course, it does not mean that all of them must know all these aspects of the medical world. Among the experts, we can employ doctors, nurses, clinic directors or managers, administration officers and patients.

The experts are responsible for preparing questionnaire, describing values of the fuzzy relations: the one between Patient Satisfaction and its areas and the second one: between areas of PS and questions, choosing methods of analyzing data and preparing results.

As mentioned before, to examine Patient Satisfaction as a fuzzy set, we will examine three fuzzy sets called Patient Satisfaction within areas $A_1 - A_3$. Thus, the experts are responsible for preparing a questionnaire for patients for examining all areas of Patient Satisfaction.

Assume that the experts prepared the questionnaire which is consisted of 19 questions. These questions examine all these three areas of PS. At first, all these questions were designed to examine mainly one area of PS, but after consideration the experts describe values of the fuzzy relation between areas PS and questions. In Table 6 there are put questions with their first relationship to areas of PS.

Moreover, assume that the experts decide that all these areas of PS are not equally important in patient satisfaction and let Table 7 contains the levels of importance of these areas in PS (fuzzy relation R_0).

On this basis of defined areas of PS the experts described the values of the fuzzy relation R_1 between areas of PS and questions. The values of fuzzy relation R_1 were put to Table 8.

Assume that this questionnaire was administrated to 10 $(P_1 - P_{10})$ patients who answered these 19 questions. Patients were asked to choose the number between 0 and 1 to indicate the level of agreement to the question.

For example, let us discuss the first question "How easy it is to make an appointment with a doctor?" The patient are asked to indicate the number between 0 and 1 which shows the level of agreement of the patient to this question, where 1 means that the patient agrees that it is really easy to make an appointment with a doctor and 0 – the patient thinks that it is really difficult to make an appointment with the

Table 6. Questions for patients defined to examine patient satisfaction

No.	Areas of PS	Symbol	Question
1	A_1	Q_1	How easy it is to make an appointment with a doctor?
2		Q_2	How easy it is to make a routing follow-up appointment?
3		Q_3	How easy it is to make appointment for physical exams?
4		Q_4	How easy it is to contact your doctor when the office is closed? At nights or during weekends?
5		Q_5	How efficient the registration service is?
6		Q_6	Is it possible to register in advance?
7	A_2	Q_7	How easy it is to speak to your doctor by telephone during office hours?
8		Q_8	How easy it is to obtain follow-up information (test results)?
9		Q_9	How easy it is to get the follow-up care (medicines, care instructions)?
10		Q_{10}	Do you like overall medical care at the doctor's office?
11		Q_{11}	Do you approve the way you are informed about improving your health?
12		Q_{12}	Do you approve the way your doctor involves other doctors and caregivers in your care when needed?
13	A_3	Q_{13}	How long does it take someone from the office to respond for the patient's call with an urgent problem?
14		Q_{14}	How long do you have to wait in the office?
15		Q_{15}	How long do you have to wait for the visit with the doctor?
16		Q_{16}	Do you like the office's appearance?
17		Q_{17}	Is the clinic convenient (location, parking, hours, office layout)?
18		Q_{18}	Are medical services available?
19		Q_{19}	Is the clinic furnished with the medial equipment?

Table 7. Fuzzy relation R_0 between patient satisfaction and areas of PS

	Area A_1	Area A_2	Area A_3
Patient satisfaction	0.6	0.8	0.7

Table 8. Fuzzy relation R_1 between areas of PS and questions

Area of PS	Number of the Question																		
	1	2	3	4	5	6	7	8	9	10	11	12	13	14	15	16	17	18	19
A_1	1	0.8	0.7	0.8	0.9	0.7	0.4	0.3	0.2	0.4	0.1	0.3	0.2	0.4	0.3	0.5	0.4	0.3	0.4
A_2	0.4	0.3	0.4	0.2	0.3	0.8	1	0.7	0.8	0.7	0.8	0.9	0.4	0.3	0.2	0.4	0.3	0.2	0.3
A_3	0.3	0.2	0.4	0.3	0.3	0.4	0.2	0.1	0.4	0.3	0.4	0.3	0.8	0.7	0.8	0.8	0.7	0.8	0.9

Table 9. Answers of patients $(P_1 - P_{10})$ to the questionnaire – the values of fuzzy relation R_2

	P_1	P_2	P_3	P_4	P_5	P_6	P_7	P_8	P_9	P_{10}
Q_1	0.5	0.7	0.4	0.3	0.4	0.2	0.1	0,1	0.5	0.4
Q_2	0.6	0.9	0.2	1	1	0.5	0.7	0,2	0.5	0.6
Q_3	0.7	0.7	0.8	0.3	0.4	0.2	0.1	0	0.6	0.4
Q_4	0.8	0.2	0.9	0.2	0.3	0.4	0.5	0	0.1	0.3
Q_5	0.7	0.8	0.3	0.3	0.4	0.2	0.1	0,3	0.7	0.7
Q_6	0.4	0.8	0.9	0.4	0.5	0.3	0.4	0,2	0.7	0.5
Q_7	0.5	1	0.2	0.3	0.4	0.2	0.3	0,2	0.9	0.2
Q_8	0.3	0.7	0.8	0.3	0.2	0.3	0.4	0,2	0.8	0.2
Q_9	0.7	0.8	0.8	0	0.1	0.2	0.3	0,1	0.7	0.3
Q_{10}	0.4	0.7	0.3	0.4	0.3	0.5	0.2	0,3	0.8	0.3
Q_{11}	0.8	0.2	1	0.5	0.4	0.3	0.5	0,2	0.3	0.7
Q_{12}	0.3	0.3	0.8	0.2	0.3	0.3	0.2	0,2	0.2	0.2
Q_{13}	0.2	0.4	0.8	1	0.2	0.4	0.4	0	0.9	1
Q_{14}	0.4	0.3	0.3	0.2	1	0.3	0.4	0,3	0.8	0.8
Q_{15}	0.3	0.2	0.9	0.4	0.8	0.4	0.2	0,1	0.7	0.9
Q_{16}	0.6	0.7	0.8	0.6	0.7	1	0	0,2	0.6	0.8
Q_{17}	0.6	0.8	0.9	0.7	0.8	0.7	0	0,2	0.7	0.9
Q_{18}	0.8	0.7	0.7	0.5	0.5	0.6	0.8	0,2	0.7	0.5
Q_{19}	1	0.4	0.5	1	0.6	0.7	0.9	0,2	0.8	0.3

doctor. If the patient wants to answer that they think that the easiness is medium or poor, then they can choose the number between 0 or 1, for example 0.5 or 0.3.

After the application of $\max\min$ composition, we can calculate the values of fuzzy relation R_3 between areas of PS and the patients. These values are put to Table 10.

Using the information from Table 10, we can say that patients are really satisfied within the areas A_1 (the range of levels of satisfaction is equal to interval [0.3, 0.8], the level of satisfaction of 5 patients is 0.8 and only of 1 patient is 0.3) and A_3 (the range of levels of satisfaction is equal to interval [0.3, 0.9], the level of satisfaction of 3 patients is 0.9 and of 6 patients is 0.8 and of 1 patient is 0.3). Thus, the director of the considered clinic does not need to improve anything within these areas.

Area A_2 is a little more difficult to analyze (the relationship between doctors and patients). The situation is not very bad because the range of levels of satisfaction is equal to interval [0.3, 1] but 4 patients are satisfied on the medium level 0.5 and 1 on the poor level 0.3.

To prepare a report with statistical methods, we transform the achieved fuzzy sets to crisp sets using the concept of α-cuts.

Since these α-cut sets are not disjoint and moreover they create a decreasing sequence of sets, we will calculate how many objects has the same grade of membership equal to α.

Table 10. Patients' levels of areas of PS : Fuzzy relation R_3

Area of PS	Patient									
	P_1	P_2	P_3	P_4	P_5	P_6	P_7	P_8	P_9	P_{10}
A_1	0.8	0.8	0.8	0.8	0.8	0.5	0.7	0.3	0.7	0.7
A_2	0.8	1	0.8	0.5	0.5	0.5	0.5	0.3	0.9	0.7
A_3	0.9	0.7	0.8	0.9	0.8	0.8	0.9	0.3	0.8	0.8

Table 11. Numbers of elements of α-cuts of PS within the considered areas of PS

α	Number of Elements of α-Cuts of PS Within the Area A_1	Number of Elements of α-Cuts of PS Within the Area A_2	Number of Elements of α-Cuts of PS Within the Area A_3
0.0	10	10	10
0.1	10	10	10
0.2	10	10	10
0.3	9	9	9
0.4	9	9	9
0.5	8	5	9
0.6	8	5	9
0.7	6	5	8
0.8	0	3	4
0.9	0	1	0

Table 12. Numbers of elements of the crisp sets for which the membership function of PS within the considered areas are equal α

α	Number of Elements of the Crisp Set When the Membership Function of Area A_1 of PS Is Equal α	Number of Elements of the Crisp Set When the Membership Function of Area A_2 of PS Is Equal α	Number of Elements of the Crisp Set When the Membership Function of Area A_3 of PS Is Equal α
0.0	0	0	0
0.1	0	0	0
0.2	0	0	0
0.3	1	1	1
0.4	0	0	0
0.5	1	4	0
0.6	0	0	0
0.7	2	0	1
0.8	6	2	4
0.9	0	2	4
1.0	0	1	0

Since we have got the crisp sets, we can use all statistical methods for calculating statistical indicators, like average, median, standard deviation and so on.

Based on the values of fuzzy relation R_0 (Table 7), the values of fuzzy relation R_3 (Table 10) and using max-min composition, we can calculate values of the fuzzy set Patient Satisfaction and these values are put in Table 11.

On the basis of the levels of Patient Satisfaction, we can calculate the α-cuts and then we can obtain statistical data as before, on which we can conduct statistical calculations.

Based on this data, we can notice that patients are pretty satisfied because the levels of Patient Satisfaction are equal to 0.7 (5 patients), 0.8 (4 patients) and 0.3 (only 1 patient).

Doctors' Survey

The most important factor for patients is communication with doctors. People like to be in a nice building, meet a kind and helpful registration officer but if they meet an incompetent and unkind doctor they will not return to the clinic. The director of the clinic is responsible for recruiting competent doctors. Hence, in this section we will concentrate on skills of communication, doctors will estimate their own level of communication and on this basis the calculations will be carried out.

Table 13. Levels of patient satisfaction: The fuzzy set PS

	P_1	P_2	P_3	P_4	P_5	P_6	P_7	P_8	P_9	P_{10}
Patient Satisfation	0.8	0.8	0.8	0.7	0.7	0.7	0.7	0.3	0.8	0.7

According to the Scottish Deans' Medical Curriculum Group, "Good communication underpins all aspects of the practice of medicine. All new graduates must be able to demonstrate effective communication skills in all areas and in all media e.g. orally, in writing, electronically, by telephone etc." (Scottish Doctor, 2011). They divided all skills related to communication into 7 groups which are put in Table 14.

Assume that the director of the clinic employed a few experts of communication between doctors and patients who described 19 questions which aim was to verify levels of communication according to each group. In Table 15 there are put question defined for verification levels of communication.

After that the experts prepare the values of fuzzy relation between groups of communication skills and questions and put them to Table 16. As before the experts must remember that these values belong to interval [0,1].

Assume now that this questionnaire was administrated to 10 ($D_1 - D_{19}$) doctors who answered these 19 questions estimating their own abilities of communication. These values were collected in Table 17 and formed fuzzy relation R_2.

When we know grades of membership of fuzzy relations R_1 between groups of communication skills and questions and R_2 between questions and doctors, we can calculate the levels of communication skills of each doctor in each group of communication skills – fuzzy relation R_3. After calculating these values using max-min composition of fuzzy relations, we put these values to Table 18.

Of course, we can calculate α-cuts, find crisps sets on the basis of fuzzy relation R_3 and compute statistical indicators like we mentioned in section "Patients' Survey".

In this section we prepare the ranking of groups of communication skills (G_1 - G_7) based on fuzzy relation R_3. Assume that the director of the clinic wants to send the doctors to the workshop on communication skills, so we will calculate the averages of grades of membership function for each groups of communication skills (G_1 - G_7) and put all these values to Table 19. The first position of the ranking is the groups of skills with the smallest value because the director of the clinic wants to improve communication skills, so the group on the first position will be the most probable the topic of these workshops.

Looking at the ranking (Table 19 B) it can be seen that the lowest levels of self-assessment are noticed in the third group of communication skills, namely "Communicating with colleagues". The most important ones (G_1 - "General principles of good communication" and G_2- "Communicating with patients / relatives") are on the 4 and 5 positions.

Table 14. Groups of communication skills

No.	Symbol	Description
1	G_1	General principles of good communication
2	G_2	Communicating with patients / relatives
3	G_3	Communicating with colleagues
4	G_4	Communicating with Police and Procurator Fiscal/Coroner
5	G_5	Communicating with media and press
6	G_6	Communicating as a teacher
7	G_7	Communicating as a patient advocate

Scottish Doctor, 2011.

Table 15. Questions defined for verification level of communication

No.	Symbol	Question
1	Q_1	Are you able to listen without interrupting?
2	Q_2	Are you able to use appropriate communication techniques during listening to the people?
3	Q_3	Are you able to gather information from the people?
4	Q_4	Are you able to deal with patient's complaints?
5	Q_5	Are you able to use telephone to gather information from the people?
6	Q_6	Are you able to give explanations and/or instructions during answering questions?
7	Q_7	Are you able to deal with aggressive patients?
8	Q_8	Are you able to break bad news?
9	Q_9	Are you able to admit the lack of knowledge or mistake?
10	Q_{10}	Are you able to request for organ donation?
11	Q_{11}	Are you able to transfer information to your colleague?
12	Q_{12}	Are you good at discharging summary and patient referrals?
13	Q_{13}	Are you able to relay appropriate information without breaking rules of confidentiality
14	Q_{14}	Are you sure who should talk to the media and press?
15	Q_{15}	Do you know how to maintain confidentiality where individual patients are concerned?
16	Q_{16}	Do you recognize what you know and do you know your own limitations?
17	Q_{17}	Do you know some basic teaching techniques?
18	Q_{18}	Do you recognize when you should be a patient advocate?
19	Q_{19}	Are you able to be a patient advocate effectively?

Table 16. Fuzzy relation R_1 between groups of communication skills and questions

Group of Communication Skills	Number of the Question																		
	1	2	3	4	5	6	7	8	9	10	11	12	13	14	15	16	17	18	19
G_1	1	0.6	0.7	0.8	0.7	0.4	0.5	0.3	0.2	0.4	0.1	0.3	0.2	0.4	0.3	0	0	0	0
G_2	0.4	0.3	0.4	0.2	0.3	0.8	1	0.7	0.8	0.7	0.2	0.3	0.4	0.3	0.2	0	0	0	0
G_3	0.3	0.2	0.4	0.5	0.3	0.4	0.2	0.1	0.4	0.3	1	0.8	0.3	0.3	0.2	0	0	0	0
G_4	0.3	0.4	0.3	0.2	0.3	0.4	0.3	0.3	0	0.4	0.5	0.2	1	0.2	0.4	0	0	0	0
G_5	0.4	0.3	0.4	0.3	0.4	0.5	0.4	0.2	0.1	0.3	0.4	0.3	0.2	1	0.8	0	0	0	0
G_6	0.2	0.2	0.2	0.4	0.2	0.3	0.2	0.3	0.2	0.5	0.3	0.3	0.4	0.3	0.4	1	0.7	0	0
G_7	0.1	0.1	0.1	0.5	0.1	0.4	0.3	0.4	0.3	0.2	0.5	0.2	0.4	0.4	0.2	0	0	0.8	0.9

Table 17. Levels of self-assessment of communication skills: fuzzy relation R_2

Questions	Doctors									
	D_1	D_2	D_3	D_4	D_5	D_6	D_7	D_8	D_9	D_{10}
Q_1	0.5	0.7	0.4	0.3	0.4	0.2	0.1	0.6	0.5	0.4
Q_2	0.6	0.9	0.2	1	1	0.5	0.7	1	0.5	0.6
Q_3	0.7	0.7	0.8	0.3	0.4	0.2	0.1	0.8	0.6	0.4
Q_4	0.8	0.2	0.9	0.2	0.3	0.4	0.5	0.9	0.1	0.3
Q_5	0.7	0.8	0.3	0.3	0.4	0.2	0.1	0.7	0.7	0.7
Q_6	0.4	0.8	0.9	0.4	0.5	0.3	0.4	0.9	0.7	0.5
Q_7	0.5	1	0.2	0.3	0.4	0.2	0.3	0.4	0.9	0.2
Q_8	0.3	0.7	0.8	0.3	0.2	0.3	0.4	0.8	0.8	0.2
Q_9	0.7	0.8	0.8	0	0.1	0.2	0.3	0.6	0.7	0.3
Q_{10}	0.4	0.7	0.3	0.4	0.3	0.5	0.2	0.3	0.8	0.3
Q_{11}	0.8	0.2	1	0.5	0.4	0.3	0.5	0.7	0.3	0.7
Q_{12}	0.3	0.3	0.8	0.2	0.3	0.3	0.2	0.9	0.2	0.2
Q_{13}	0.2	0.4	0.8	1	0.2	0.4	0.4	0	0.9	1
Q_{14}	0.4	0.3	0.3	0.2	1	0.3	0.4	0.5	0.8	0.8
Q_{15}	0.3	0.2	0.9	0.4	0.8	0.4	0.2	0.8	0.7	0.9
Q_{16}	0.6	0.7	0.8	0.6	0.7	1	0	0.4	0.6	0.8
Q_{17}	0.6	0.8	0.9	0.7	0.8	0.7	0	0.5	0.7	0.9
Q_{18}	0.8	0.7	0.7	0.5	0.5	0.6	0.8	0.7	0.7	0.5
Q_{19}	1	0.4	0.5	1	0.6	0.7	0.9	0.8	0.8	0.3

Table 18. Levels of doctors' self-assessment of communication skills: Fuzzy relation R_3

Groups of Communication Skills	Doctors									
	D_1	D_2	D_3	D_4	D_5	D_6	D_7	D_8	D_9	D_{10}
G_1	0.8	0.7	0.8	0.6	0.6	0.5	0.6	0.8	0.7	0.7
G_2	0.7	1	0.8	0.4	0.5	0.5	0.4	0.8	0.9	0.5
G_3	0.8	0.4	1	0.5	0.4	0.4	0.5	0.8	0.4	0.7
G_4	0.5	0.4	0.8	1	0.4	0.4	0.5	0.5	0.9	1
G_5	0.4	0.5	0.8	0.4	1	0.4	0.4	0.8	0.8	0.8
G_6	0.6	0.7	0.8	0.7	0.7	1	0.4	0.5	0.7	0.8
G_7	0.9	0.7	0.7	0.9	0.6	0.7	0.9	0.8	0.8	0.5

Table 19. Averages of grades of membership function of fuzzy relation R_3

A) Before Preparing the Ranking		B) The Ranking		
Groups of Communication Skills	**Averages of Grades of the Membership Function**	**Position in the Ranking**	**Groups of Communication Skills**	**Averages of Grades of the Membership Function**
G_1	0.68	1	G_1	0.59
G_2	0.65	2	G_2	0.63
G_3	0.59	3	G_3	0.64
G_4	0.64	4	G_4	0.65
G_5	0.63	5	G_5	0.68
G_6	0.69	6	G_6	0.69
G_7	0.75	7	G_7	0.75

RESULTS AND CONCLUSION

The application of fuzzy relations let the researchers use grades (numbers belonging to interval [0,1]) of the agreement to the specific question.

Typically when there are a few examined areas, the questionnaire designers define questions for each area separately. When the group of the experts is employed, they can describe levels of relation between examined areas and questions what may cause the reduction of the questions and more detailed information.

Instead of finding the values of the relation between examined areas and people, it is easier to produce two fuzzy relations: the first one between examined areas and questions and the second one between questions and people, and then using the max-min composition calculate the relation between examined areas and people. This method can be used to calculate the levels of Patient Satisfaction and levels of communication skills of doctor.

After finding, for example levels of Patient Satisfaction, using the α-cuts, the crisp sets can be found and on this basis, the statistical analysis may be performed. Because there may be a lot of data, so the expert system may be designed to help analyze this data.

REFERENCES

Encyclopedia Britannica. (n.d.). Information system. Retrieved 09.04.2017 from http://www.britannica.com/EBchecked/topic/287895/information-system

Encyclopedia of Mathematics. (n.d.). Set. Retrieved 25.04.2017 from https://www.encyclopediaofmath.org/index.php/Set

Kabengele Mpinga, K., & Chastonay, P. *Patient Satisfaction Studies and the Monitoring of the Right to Health: Some Thoughts Based on a Review of the Literature*, Global Journal of Health Science, Vol. 3, No. 1; April 2011, Retrieved 08.05.2017 from http://www.ccsenet.org/journal/index.php/gjhs/article/viewFile/8093/7143

Kotarbiński, K. (1985). *Wykłady z dziejów logiki* (2nd ed.). Warszawa: PWN.

Kravitz, R. (1998). Patient Satisfaction with Health Care. Critical Outcome or Trivial Pursuit? *Journal of General Internal Medicine*, *13*(4), 280–282, Retrieved 07.052017 from https://www.ncbi.nlm.nih.gov/pmc/articles/PMC1496942/

Lisowska, B. (n.d.). Zmiany w służbie zdrowia: Wizyta w kwadrans, kolejki przed gabinetami. *Gazeta prawna.pl*. Retrieved from http://serwisy.gazetaprawna.pl/zdrowie/artykuly/862915,zmiany-w-sluzbie-zdrowia-wizyta-w-kwadrans-kolejki-przed-gabinetami.html

Masić, I., Ridanovic, Z., & Pandza H. (1995). Medical expert systems. *Med. Arh.*, *49*(3-4), 107-112.

Peeva, K., & Kyosev, Y. (2004). *Fuzzy relational calculus, theory, application and software. In Advances in Fuzzy Systems – Applications and Theory* (Vol. 22). Singapore: World Scientific Publishing.

Piegat, A. (1999). *Modelowanie i sterowanie rozmyte*. Warszawa: Akademicka Oficyna Wydawnicza EXIT.

Plentara, R., Knyszyńska, A., Bażydło, M., Zabielska, P., Klim, A., Kotwas, A., . . . Karakiewicz, B. (2015). Satysfakcja pacjentów podstawowej opieki zdrowotnej z opieki medycznej i psychospołecznej [Patient satisfaction measure of the quality of primary health care]. *Pomeranian Journal of Life Sciences*, *61*(3), 335–340. Retrieved 08.05.2017 from https://www.pum.edu.pl/__data/assets/pdf_file/0014/111038/PomJLifeSci_61-03_335-340.pdf

Prakash, B. (2010). Patient Satisfaction. *Journal of Cutaneous and Aesthetic Surgery*, *3*(3). Retrieved 02.05.2017 from ncbi.nlm.nih.gov/pcm/articles/PCM3047732

Rabin, R. C. (2014). *15-Minute Visits Take A Toll On The Doctor-Patient Relationship*. Keiser Health News. Retrieved 07.05.2017 from http://khn.org/news/15-minute-doctor-visits/

Rynekzdrowia.pl. (2009). Ile-minut-lekarz-powinien-rozmawiac-z-pacjentem. Retrieved 07.05.2017 from http://www.rynekzdrowia.pl/Uslugi-medyczne/Ile-minut-lekarz-powinien-rozmawiac-z-pacjentem,11641,8.html

Shortliffe, E. H. (1986). *Medical Expert Systems—Knowledge Tools for Physicians,* Western Journal of Medicine, *145*(6). Retrieved 06.05.2017 from https://www.ncbi.nlm.nih.gov/pmc/articles/PMC1307157/

Shu-Hsien, L. (2004). Expert system methodologies and applications—a decade review from 1995 to 2004. In *Expert Systems with Applications*. Retrieved 19.09.2012 from http://www.dca.fee.unicamp.br/~gomide/courses/EA072/artigos/ExpertSystemMethodologiesApplicationsReview1995to2004Liao2004.pdf

Shusaku, T., & Hiroshi, T. (1996). Automated Discovery of Medical Expert System Rules from Clinical Databases based on Rough Sets. In *Proceedings of KDD '96*. Retrieved 06.05.2017 from http://www.aaai.org/Papers/KDD/1996/KDD96-011.pdf

Stanford Encyclopedia of Philosophy. (n.d.). Logic classical. Retrieved 25.04.2017 from https://plato.stanford.edu/entries/logic-classical/

The Scottish Doctor. (2011). *Outcomes for Communication*. Retrieved 20.04.2017 from http://www.scottishdoctor.org/node.asp?id=0501010000

Tvp.info. (2015). 90 pacjentów w siedem godzin. „Średni czas wizyty to 4,5 minuty. Retrieved 08.05.2017 from https://www.tvp.info/18329897/90-pacjentow-w-siedem-godzin-sredni-czas-wizyty-to-45-minuty

White, B. (1999). Measuring Patient Satisfaction: How to Do It and Why to Bother. *Family Practice Management*. Retrieved 08.05.2017 from http://www.aafp.org/fpm/1999/0100/p40.html

Zadeh, L. A. (1965). Fuzzy sets. *Information and Control*, *8*(3), 338–353. doi:10.1016/S0019-9958(65)90241-X

Chapter 12
Building Relationships Within a Therapeutic Team

Agata Pasternak
High School Economy, Poland

ABSTRACT

This chapter describes how a therapeutic team is a term defining all qualified healthcare workers, who are actively participating in the treatment, care and rehabilitation processes of a patient. Depending on the type of department or institution where a patient is staying, he can come across numerous therapeutic teams. A therapeutic team consists of a group of people, who fulfil a treatment process together. Their cooperation may result on the most effective strategy to provide care, due to every member of a team being a source of information about the patient and his afflictions. Professional development of every member of a therapeutic team is an important component in improving quality of provided services, which effects the increase of a patient's satisfaction level. Therefore, its role is incredibly important. Moreover, professional development is a process that takes place during a human lifespan and is associated with activities, achievements, but also with existence, expression and self-realization.

INTRODUCTION

The role of a therapeutic team is, integrally, a complex care of a patient, with consideration of all the aspects of patient's condition. At the basis of a teamwork lies the holistic philosophy, which is defined in medicine as a comprehensive treatment of a patient as a bio-psycho-social unity. According to this, a man is able to come to a health welfare only by undertaking a complex care with a consideration of all the elements affected by the disease. Therefore, holism implies cooperation, not a misconception associated with a responsibility, that in all circumstances I can deal 'with my patient' on my own (Szary & Knotowicz, 2014)

The history of medicine shows, that until not so long ago, a doctor decided about the whole care and treatment process, and the other people related to a patient care remained to doctor's disposal and their role was limited to execution of commands without ability to make their own decisions.

DOI: 10.4018/978-1-5225-3946-9.ch012

Nowadays, there is a tendency to let all the therapeutic team members make their own decisions in consultation with each other and in their own field of professional competencies, while the doctor remains a core of a treatment process. In this conception, it is important to develop an individual specialization, but multidisciplinary meetings are also important, because the essence of medicine and its roots claim that, if possible, one should effectively help an ill and suffering man, and this implies an open attitude, an ability to work within a therapeutic team, having a proper life philosophy, professionalism and the ethics (Szary, 2013).

Is this type of working with a patient system really commonly used? From experience, creating a good therapeutic team with proper relationships within and in which decisions are made without unnecessary conflicts - is possible, but difficult.

In a social awareness, doctor appears as the main decision maker and this picture is so ingrained that the other members of a therapeutic team tend to accept this conjuncture, despite of the autonomy of their own professions. The patients also look forward to the doctor to make all decisions in their recovery process, lessening the role of the other members of a therapeutic team.

This conjuncture may cause conflicts and have a bad impact on relationships within a team, and hence on a treatment process and care of a patient.

Conflicts are integral components of a human life and it is not only a negative situation. Conflicts indicate lack of consent on present conjuncture and ambition of development. Despite that fact, conflicts are usually treated as something undesirable. That is a result of lacking the ability to deal with them.

It is worth to emphasize that in recent years the views on conflicts in organizations essentially changed. Stephen P. Robbins have noticed an important difference between a traditional and current view on conflict – which he calls an interactive conflict. (Robbins, 2001).

Today it is considered that conflicts are inevitable, and often even necessary. Their occurrence is a natural phenomenon. Large number of conflicts are negative: they may impede achieving team's goals and even harm individuals. However, some of them are positive: they may cause work of a team to be more effective. Conflicts are often tools of innovation and change, they lead to finding new resolutions. The purpose of this publication is to see into the process of building positive relationships within a therapeutic team and functional use of appearing conflicts.

THE MEMBERS OF A THERAPEUTIC TEAM AND THEIR ROLE IN TAKING CARE OF A PATIENT

Working at the health service in the atmosphere of cooperation and professional co-responsibility, results in many positives for a patient. None of professional groups in a medical care cannot work individually, considering bio-psycho-social approach to an ill man (Kapała, 2007).

Modern model of a holistic care of a patient requires cooperation and professional co-responsibility of every member of the therapeutic team (Fejfer-Wirbał, Gładczuk, &Marcinowicz, 2013).

A therapeutic team is a term defining all qualified healthcare workers, who actively participate in a treatment process, care and rehabilitation of a patient. According to B. Jankowiak and A. Bartoszewicz 'a therapeutic team is a group of people jointly implementing the treatment process', whereas features of the team are:

- A common goal and a responsibility of its realization,
- A common establishment of the fields of actions and individual responsibilities and privileges related to them,
- An efficient flow of information (Kapała, 2007).

Depending on the type of department or institution, where a patient is staying, he can come across more or less numerous therapeutic teams. A therapeutic team consists of a group of people, who fulfil a treatment process together. Its cooperation may result in elaborating the most effective activities, because every member of a team is a source of information about the manifested in a patient:

1. Symptoms,
2. Behavior,
3. Needs,
4. Progress in an adaptation process.

Care that is offered by multidisciplinary team should be comprehensive and scheduled. Its members with a different vocational training are fulfilling a common goal supervised by a group's coordinator – the leader.

A composition of a team includes:

- A medical doctor,
- A nurse,
- A psychologist, a dietician, a physiotherapist, a medical caregiver, an occupational therapist,
- A social worker, a priest, a family of the patient and others.

A composition of a multidisciplinary team may be diverse and it mostly depends on the problems of a patient, but also on a place where the care is provided.

Primary members of a therapeutic team are medical doctors and nurses. Those two occupational groups are accompanying a patient throughout almost the whole stay in the hospital.

A doctor in a therapeutic team makes the most important decisions about the treatment of an individual patient. Generally, a patient has his own main doctor, who coordinates all the actions taken by the doctors on duty. Work of all the doctor of a specific department is coordinated by a head of that department, therefore his role in a therapeutic team seems to be important.

Doctors of the department in a treatment process may order consultations from doctors of other specialties, ipso facto including them into work of a team. Only an efficient cooperation and an exchange of experiences guarantee effective treatment process.

A role of a nurse in a therapeutic team is associated with taking care of a patient in every possible aspect. Moreover, she collaborates with a doctor in a treatment process (among others by participating in diagnostic tests, executing commands, observing the condition and parameters). She also cooperates with other members of a team in a necessary range for a good of a patient. Nowadays, a nurse by fulfilling a professional role, makes independent functions, such as: care, nurture, management or dependent on other professionals, e.g., health promotion, rehabilitation, prevention, but she also has a therapeutic function, which depends on a doctor (Glińska & Lewandowska, 2007).

It's worth to emphasize that a therapeutic team provides proper care and protection for the ill, only when its members co-work professionally, have mutual trust and are able to cooperate with a patient and his relatives (Werachowska, Damps-Konstańska, Janowicz & Krakowiak, 2013).

The Sources of Conflicts

By analyzing the definitions that appear in the publications of social psychologists – a conflict means a divergence of interests or belief that certain aspirations of its parties cannot be fulfilled at the same time. A conflict is an unsolved, or solved in a way that is incompatible with social expectations or objective conditions, contradiction between groups or individuals (Januszek & Sikora, 1997).

Considering those two mentioned definitions, it can be said that a conflict is a social process that is going between individuals or groups, causing tensions and negative emotions between them. Therefore, it is a struggle and its causes can be found in contradiction of interests, goals, views and responsibilities. A conflict is a divergence in understanding, an approach, a preference, an orientation, ways of perceiving reality, a morality and a cultural level.

Looking at the term from a theoretical side, it can be clearly shown that the more opportunities for communication between people exist, the more opportunities for existence of conflict are created. On the other hand, from a practical side, it is known that a conflict is created with a participation of communication, but it does not necessarily mean that its main cause is the exchange of information or views in a working environment (Marciniak, 2011).

The causes of a conflict in a team have a varied background and it is worth to try to describe them.

The Scope of Duties

The scope of duties is different for individual members of a therapeutic team. However, it does not mean that people with a smaller scope of duties have also smaller role in a whole treatment process.

Members of a therapeutic team are important cells on a particular stage in a health recovery process, which are often the most important at a certain stage. A scope of duties cannot be a factor that lessens significance of individual members of a therapeutic team.

However, the reality of a hospital can be opposite. People with a large scope of duties, e.g. a doctor, a nurse may – consciously or not – put themselves as decision makers and impose their opinions. Such situation may be a source of a conflict, making the other members of the team feel underestimated.

The Level of Education

The education is an important factor that has an impact on a position of individual members in a therapeutic team. Usually teams include people with a different level of education: it may be graduates of medical studies, bachelor and master degree studies in health sciences, as well as technicians of individual specialties. The level of education is usually adequate to the role that a person has to fulfil while taking care of a patient. However, it is one of the causes of conflicts. Different educational backgrounds may determine an existence of informal hierarchy in a team and cause that opinions of people with a lower level of education might be challenged.

A Salary

A salary is an important element impacting on relations between individual members of a therapeutic team.

In a current reality Polish healthcare system disproportions between earnings of individual employees may be significant. It is impacted by a remuneration policy in a certain institution, as well as a form of employment of individual employees.

The difference in earnings in relation to a workload and many other factors may be the background of frustration and may cause a feeling of underestimation in those who earn less. Moreover, a salary as a motivational element may have an impact on the involvement in fulfilling assigned tasks. Members of a therapeutic team that, in their opinion, are not rewarded enough, may be less engaged in realizing their responsibilities, encouraging co-workers to criticize.

A Team's Style of Work

A therapeutic team is a collection of individuals participating in a treatment process. Each of its members has his own tasks to manage, but only an efficient cooperation can guarantee an expected effect. A team can take on different styles of work.

It is important that each member prefers the same style of work, because it makes communication easier and restricts causes of conflicts.

Generally speaking, there can be distinguished several styles of work in the team. One of them is a focusing on realization of the tasks. This style of work may be dangerous for a team, if its members focus only on their tasks, in the meantime neglecting communication and an exchange of information. It may lead to misunderstandings and have a negative impact on realization of expected results.

Another form of working style in a team is a focusing on a leadership. In this case, team's individual members try to take a role of a leader and enforce the way of a task realization on others. Leaders may create a concept and inspire others to work, but they also may restrict them and discourage self-reliance.

In some teams, their members may take the style of work focusing on building proper relationships. They work hard to create a good atmosphere within a group and to compromise conflicts. People focused on relationships may not deal well with work that requires more attention. Left to themselves, they take care of the good of a team, but their work may be less effective.

One of the working styles is a style focused on learning. This kind of workers like to know the problem precisely, with all its nuances. They are disciplined and tend to think more strategically than most people. However, without a good squad, they are unable to put their excellent plans into life. Their work is directly related to challenges ahead them – specifically from a real, not from a theoretical solution.

Each of these different styles works in association with the other ones. Only thanks to a mutual support, every member has a chance to show his true potential.

The Cultural Differences

In the age of globalization and free flow of workers, teams culturally differentiated became standard. It seems that this type of difference should not have an influence fulfilling professional tasks.

However, the cultural differences play a big role in a work of a team and they should not be trivialized. Unfortunately, these differences may be a source of a conflict – it happens mainly as a result of misunderstanding and lack of established universal principles.

The three interfering and disturbing communication factors that have their roots in the cultural differences from which the participants of the communication come are, as follows: ethnocentrism, prejudices and stereotypes (Mikułowski, Pomorski, 2003).

Different cultures mean different views on many issues, customs and schemes of conduct. They mean also many worries and prejudices that result from an ignorance and lack of will to know.

It is important that a professionalism, an actual medical knowledge and the good of a patient were set above the cultural prejudices. The members of a therapeutic team should be aware of these differences and, if possible, get to know and use them. Only thanks to differences optimal solutions can be created.

The members of a team strive for a common goal and are jointly accounted for achieving that goal. Their interaction with each other has an impact on achieving that goal, therefore it is their responsibility to integrate with each other (Mohrman, Cohen, &Mohrman, 1995).

Personal and Interpersonal Competencies

Main Personal Competencies:

- Responsibility/ self-discipline
- Involvement
- Striving for results
- Self-reliance
- Flexibility and adaptability
- Being open to learning
- Loyalty and willingness to commit to a company for a longer period of time
- Ability to work under the pressure of time
- Proper self esteem
- Ability to make decisions

Main Interpersonal Competencies:

- Effective communication
- Ability to work in a team.

Interpersonal abilities belong to a group of soft psychosocial skills. Repeatedly they tend to be immeasurable and difficult to precise estimation. However, they are a key element of professional competencies that help employee to fit himself in a therapeutic team, and to help a team realize set goals. The assimilation of interpersonal skills is not a sufficient condition to be interpersonally efficient. It is indispensable to have social knowledge to enable the analysis of situation and application of an adequate strategy of action and a proper interpersonal attitude characterized by a positive approach to self and others.

Each of the members of a therapeutic team is different with his skills, experience and knowledge. Each of them has also a different character and range of interpersonal and social skills. Despite of these differences, all the members of a team have one common, noble goal, which is the good of another human being. Therefore, continuous development and upskilling are core qualities of the effective professional.

Leader in a Therapeutic Team

A team – a group of people working together and aiming to achieve a common goal – needs a leader. The leader is coordinating manager and supervising work of a specific team of employees in a firm, company or institution. It is his duty to assign current and long-term tasks for individual members of a team, to verify their progression, to reward and to draw consequences, to motivate to an action. The leader is responsible to the management for results achieved by the team, since he is the most experienced one in a certain field. A good leader does not restrict himself only to issuing commands. A good leader – motivates, gives advices, analyzes potential and capabilities of employees, adjusts the scope of duties to their predispositions and aptitudes. Team leader's actions are supposed to lead to achieve the highest possible efficiency and maximization of the profits, but also to professional development of the 'proteges'.

A therapeutic team is a specific type of a team. It consists of many specialists, which role on a certain stage of a treatment process may change. A doctor, who is important during a surgical procedure, on the subsequent stages transfers a patient to another specialist, so he could finally end up being taken care of by a physiotherapist. Additionally, he is being taken care of by nurses, guardians and other employees. The selection of a leader may be difficult for all the members of a team, but it is not impossible. If the treatment process takes place within one ward, the main doctor that coordinates a patient from admission to discharge from a hospital may become the leader. He may supervise a fluency of all processes, a flow of information and an efficiency of actions. The situation looks differently, if a patient's treatment process includes staying in different departments. In that case, the role of a leader may be entrusted to another person.

Being a leader of a therapeutic team is a difficult, responsible task and an inadequate approach to this role may become a source of conflicts and misunderstandings.

A good leader coordinates, supports, motivates. A bad one enforces his opinions, undermines the competencies and interferes in the autonomy of individual specialists who work with him. An improper approach to the role of the leader may cause aversion, feeling of underestimation or even protests in a team.

A leader of a therapeutic team should have such features as: the ability to make contacts, a self-confidence, self-discipline and high interpersonal competencies. He has to be an experienced person, who is respected and trustworthy. When the health and life of another human being is a subject of a work of a team, an extreme gentleness and concentration in making any decision is required.

It is not unusual, that the members of a team may be higher in the hospital hierarchy than its leader. It is important, that he was able to motivate and coordinate work of people who are more educated, titled, being prominent specialists in specific fields. An attitude of a leader needs to be adamant if he is convinced about his right.

Does an ideal way of leading a therapeutic team exist? The answer is: no. The style of leading is determined by three factors: a quality of relations between the leader and the group, a structure of a task and a power held by a leader. Every patient has a different history, needs and emotions. A therapeutic team needs to change and adjust to a specific situation. The style of leading a team is a resultant of many factors, and a good leader is able to adjust to a changing situation.

The Methods of Resolving Conflicts

A conflict is an inevitable occurrence, because people differ from each other in personality features, views and culture (Reetz-Wasielewska, Kretowicz, & Zarzeczna-Baran, 2016).

A therapeutic team is a group of people, specialists in various fields, qualified workers, who have one mutual goal – the good of a patient. It would seem that with such a noble goal, a team could unite and strive together to achieve it. However, where a group of numerous and differentiated people works, there may arise a conflict. It is a natural phenomenon, normal in the reality of group work. The basis of an effective team cooperation should be its members' awareness of their range of competencies, roles and tasks, because a properly working team with clear goals and rules of action may contribute to improving the quality of taking care of a patient and his family (Babska, Tkaczyk, &Nowicki, 2008).

There may Occur Positive Results of Conflicts, such as (Leslie, 1983):

- A verification of adopted methods and practices
- Better understanding of needs and motivations of other departments
- Lessening tension between coworkers
- More flexibility and ability to answer to the market needs
- Improving a morale and a satisfaction from work

The positive results of conflict may also include (Rogoda, 2013):

- **A Motivation for Achievements:** A competition favors the development
- **Informing About Abnormalities:** During conflict that requires mobilization of the forces, may occur errors in the functioning of the organization
- **A Motivation for Changes and Innovations:** A mobilization of forces favors searching and implementing innovations, when current solutions do not provide an advantage over the opponent
- **An Awareness Raise of Involved Parties:** A conflict motivates to analyze the situation, to verify allies and opponents
- **An Increase of the Team Integration:** An external threat favors tightening bonds
- **A Selection of an Efficient Leader:** An employee who won the competition with internal opponents, probably has features such as: a professional competency, an ability to work hard, an ability to gain allies and patrons, a stress resistance

Conflicts in a therapeutic team may also lead to negative consequences, as well for patients, as for members of the team. An improper course of treatment or rehabilitation process may be its consequence.

Therefore, members of a team and top management cannot be indifferent to conflicts and should try to resolve them.

Regardless of a method, process of resolving conflicts is complex and multistage.

According to Kilmann and Thomas there are several ways of resolving conflicts.

They defined them as (Kilmann & Thomas, 1974):

1. **Avoiding Conflicts:** The essence of this approach is a renouncement of cooperation with a person, who is a source of a conflict. This style of resolving conflicts is used by people with a weak emotional construction, who think that other resolutions are impossible. The cause of such state is disproportion between positions of individual members of the team. A person with stronger, more established position, being a greater authority may be an insurmountable barrier for individuals conflicted with that person. When one side of an argument is stronger – the other one withdraws and gives up the realization of its own rights and interests. Analyzing this method it is worth to

emphasize, that in situation when the health of a patient is a superior good, an avoiding is not a promising solution. Running away from a solution of a problem through avoiding interactions may disrupt the work of a therapeutic team and postpone achieving a goal.

2. **An Indulgence:** Adequately to the way described above, an indulgence also is caused by disproportions between positions of individual members of the therapeutic team. It is the most commonly used a resolving conflicts method of using a stronger member of his position. An indulgence is not a constructive way of resolving conflict, because demands of its weaker party are not realized. This style, generally speaking, consists in proceeding in accordance with the interests of the opposite party. Also in this case, a broadly understood good of a patient may be violated.
3. **A Rivalry:** In this case both sides of a conflict are pushing their opinions in every possible way, trying to involve uncommitted persons in the conflict. This style is characterized by the fact that in order to achieve its goal, a party of a conflict puts a lot of energy and uses many resources, including manipulation and instrumental treatment of other people. Such approach to a conflict may cause that individual members of a therapeutic team focused on rivalry, will pay too little attention to the essence of their activity, which is the good of a patient.
4. **A Compromise:** When choosing a way of a compromise, it is possible to partially satisfy the interests of both parties. However, everyone is losing and gaining something. It is worth to take a compromise under consideration, when it is necessary to quickly resolve a problem. This solution is used when conflicted parties are equally strong, have similar authority, knowledge and experience.
5. **A Cooperation:** This style is a result of an assumption that one can always find a solution that satisfies both parties of a conflict. This is the one of the most effective styles of resolving conflicts. It is particularly useful in situations when, when both sides have a common goal and a real cause of a dispute is incorrect communication or lack of it. Parties with a mutual effort are trying to find solutions that erase causes of the conflict. It is acting according to assumption, that one can always find a solution that satisfies both sides of a conflict.

One of the forms of positive resolving conflicts may be the constructive dispute. According to S. Kratochvil it is a way that leads to positive resolution of a conflict, thus both parties achieved their goals and did not suffer excessive loss (Kratochvil, 2016).

The rules of the constructive resolution of a problem are as follows:

- The location and time of the conversation should be determined in a way that members of a team would not be bothered by a communication noise and interference by third parties.
- It is important to distinguish emotions from the real core of a dispute, so it did not have an impact on the resolving process.
- It is important to define one's reasons, clearly determine one's expectations.
- The principle of fair play should be remembered, i.e. one should always honestly handle the dispute – the arguments not associated with the case should not be used. One should not bring back to the argument already solved problems, disputable problems (a reproach), one should not blackmail, pin down, attack things or people of a special meaning to the interlocutor, use generalizations (*you always…*), threaten with the consequences inadequate to the situation.

An advantage of a constructive resolution of dispute is achieving set goals in a way that does not impact on the good of a patient.

In the 70's an American writer, a clinical psychologist Dr. Thomas Gordon created a program called 'Parent Effectiveness Training', in which he presents ways of resolving conflicts and problems, pointing to the types of communication that create in a child self-reliance, responsibility and ability to make proper choices attitude (Gordon, 1998). This program primarily refers to resolving disputes between parents and children. In may be also used in every interpersonal conflict situation. Considering the fact that conflicts in a therapeutic team are a delicate matter and are burdened with the risk of impacting on health and life of a patient, one may try to transfer assumptions of 'effectiveness training method' on a hospital field.

The goal of this is mutual creation of such a solution of the conflict, in which there will be two winners – with no losers, both parties benefit from this solution. A condition for its success is a good interpersonal communication, active listening and informing about one's own needs and feelings.

According to T. Gordon the important element of an optimal contact is to show acceptance to the other person. The acceptance has a positive impact on creating self-esteem, enables becoming a self-reliant, better person and allows development, constructive changes and learning to resolve one's own problems.

While using this 'Effectiveness Training' method, its creator – Thomas Gordon suggests to make six important steps. When implementing Gordon's theory on therapeutic team, one should:

- **Recognize the Conflict and Name It:** It is the first and deciding phase. One should precisely define a conflict that needs to be resolved together. Feelings and unfulfilled desires should be expressed. The speeches should be in the first person, i.e. 'I'. The sentences humiliating or lowering the value of the other person should be avoided. It needs to be clearly shown that both parties of a conflict should try to find such solution that will satisfy all the needs and to find a solution in which will be no defeated ones.
- **Find a Possible Resolution:** A key to this stage is a relatively large quantity of a possible solutions. They should be proposed by both sides of a conflict. In this stage one should not judge any ideas and do not express contempt. Its core value is to find solutions that will be judged in the next stages.
- **Critically Judge the Propositions of Solutions:** In this stage one judges the submitted proposals. It is important to clearly explain, why one makes a specific assessment, what is possible to achieve, etc.
- **Decide on the Best Solution:** After careful assessment, one should make a decision which of the conflict solving methods is appropriate and possible to achieve.
- **Execute Made Decisions:** After choosing the solution that is optimal for all, one should take up the implementation of the solution in practice. In this stage roles, scope of duties and time for implementation are clearly defined.
- **Further Critical Assessment:** This is the last of the stages of resolving the conflict.

This method requires cooperation of all the people involved in resolving the problem. A condition of its success is a good interpersonal communication, active listening and expressing one's own needs and feelings. During the time of solving a problem may occur strong emotions both on one and the other side, therefore an active listening is important for expressing one's feelings and dealing with them. This method provides an opportunity of finding a creative and the best possible solution of a conflict. It also develops thinking skills.

The Negotiation

The negotiation is a bilateral communication process, which aims to achieve an agreement.

The negotiation are based on communication of parties, when they expect that an agreement may provide a greater benefit than acting without an agreement.

The negotiation is a process in which participates at least two parties representing incompatible positions that are an obstacle to their interests; actions that are undertaken by the parties are aimed at achieving an agreement that will result in establishing positions (Osika, 2000).

The essence of negotiations is to achieve such resolution of a conflict that will satisfy both sides. By negotiating, one should be ready to give up some of his postulates in favor of realization of others.

The negotiation is a complex, dynamic cognitive-emotional process in which the stake is not only achieving set goals, but often also a self-esteem, ambitions, likes and dislikes. It is also a process of collecting information, matching partners and finally – convincing each other. The negotiation is a common phenomenon. Politicians, traders and unionists are negotiating.

The negotiation consists of two components: a negotiating position and an interest.

The position is the demand for something measurable, while the interest is a reason that led to taking the position. It is worth to emphasize the fact that the interest is overriding to the position. The worst failure of both parties is to break up the negotiation, which leads to even greater conflict.

In the case of conflict in the therapeutic team, interest of each of the parties may be equal with the interest of a patient, which is his health, and sometimes even life. Therefore, in this case the process of negotiation should be led in a well-thought and responsible way.

Participants entering the negotiations usually have a prepared scenario, a vision of the way of realization of their needs, but they need to remember that during negotiation those propositions will be verified, because the offers submitted by the parties are only one of possible ways of realization of their needs, and an agreement is possible only when it concerns these needs itself, not the original assumptions related to the way of their realization (Osika, 2000).

The basic factor that initiates the negotiation are needs, their types and power of motivation. The negotiation on saving human live will look differently than a negotiation on buying a new car. When parties in negotiation want to realize individual need we talk about an interpersonal negotiation, but when they are the representatives of the group interest, we call it an intergroup negotiation.

The style of negotiation strictly depends on the strength and attitude of the partners towards each other. Considering a mutual trust of the partners and an attitude of the parties to negotiation, we may distinguish a cooperating and a fighting style. In reality, a negotiation attitude oscillates between four basic strategies: domination and submission & cooperation and fight (Nęcki, 1995).

The Mediation

A difference between the negotiation and the mediation is that in negotiation parties are resolving the conflict by negotiating with each other on their own. In mediation parties ask a mediator for help. It may be said, that a mediation is a negotiation managed by a mediator.

The mediator is usually an impartial person, whose role is to ensure the progress on the way to agreement of the negotiating parties.

The mediator needs to be accepted by both sides of the conflict, respected by them, and it is not unusual for him to be an authority.

The parties of the conflict need to be ready to trust a mediator and let him interfere, when it is needed.

In a therapeutic team the role of a mediator may be fulfilled by a person that cooperates with it, well orientated in a nature of the problem, rich in experience, knowledge and skills. It may be a doctor, a nurse, physiotherapist or any other specialist, who is trusted by the parties of a conflict and may be entrusted with their doubts.

The attitude of a mediator is primarily an impartial attitude. It would be the best if all the parties agreed on choosing a neutral person, who will facilitate achieving an agreement. The mediator should also be careful of making his behavior to be interpreted as biased.

The rules that guide the mediators in their everyday work have their roots in different schools of mediation, however there exists some common rules. Waszkiewicz (2009) mentions such as:

1. **A Voluntariness:** Understood as a lack of pressure coming from the outside. Conflicted persons are deciding on their own about joining mediation, and in every moment, they can give it up without any consequences.;
2. **An Impartiality and Neutrality of the Mediator:** He needs to be an equal ally of both parties of a dispute. A mediator never favors anyone, even if he feels compassion for one of the parties. He cannot be biased, he should not show his emotions. Moreover, he should be neutral, thus he should not have any interest in any result of a dispute.
3. **A Confidentiality of Mediation:** This rule guarantees a sense of security for the participants of mediation by keeping secrecy and excluding third parties.
4. **Other Rules:** A selflessness which implies that a mediator does not get any material benefits from what is the subject of negotiation between the parties. Another rule is a respect – a mediator needs to secure the conditions of the conversation in a way that allows the parties to feel respected. On the other hand, the rule of professionalism is a kind of guarantee of continuous professional development of the mediator.

The role of mediator includes also support for the parties:

- By asking questions, that may help parties to organize their own expectations;
- They let the parties see elements, which they haven't notices earlier.

The mediator may also:

- Probe the convergence of their interests and try to force them to make concessions in common and individual meetings.
- Organize and direct a conversation.
- Encourage parties to search for creative solution to a problem.

The help of a neutral third party in achieving an agreement between conflicted sides, was used in different historical periods, different countries and cultures. Nowadays, the mediation is becoming more popular and is getting a status of a separated procedure of solving conflicts. It is highly helpful in achieving an agreement in situations where it is needed and it determines an effective care for the patient. It also gives a possibility of establishing principles for a conflict-free relationship in the future.

The Barriers in Communication

To make the actions in a healthcare center more efficient, necessary is not only a 'good' communication based on showing positive emotions, but primarily the precise communication, accepted and used by workers that enables them the transmission of both positive and critical information (Stankiewicz, 1999).

The therapeutic team consists of a group of people differentiated in their experience, level of education, knowledge, competencies and many other features. The efficient realization of set goals, in this case – the treatment process of a patient, is conditioned by a proper communication and an efficient flow of information between all the members of the team. The exchange of information relevant for the help to the patient is important, because it is the basis of the complete understanding his situation, and also it enables to plan a proper actions for the benefit of the patient. It is definitely a complex process that requires great skills and involvement. Otherwise, relevant misunderstandings may appear and have an impact on the health condition of the patient.

The communication is defined as intentional exchange of verbal and non-verbal signs (symbols) undertaken for the improvement of cooperation or for sharing meanings between partners or as a process of transmitting information from one person to another (Czerw et al, 2012)

In order to enable the communication process to exist, it is necessary to have its necessary and interrelated elements. Those components are: participants, context, statement, channel, feedback and noise (Dobek-Ostrowska, 1999).

The barriers in the interpersonal communication are not only a reason to frustration. They are also an obstacle in achieving one's goals.

We communicate since forever. The sender encodes his content, sends it through the communication channel of the receiver, who is going to decode it and send a feedback in response to a received content. Formalized contacts between members of the organization enforce a formal and official way of communication. Communicating with each other is primarily about realizing assigned tasks and responsibilities and compliance according to legal rules and habits of the organization (Dobek-Ostrowska, 1999).

The communication needs of members of a therapeutic team are mainly created by tasks assigned to them. Considering the fact that a team consists of people, they are also a social structure, in which a specific role division and assigned hierarchy is developed. This structure is characterized by a specific culture that has an impact on communication processes that take place in a team.

In each team specific lingual procedures defined by many factors and a characteristic dictionary of messages are created.

It is worth to emphasize that the acts of communication are determined by a grid of dependencies between individual members of a therapeutic team.

An important aspect that is worth consideration refers to the modern conditions. Changes that are happening in a way the medical industry is functioning, are the result of the progressive globalization that causes specific consequences for communication processes.

More clearly defined differences in human resources in terms of the character and persistence of participation in the organization and intercultural differences between individuals cause that communication is burdened with serious problems.

As a result of a more noticeable trend of temporary employment, the involvement of employees towards workplace and the need of integration are continuously declining, what causes that individuals are less likely to engage in the group's communication.

Communicating in every, even the most technologically advanced way, is a bilateral process. A process characterized by its dynamics. When the communication is effective? Only when the receiver understands what messages are sent to him by a sender.

The effectiveness of a communication in a team may be affected by such factors as:

1. **Differences in Perception:** Differences in perception may be a resultant of different levels of knowledge and experience. A therapeutic team consists of people of differentiated professional and social experience. Its members' level of education may also be differentiated. Despite of a common goal, each member of a team has a right to look at how it is achieved from different angle.

These differences in perception may be affected by many factors connected as well with the characterological features of communicating people, as with their experience.

In order to improve the communication process in a therapeutic team, it is necessary to explain the message in such way to make it understandable for people with different views and experience. It is useful to perceive from the speaker's point of view and to postpone reactions to the time of considering the relevant information. It is essential to ask questions and wait for the feedback answer.

2. **Differences in Language:** This factor is a main cause of misunderstandings in communication between members of different cultures that speak in different languages. The source of frustration is an insufficient and often superficial knowledge of the language that is used to communicate (Mikułowski, Pomorski, 2003). It may happen in, e.g. semi-official political or business contacts when invited guests try to converse in the native language of the host. However, even in organizations functioning within the same culture, composed of people using the same language, not always the same words have the same meaning for both sender and receiver. This situation may happen when an employee jargon or specialized terminology known only to a narrow group is used (Sobkowiak, 1998).

Differences in language may be a barrier in a therapeutic team, which consists members representing different, distant disciplines. The medicine and health sciences, despite of a common base, which is the care of human's health, are combined of many areas. The specialist vocabulary used by the representatives of individual fields of medical science may be not understandable for the other members of a team. Moreover, in the age of globalization and multicultural therapeutic teams the language barrier, accent or regional language accretions are significant. During the process of overcoming barriers in communication the explanation of the unconventional or specialized terms is required. One should use a simple, direct and natural language. Also the ability to rephrase (to repeat in own words) in order to check the understanding of the message is important.

3. **The Communication Noise:** The communication noise is a wide term, involving every factor that impedes and jam the message. In a hospital reality there are many of these factors. A conversation in front of patients, families or other workers carries a risk of misunderstanding, especially when it takes place in the corridor or in a lounge full of people. Emergency situations of any kind, fuss in a ward, working equipment – these are also the sources of the noise. It might seem that the importance of this factor is not that big, but a huge amount of overlapping causes of the noise may become a relevant barrier in a communication process of a team.

The noises should be eliminated. One could, e.g. turn off a working device that makes the conversation difficult or move to another location. When the noise cannot be avoided, greater transparency of the message should be ensured.

4. **Emotions:** The professional attitude should exclude emotions. This is one of the most difficult barriers to overcome in a communication process.

Emotional reactions – anger, feeling of liking, defensive impulses, hate, jealousy, anxiety, embarrassment – they may have an impact on understanding of messages and on how the messages affect the others. The specifics of working with a patient, a contact with suffering and death may affect the communication process. Moreover, working under the pressure, large scope of duties, influence on the appearance of unexpected emotions.

The first step to overcome negative effects of emotions is to get to know them better. Being sensitive to one's own moods and the awareness of how they can affect the others before they receive the message, facilitate an effective communication. It is useful to try to better know the emotional reactions of other people, and to be prepared to deal with them. Developing trust, confidence and openness leads to secure communication without unnecessary emotions and defensive attitudes.

5. **Incompatibility of Messages:** When a verbal (words) message is incompatible with non-verbal (body language) message it brings confusion to a communication process. This type of barriers may appear regardless of the will of communicating people, and its source may be, among others, the suppressed emotions. Inadequate gestures, body posture, face expression is the basis for the misunderstanding and impede the proper reception of the message.

In the medical environment a very relevant element that may cause an incompatibility of messages is the outfit. It is a kind of label that defines the role of an individual member of the team. Wearing a uniform inadequate for the role may affect the authority or incorrect targeting of messages. The basis for eliminating these incompatibilities is being aware of them and avoiding sending false messages. Gestures, outfit, posture, face expression and other significant non-verbal messages should be compatible with the verbal ones.

6. **Distrust:** The credibility of a message mostly is determined by the credibility of the sender (knowledge, honesty, mutual relationships). The sender who has previously distinguished himself with a lack of professionalism or has not stood up to his role may cause that his message would not be received in a proper way. Overcoming distrust relies mostly on building trust. The credibility is a result of long-term process in which people respect honesty, justice and good intentions of a person.

The Styles of Communication

We distinguish basic communication styles: introversive, extroversive, defensive, bargaining and effective communication style.

The introversive style is represented by people who are trying to limit communication with others, who are withdrawn, not interested in opinions, attitudes and emotions of other members of the organization. If the leader represents this style of communication – it may be seen in autocratic style of leadership; if several introverts meet together, we can expect a little creativity of team's members and low efficiency of work.

The extroversive style is represented by people focusing on their own ideas and feelings wanting to show them to the others, but at the same time not being open for other people's suggestions. Leaders representing this style of communication are concentrating all the attention on themselves, they are unable to listen what other members of a team have to say and they do not like criticism that is aimed to them. This communication style may lead to insecurity and be threatening to the members of the team.

The defensive style is presented by people who attempt to test and judge the others, but do not let other people to know their feelings and views. This style creates the atmosphere of distrust amongst members of the team.

The bargaining style is represented by the people who receive the feedback information, are open to the others but at the same time expect reciprocity. This style may cause anxiety and limit coworkers.

The effective communication style is represented by flexible people that are open to others. Such persons are able to accept criticism of own actions and gain experience with feedback. They are great members of a team and wonderful leaders.

The Rules of Efficient Communication in Therapeutic Team

The effectiveness of communication depends on similarity of communication skills, attitudes, level of education, social experiences and cultural aspects of the participants of that process. The bigger differences between mentioned features, the bigger probability of failure in communication. Ineffectiveness of communication imply that the meaning of a message created by a receiver will be different from the meaning established by a sender. Effective communication is determined by proper understanding of the message. Despite the specific organization of Polish healthcare, it needs to be repeated that an extensive network of contacts makes communicating and resolving problems many times easier. Situational requirements (e.g. the presence of the patient) often cause external stiffening and formalizing communication between the people from the same group of friends that are on different levels of the professional structure. This 'formality' of communication is supposed to present workers as professional and competent persons in order to create in a patient the feeling of trust and security. We can speak about an effective communication within a therapeutic team, when all the members understand messages transmitted by the rest of the group and are able to communicate with each other in an understandable way. Achieving success in this field depends only and exclusively on understanding rules controlling the process of communication, and on implementing those rules into real life by all team members. The base of a proper attitude towards colleagues from a team is achieving an emotional maturity and proper self-esteem. It results in healthy and adequate reactions (Motyka, 2010).

In the effective communication words are the main substance of a message, but the body language, timbre of voice, gestures and the body posture are the context in which the message is embedded.

It has a special meaning in situation when communication takes place in inconvenient conditions, such as in a hospital ward, and messages refer to incredibly important matters from a point of view of a patient's good.

When the goal of communication is to achieve an agreement in such relevant matters as health and life of a patient, the members of a therapeutic team should upskill at various levels the techniques of communication and react to every problem by implementing corrective action.

The term ‘motivation’ has a lot of meanings. It means willingness and readiness to undertake an action. The motivation is a complex and complicated process. It is the result of the fact that every person has different needs and goals. Motivational factors in medical professions, thus the amount of remuneration, the ability to upgrade one’s qualifications by participating in courses, trainings and many other forms of upskilling, the working conditions and cooperation in an interdisciplinary team, may be individual. The employee’s needs analysis carried out by team leaders allows to create proper working conditions, motivates the employee and thereby improves the quality of provided services and the image of the workplace.

About positive relationships within a therapeutic team also decides a motivation system: homogeneous, fair and transparent. It is unacceptable to favor one employee to another. Obviously, there will be disproportions resulting from the level of education or responsibilities (e.g. difference in earnings), but it should be adequate to the role.

The feeling of injustice may be raised by an unjustified inequality in an access to such motivators as the ability of upgrading qualifications, attractive working conditions or even appreciation and respect of others.

The members of a team that feel underestimated in any aspect may less effective in realizing their responsibilities or cause conflicts. Similarly, a properly constructed motivational system encourages all the members of a therapeutic team to greater commitment, builds a sense of responsibility in them and makes the team focus on achieving set goals. Speaking of medical and medically related professions it is worth to remember about internal motivators that are results of emotions, such as internal needs, will to help others or the need to do good. If the members of a therapeutic team consider such motivators as important element that determines realization of professional responsibilities, one can be sure that these responsibilities will be executed with the utmost care.

The Motivation as the Basis for Effective Cooperation

The motivation in every profession is an important element building involvement to realization of assigned duties. The ready recipe for choosing ideal motivators does not exist, because everyone is motivated to work by different factors. The views on motivation have evolved as people learn about nature and mechanisms contributing to specific behaviors. This was the subject of discussion for representatives of many sciences, starting with psychology, philosophy, theology, sociology and ending at management (Król & Ludwiczyński, 2007).

The key to satisfaction and at the same time to increasing internal motivation is the knowledge of individual needs of employees and the adjustment of proper tools to particular people. Every organization should have its own motivational system that would have an efficient impact on its employees, encourage to beneficial behavior and discourage to negative actions. The lack of such system results in restriction of professional activity, because there is no encouragement, motivation and a punctual reception of salary becomes the main goal for the employee (Pagórski & Markiewicz, 2015). In medical professions the motivational system may be slightly different from the other professions and it often refers to a possibility of fulfilling the need to help others.

The members of a therapeutic team despite of financial motivators also value the appreciation of patients and top management, a good atmosphere and communication at work, possibilities for development and promotion. However, it is impossible to hide the fact that the remuneration is necessary to meet the basic needs of employees. Even the most sophisticated motivational system will not be effective, if the employee feels that his remuneration is lower than he deserves.

Therefore, when implementing motivational factors, it is worth to remember that the non-financial motivation should always go together with the financial one.

Unfortunately, the disproportions in earnings of particular members of therapeutic team are visible and substantial. Despite the fact that the basis of their work is a common goal – the health of the patient, the role of each team member is different and differently paid.

Big differences in earnings may be a source of conflict and make the less paid employee feel underestimated, what may have a direct impact on involvement in realization of entrusted responsibilities. Financial disproportions may be balanced by the non-financial motivators. There is a wide range of them.

These valued the most by employees are: recognition and appreciation of work by superiors and other members of the group, optimal workplace equipment, and possibility of professional upskilling in a form of subsidized courses, trainings or conferences. Also, the atmosphere in the workplace, sense of community and co-responsibility are very important.

The motivator that enables the whole team to unite is mutual defining of the goal and building a strategy that will lead to its realization. Members of the team that participated in defining the goal are more engaged in work because they feel responsible for their decisions.

The level of motivation should be raised regularly by using different tools. The employees are getting used to applied mechanisms and are able to fully appreciate them only twice: when they get them and when they lose them. Therefore, using the same impulses on should try to increase their dose in order to maintain their motivating influence. The best option is, however, to differentiate used motivators.

The Possibility of Professional Development of Team Members: The Role in Building Proper Relationships

The signs of our times are ongoing changes in a social and economic life. In each field can be observed faster pace of development and it translates to important changes in a social awareness.

A care for high qualifications of the employees became noticeable and it guarantees the development of institution. A whole healthcare system submitted to these trends. In the old days, the purpose of health services was to help the ill members of society, what is included in the term of 'service'.

Nowadays, this term went out of date and is replaces with 'healthcare system'.

The efficient functioning of that system is possible thanks to implementing mechanisms that are used in every large organizations.

Healthcare facilities are, nowadays, companies guided by the rules of the regulated market, whose purpose is the provision of diagnostic, preventive and therapeutic services. The patient is a client with a greater awareness, which means that his requirements towards a service provider (the hospital) are raising. In order to meet the requirements of a patient-client it is essential to improve qualifications of every member of a therapeutic team.

Professional development of every member of a therapeutic team is an important component in improving quality of provided services, which affects increase of a patient's satisfaction level, therefore its role seems to be incredibly important.

Moreover, professional development is a process that takes place during a human life-span, and is associated with activities, achievements, but also with existence, expression and self-realization.

The possibilities of professional development stem from certain individual characteristics, self-motivation, but also from the conditions offered by the employer to the employee.

With a term of professional development is assigned the issue of the vocational training, which – if is properly realized - extends competence and skills of the employee (Brudecka, 2007).

Everyone with broad knowledge significantly influences the quality and effectiveness of the organization.

In the aspect of the team members vocational training the postgraduate education should be mentioned. It includes all strictly defined forms of the vocational training regulated by the legal rules. The vocational training is a broad term that includes postgraduate education and also other forms of gaining knowledge (not necessarily institutionalized ones) (Stychlerz, 2008).

The main goal of the postgraduate education is to improve the skills of quick and flexible accepting new tasks and adjusting them to social needs, such as: filling in the gaps resulting from the progress of medical and common knowledge, developing organizational skills, ability to resolve professional problems, intellectual and educational skills, development of proper ethical attitudes (Ksynkiewicz-Dorota, 2005).

One should also remember, that despite of the 'formal' vocational training resulting from the legal rules (such as: training, specialist, qualification courses and specializations) exists also informal training.

An example of such training may be an intra-company training or any kind of conference organized outside of the workplace. Altogether it creates perfect conditions for the development and the vocational training of therapeutic team members.

In all the forms of vocational training the emphasis is on the ability to self-study. It is a complex activity that consists in a self-gaining of knowledge and skills, but also in changing attitudes and behaviors.

Regardless of the position of education in the structure of professional activity, an individual ability to self-study is very important. In situation where the access to courses is difficult (a price, a profile) self-education – organized and individual – may satisfy the need for a professional improvement. Self-education is not only a self-access to the source of knowledge, but also an action enhancing knowledge acquisition skills (Felcenloben, 2007).

The undertaking of vocational training is associated with dedication of time and other material and non-material means.

Workplaces expect from an employee a continuous upskilling, but often they do not want to share responsibility for that process.

The members of a therapeutic team in order to meet those expectations and professionally develop, are often forced to bear all the costs associated with the vocational training. Workplaces are not obliged to share the costs of courses and trainings chosen by employees. Hospitals deal with these issues individually, depending on the fund they have and the level of usefulness of particular forms of employee training for the functioning of the institution.

For the members of a therapeutic team that are working on professional development an important matter, except holidays, vacations, days off and financial support, may be an access to resources collected at workplaces.

They may include: electronic resources, literature, scientific aids or other teaching aids. Also, very important is help of the superiors and other, better educated coworkers.

Nowadays a lot of hospitals has a bibliographic database, in which a scientific literature is collected. An access to it gives an opportunity to continuous broadening of knowledge.

Workplaces may also contribute to a professional development by allowing participation in conferences, symposia and trainings organized by scientific institutions.

Each of these forms of support affects an educational activity of employees. The bigger support is, the more evident is the increase of interest in individual vocational training.

The benefits for members of the team that are participating in vocational training are mostly the personality development and meeting the needs of self-realization. Moreover, their competences and professional abilities are broadening, which results in better contacts with a patient and his family. But most of all the relationships within a team are improving. The material aspect of vocational training is also relevant, because there exist healthcare facilities that reward learning employees with different kinds of cash bonuses.

The structure of medical environment in particular healthcare facilities is highly hierarchized both formally and informally.

From all the factors that change the position of the team members at the workplace, the level of education seems to be highly relevant.

For the workplace the broad knowledge and skills of the employee are resulting in improvement of the quality and effectiveness of work, fast adaptation to the environment and also elimination of the rivals.

Vocational training allows also better cooperation of particular members with the whole therapeutic team.

Well educated coworker that has broad knowledge become an equal partner in a treatment process.

It is worth to emphasize that the most important addressee of services provided by the therapeutic team is a patient. He is the one who takes full advantage of the fact that the members are continuously upskilling.

Thanks to that they can quickly recognize the health needs of their patient and understand his situation thoroughly. This increases the quality of care taken over the patient and changes the subjective assessment of received services.

SUMMARY

The treatment process of a patient requires involvement of many people - in medicine it is called a therapeutic team. At the basis of a teamwork lies the holistic philosophy, which is defined in medicine as a comprehensive treatment of a patient as a bio-psycho-social unity.

The efficiency of team's actions as a whole, as well as each individual member is conditioned by proper relationships in a team.

When there are interactions between team members, conflicts are inevitable. There are many causes of conflicts and often they are difficult to define. It is important to resolve the conflict in a constructive way, so it could not affect a treatment process and the good of the patient.

The key role seems to be the role of a team leader, who is supposed to motivate and lead the team to the resolution of the conflict. It may be done by negotiating, mediating or other adequate methods.

A good therapeutic team is the one with the proper communication patterns, which enable mutual understanding and more clear flow of information.

The team motivational system that is transparent and fair for all the members is also relevant for building positive relationships within a team. It raises the morale and encourages all members to more effective work with the benefit of the patient.

It is also worth to emphasize that a good team is the one that has a chance to develop, improve on a professional and social fields and such possibilities should be created for the team.

REFERENCES

Aniszewska, G. (2007). *Kultura organizacyjna w zarządzaniu* (p. 23). Warszawa: Polskie Wydawnictwo Ekonomiczne.

Babska K., Tkaczyk M., & Nowicki M. (2008). Współpraca w zespole terapeutycznym – Podstawowa zasada profesjonalnej opieki nad chorym dializowanym otrzewnowo – założenia a rzeczywistość. *Pol Merk Lek*, *14*(12 Suppl. 4), 12-14.

Bodak, A. (2007). Skuteczność w komunikacji wewnętrznej we współczesnych zespołach pracowniczych. In S. Rudolf (Ed.), *Perspektywy rozwoju partycypacji pracowniczej w Polsce w warunkach Unii Europejskiej*. Wydawnictwo Uniwersytetu Łódzkiego.

Brudecka, B. (2007). Rozwój kształcenia pielęgniarek. *Magazyn Pielęgniarki i Położnej*, *6*, 13–14.

Czerw, A., Religioni, U., Matuszna, A., Lesiak, K., Olejnik, A., & Śniadała, D. (2012). Principles of effective communication in medical entities. *Hygeia Public Health*, *47*(3), 247–253.

Dobek-Ostrowska, B. (1999). *Podstawy komunikowania społecznego*. Wrocław: Wyd. Astrum.

Fejfer-Wirbał, E., Gładczuk, J., & Marcinowicz, L. (2013). Relacje lekarz-pielęgniarka w polskiej literaturze medycznej. *Medycyna Rodzinna*, *1*, 19–22.

Felcenloben, M. (2007). Samokształcenie pielęgniarek i położnych. *Magazyn Pielęgniarki i Położnej*, *4*, 13–14.

Frydrychowicz, S. (2009). Komunikacja interpersonalna w zarządzaniu, *Wydawnictwo Forum Naukowe Poznań*, 17.

Glińska, J., & Lewandowska, M. (2007). Autonomiczność zawodu pielęgniarskiego w świadomości pielęgniarek z uwzględnieniem pełnionych funkcji zawodowych. *Problemy Pielęgniarstwa*, *15*(4), 249–253.

Gordon, T. (1998). *Wychowanie bez porażek w praktyce*. Warszawa: Instytut Wydawniczy PAX.

Greenhalgh, L. (1986). Managing conflict. *Sloan Management Review*, *27*(4), 45–51.

Grzesiuk, L. (2001). *Umiejętności menedżera. Psychologia stosowana dla menedżerów, Wydawnictwo Wyższej Szkoły Handlu i Prawa im.* Warszawa: Ryszarda Łazarskiego.

Jankowiak, B., & Bartoszewicz, A. (2003). Komunikowanie się w obrębie zespołu terapeutycznego In A. Kwiatkowska, E. Krajewska – Kułak, C. Czabała et al. (Eds.). Komunikowanie interpersonalne w pielęgniarstwie (pp. 117-126). Czelej, Lublin: Wyd.

Janowska, J. (2016). Cztery wymiary komunikowania się w organizacji. *Marketing i Rynek*, *3*, 252–262.

Janowska, Z. (2014). The role of management in the adaptation of multicultural work teams. *Prace Naukowe Uniwersytetu Ekonomicznego we Wrocławiu*, *349*, 120-129.

Januszek, H., & Sikora, J. (1997). *Podstawy socjologii* (p. 37). Poznań: Wyd. AE.

Jasiński, Z. (2016). Decisions made by organizer of an employees' teams making their functioning difficult. *Prace Naukowe Uniwersytetu Ekonomicznego we Wrocławiu*, *421*, 199-204.

Kapała, W. (2007). Lekarze i pielęgniarki – w stronę aktywnego współdziałania. *Nowoczesne Pielęgniarstwo i Położnictwo*, *1*, 1–14.

Kilmann, R., & Thomas, K. W. (1974). *Thomas-Kilmann Conflict Mode Instrument. Xicom*. Tuxedo.

Kratochvil, S. (2016). *Terapia małżeńska* (p. 123). Gdańsk: Via Medica.

Król, H., & Ludwiczyński, A. (2007). Zarządzanie zasobami ludzkimi. Tworzenie kapitału ludzkiego organizacji. Warszawa. *PWN*, *31*, 336.

Ksynkiewicz-Dorota, A. (2005). *Zarządzanie w Pielęgniarstwie*. Lublin: Czelej.

Leslie, R. C. (1983). Management of Conflict. *Industrial Management & Data Systems*, *83*(1/2), 77. doi:10.1108/eb057300 PMID:6551214

Marciniak, J. (2011). *Mobbing, dyskryminacja, molestowanie – zasady przeciwdziałania* (p. 59). Warszawa: Wolters Kluwer Polska.

Meller, D., & Milik, A. (2014). Komunikacja interpersonalna w zakładach opieki zdrowotnej. *Zarządzanie i Finanse Journal of Management and Finance*, *12*(2), 133–144.

Mikułowski Pomorski, J. (2003). *Komunikacja międzykulturowa. Wprowadzenie*. Kraków: Wyd. AE.

Mohrman, S. A., Cohen, S. G., & Mohrman, A. M. (1995). *Designing team based organizations: New forms for knowledge work*. San Francisco: Jossey-Bass.

Motyka, H. (2010). Komunikacja interpersonalna w opiece medycznej. *Medycyna Rodzinna*, *4*, 124–128.

Nęcki, Z. (1995). *Negocjacje w biznesie*. Kraków: Wydawnictwo Profesjonalnej Szkoły Biznesu.

Osika G. (2000). Negocjacje-charakterystyka problemu *Organizacja i zarządzanie. Zeszyty naukowe politechniki śląskiej, 1467*(1), 55-65.

Pagórski P., & Markiewicz D. (2015). Motivating employees of some hospital with a particular emphasis on nurses. *Pielęgniarstwo polskie, 2*(56),216-224.

Pawlak, J. (2015). The Influence of Subjectivity and Employee Participation on Team Involvement and Responsibility during Times of Change. *Zeszyty Naukowe Uniwersytetu Ekonomicznego w Krakowie*, *944*(08), 57–67. doi:10.15678/ZNUEK.2015.0944.0805

Potocki, A., Winkler, R., & Żbikowska, A. (2011). Komunikowanie w organizacjach gospodarczych. *Wydawnictwo Difin Warszawa,* 16-18.

Prawelska-Skrzypek, G., & Lenartowicz, M. (2013). Badanie organizacji i zarządzania na gruncie humanistyki. *Problemy Zarządzania*, *11*(4), 45–57. doi:10.7172/1644-9584.44.4

Reetz-Wasielewska, A. E., Kretowicz, K., & Zarzeczna-Baran, M. (2016). Konflikt w zespole pielęgniarskim. *Problemy Pielęgniarstwa*, *24*(2), 125–130.

Robbins, S. (2001). *Zasady zachowania w organizacji*. Poznań: Zysk i S-ka.

Rogoda, B. (2013). Zarządzanie konfliktem i przeciwdziałanie mobbingowi a intensyfikacja procesów innowacyjnych. *Nierówności Społeczne a Wzrost Gospodarczy*, *46*(2), 289–301. doi:10.15584/nsawg.2016.2.16

Rozkwitalska, M. (2011). *Bariery w zarządzaniu międzykulturowym*. Warszawa: Wolters Kluwer Polska.

Rzeźnik, M. (2011). *Zarządzanie komunikacją w zespole projektowym. Warszawa: Wydawnictwo PJWSTK.*

Śmiatacz, K., Michalska, A., & Samek, K. (2014). Rola komunikacji w unikaniu błędów menedżerskich. *Marketing i Rynek*, *10*, 484–489.

Sobkowiak, B. (1998). Procesy komunikowania się w organizacji. In B. Dobek-Ostrowska (Ed.), *Współczesne systemy komunikowania* (pp. 22–40). Wrocław: Wyd. UW.

Stanisz-Busch, E. (2010). *Podstawy zarządzania marketingowego w placówce Medycznej*. Poznań: Wolters Kluwer.

Stankiewicz, J. (1999). *Komunikowanie się w organizacji*. Wrocław: Wyd. Astrum.

Stewart, J. (2010). *Mosty zamiast murów. Podręcznik komunikacji interpersonalnej*. Warszawa: Wydawnictwo Naukowe PWN.

Stychlerz, A. (2008). Dyplom to nie wszystko. *Magazyn Pielęgniarki i Położnej*, *1-2*, 15.

Świątek, W. (2016). Rola lidera w innowacyjnej organizacji. *Zarządzanie Zasobami Ludzkimi*, *1*, 9–23.

Syrkiewicz, O., Ewitała, M., Holecki, T., & Kotowski, P. (2012). Koncepcja marketingowego zarządzania organizacją świadczącą usługi medyczne. *Zarządzanie i Edukacja*, *82*.

Szary, S. (2013). Nowoczesna medycyna w służbie człowiekowi. *Hygeia Public Health*, *48*(1), 17–20.

Szary, S., & Knotowicz, J. (2014). Different aspects of holism in medicine and physiotherapy. In Fizjoterapia wobec nowych wyzwań (pp. 7-17). Poznań: Wydawnictwo WSEiT.

Targosz-Krysik, B. (1997). *Urzeczywistnienie zasad demokratycznych w uczącej się organizacji*. Edukacja Dorosłych.

Tomaszewska M. (2008). Możliwości doskonalenia zawodowego pielęgniarek – potrzeby a rzeczywistość. *Problemy pielęgniarstwa*, *16*(1-2).

Trippner-Hrabi, J. (2014). Etapy rozwoju zespołów zadaniowych w organizacjach. *Przedsiębiorczość i Zarządzanie*, *15*(6), 189–2001.

Walton, R. E., & Dutton, J. M. (1969). The management of interdepartmental conflict: A model and review. *Administrative Science Quarterly*, *14*(1), 73–84. doi:10.2307/2391364

Waszkiewicz, P. (2009). Zasady mediacji. In E. Gmurzyńska & R. Morka (Ed.), *Mediacje. Teorie i praktyka* (pp. 91-105). Warszawa: Oficyna a Wolters Kluwer business.

Werachowska, L., Damps-Konstańska, I., Janowicz, A., & Krakowiak, P. (2013). Medical caregiver as a new member of the therapeutic team for chronic ill and elderly patients. *Problemy Pielęgniarstwa, 21*(2), 235–241.

Włodarczak, W. (2009). Pielęgniarstwo w Polsce i na świecie. Kompendium wiedzy dla studentów pielęgniarstwa. In *Państwowa Wyższa Szkoła Zawodowa im. Stanisława Staszica w Pile.* Wyd. Tekst Bydgoszcz.

Wolniak, R. (2012). *Wymiary kulturowe polskich organizacji a doskonalenie zarządzanie jakością.* Warszawa: Ce-DeWu.

Żuchowski, I. (2009). Wybrane aspekty procesu szkoleniowego w praktyce działalności małych i średnich przedsiębiorstw. *Przegląd organizacji*, 7-8.

Chapter 13
Managed Healthcare:
Doctor Life Satisfaction and Its Impact on the Process of Communicating With the Patient

Anna Rosiek
Ross-Medica, Poland

Aleksandra Rosiek-Kryszewska
Nicolaus Copernicus University, Poland

ABSTRACT

Satisfaction with life is very important for a doctor, as it affect his clinical practice. The aim of this chapter is to analyze doctor satisfaction with life, its influence on the communication process and the doctor's daily job activities. Data was collected from a group of 40 doctors from the Kuyavian-Pomeranian Voivodeship surgical ward and the non-surgical division. The satisfaction with life depends on the gender of the doctor ($p < 0.05$). The life satisfaction results, remained statistically significant, based on the average correlation value to the communication process with the patients ($p < 0.05$). A higher level of life satisfaction was observed in the group of doctors from non-surgical wards.

INTRODUCTION

Life satisfaction is of great importance for a doctor, as it influences clinical practice. It affects the mental hygiene, general physical well-being, social relationships and raises or lowers the quality of their occupational activities (Surman, 2015). Satisfaction with life remains in correlation with positive emotions, such as happiness or sense of knowing own place in the world (Yoshiaki, 2015; Coomber, 2007): the concept of oneself, acceptance of own limitations and values are all affecting the general concept of life satisfaction. Both the overall life satisfaction and satisfaction with such an important element like the occupational activity may be an important psychosocial resource, significantly conditioning the quality of occupational duties. Since work is an important part of our lives, it must be rewarding and give the

DOI: 10.4018/978-1-5225-3946-9.ch013

opportunities for development (Bhatnagar, 2012). In literature you can rarely find anything about the relationship between the doctor's overall satisfaction with life and performed activities, like the process of communicating with the patient.

Effective Clinical Communication

Effective clinical communication is a key element in the medical services. Effective communication is dependent on communication skills, attitudes, education and social experiences of people who communicate with each other. Differences within the characteristics or behavior can lead to failures in the communication process. Effective communication takes place, therefore, if the message is properly communicated and understood by the recipient.

Contact with a person who is ill is a specific relationship. Massages communicated to the patient must be tailored to his abilities and also take into account other restrictions such as difficulties with hearing, sight or speech. Getting to know the patient via his needs and expectations forms the basis for establishing a therapeutic communication (Jopkiewicz, 2011). Patients and their families expect safe care during treatment. Communication cannot be one-sided, mechanical; there must be an exchange of information that will be interpreted by all participants in the process. Such communication is therefore a positive action.

Many researchers analyzing the issue of clinical communication draws attention to the joint decision model (Shared Decision Making - SDM). It occurs when patients and physicians work together to reach a decision medical adjusted to the values and expectations of the patient. Shared decision-making model is also important for patients of ethnic minorities, as it contributes to the reduction of cultural barriers and mistrust towards the patients and staff of the proposed treatment methods. The main objective is, however, security and building trust (DeMeester, 2016). Particular importance of model plays in treatment of the terminal. Effective communication between the patient, family and team of medical care is very important in the care of the sick. Patients with cancer have special communication needs. Both the patients and their families want to get as much medical information from doctors and medical staff to make choices and make the right decision on how to treat and care for the sick (Teutsch, 2003).

Interesting look at effective communication proposed L. Gordon Moore and John H. Wasson. The researchers presented one of the ideal model of medical practice (Ideal Medical Practice Model-IMP), which aims to strengthen the doctor-patient relationship, and also extend the time of direct contact between doctor and patient, vaccinate patients a sense of responsibility for their health and to lower total healthcare costs (Gordon Moore). Therefore, wanting to enable effective interaction of physicians, patients and health care workers must create the right conditions for the free flow of information, ie. to facilitate the patient to express themselves, be heard no objection, in concentration, understanding and acceptance (Maciąg, 2004).

Effective communication exists when compliance with the following attitudes exists: authenticity, acceptance, empathy, assertiveness and when communication goals are defined:

1. Establishing and maintaining relationships
2. Determining the nature of the problem and monitoring of the progress
3. Provisioning of information about treatment plans and implementing a method of treatment

Combining the main objectives of effective communication of clinical propose Model Effective Clinical Communication (ECC Model). This model assumes minimize the distance that exists between doctor and patient and health professionals through support, respect and understanding of the situation in which he found the patient. From these factors depends on whether you developed mutual trust between the healthcare provider and the beneficiary of medical service.

Effective Communication Model (ECC Model) is shown in Figure 1.

- **Development of Relationship:** Building a relationship that safe for the patient; friendly and courteous atmosphere during medical interview; getting the patient to cooperate
- **Understanding:** Listening to the patient, expressed understanding for his emotions
- **Assistance:** Striving to meet the needs of the patient, signaling the willingness to talk about any subject directing patient's behavior- changes to his lifestyle, reducing anxiety and uncertainly
- **Respect:** Honoring patient's decisions, preservation of intimacy

While looking for ways to communicate effectively in the treatment process, it should be noted that the interest of both parties is common. Each side wants to achieve the success, that is to smoothly lead to a situation where the patient will once again enjoy good health.

Responsibility for the effectiveness of treatment lies on both sides- the doctor and the patient.

Doctors have, in the eyes of patients, extraordinary power. All the good and bad things happening during the treatment process are ascribed to the doctor: the rate of recovery, the length of waiting for a medical examination or availability the doctor however has limited influence on many of those things. The attitude to the patient is however well within the doctor's sphere of influence. Therefore, it is worthwhile to build partnership relations based on the presented model of effective communication. But to achieve this, the expectations must be clearly defined and expressed with respect to the other person. Meanwhile, as indicated by the opinions of patients and authors' own observations, contact between a doctor and a patient is predominantly diagnostic. The doctor should try to meet the patient's expectations both spheres: informational and emotional, which is particularly important for treatment of a chronic disease.

Figure 1. Effective Communication Model (ECC Model)

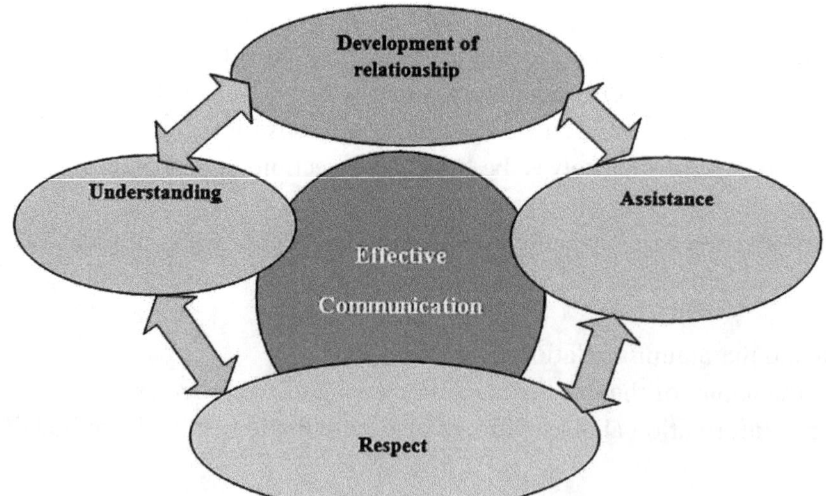

Clinical Communication in the World

From the time of its birth medicine has changed dramatically. Access to information and new technologies has shaped the modern medicine. It is difficult to be surprised by the growing public interest in communication in health care in the world. Especially in the United States there is intensive development in clinical communication, which is widely understood and practiced. It is especially important today, when the age-old forms of communication - through direct contact "face to face" are complemented by various media.

The authors have reviewed databases. Keywords used: doctor-patient communications and effective communications skills. Overview of the international literature and a number of studies conducted in this area show that negative experiences related to the lack of communication and stress associated with a visit to the doctor's office can be transformed into a positive therapeutic effect when the doctor and medical staff are empathetic and apply effective communication (Di Blasi, 2001; Rider, 2006; Yagil, 2015; Klakovich, 2006). Similar evidence can be obtained from the experiment conducted by psychologists under the direction of G. Lester, who confirmed the hypothesis that inadequate interpersonal communication between doctor and patient increases the risk of a claim for damages, and also means that the doctor is rated as less competent. Researchers around the world, including Poland, recognize the fact that a medical visit is a special form of interpersonal communication. As demonstrated by Cacioppo and colleagues each meeting of two people causes psychological responses (Cacioppo, 1990). The reaction is even stronger in medical meetings, since they bring together people of different social status. Thus, the researchers perceive the need to introduce worldwide effective clinical communication to make a substantial reconstruction in the doctor-patient relationship, at least to an extent that "modern medicine" is not a substitute for traditional relations in the field of communication.

Proper communication between doctor and patient during treatment process in a hospital ward plays an important role for especially for the patients, because it helps to understand the medical information submitted to them (Kissane, 2012; Williams, 2007; van Woerkum, 2003). It is essential to better understand the needs and expectations of the patient, because it allows the physician to control patients emotions resulting from illness (Duffy, 2004; Weiner, 2004; Street, 2009). Life satisfaction studies were conducted among doctors to gain knowledge about the factors of better communication with the patient. Detailed analysis of the collected data answers the question whether there is a link between the overall life satisfaction of a doctor and his ability to communicate with the patient. The results of the research are important for filling the knowledge gap, because the relationship between life satisfaction perceived by physicians and the perception of their professional role involves both the medical aspect associated with taking care of the patient, professional contacts in the workplace, as well as external influences from the work environment. This aspect also has never been studied in Polish population. This study fills the gaps in the literature and needs to be highlighted.

Material and Methods

The study has enrolled 40 doctors divided into two groups – from non-surgical wards (20 doctors) and surgical wards (20 doctors). After hearing the form and course of the research from presented instructions, testing and checking the understanding of the commands contained within, everybody completed the questionnaire. The study used Satisfaction with Life Scale (SWLS). The scale SWLS is designed to test adults, both healthy and ill (Larsen, Diener, Emmons, 1985). The scale of satisfaction with life contains five statements. The test assesses the degree to which any of the claims refers to its present life. The result of the measurement is the overall sense of satisfaction with life. The results of SWLS in the study were converted into sten scores. (The Sten (standard ten) is a standard score system commonly used with personality questionnaires. Stens divide the score scale into ten units. Each unit has a band width of half a standard deviation except the highest unit (Sten 10) which extends from 2 standard deviations above the mean, and the lowest unit (Sten 1) which extends from 2 standard deviations below the mean (Juszczyński Z., 2009). The results within 1-4 represent the results stens low value, sten 5 and 6 are regarded as the results of the average, and from 7 to 10 as a high stens (Table 1).

In addition to obtain information on the factors of better communication between doctor and patient, authors checked whether there is a correlation between satisfaction with life and the performance of his/her professional activities. Doctors were asked about issues such as: being available for patients, are the recommendations understandable for the patient before the end of medical consultation or what is the biggest difficulty in effective communication with the patient. The physicians were asked 22 questions about their professional activities. Then the correlation of every question with the general life satisfaction was checked.

Spearman's rank correlation coefficient was used for the calculation of the strength of relationship in analyzed categories. The strength of the correlations (R Spearman) was determined according to the following criteria:

below ± 0.2 → slight correlation (almost negligible relationship)

from ± 0.2 to ± 0.4 → low correlation (definite relationship)

from ± 0.4 to ± 0.6 → moderate correlation (substantial relationship)

from ± 0.6 to ± 0.8 → high correlation (marked relationship)

from ± 0.8 to ± 0.9 → very high correlation (very dependable relationship)

Table 1. Point values and sten SWLS

Stens Value	Point Value	Results
1	5-9	Low value
2	10-11	
3	12-14	
4	15-17	
5	18-20	Average value
6	21-23	
7	24-26	High value
8	27-28	
9	29-30	
10	31-35	

from ± 0.9 to ± 1.0 → practically complete correlation

Scatter diagrams which show the cardinality of concurrent points with coordinates determined by two variables in order to emphasize the different weights of the points were used for the presentation of parametric dependence.

The study were approved by the Bioethics Committee of the Collegium Medicum in Bydgoszcz.

The results of the study were analyzed statistically using the non-parametric Spearman test with Spearman's rank correlation coefficient, Mann-Whitney U test, because the variables are qualitative. The minimum confidence level is determined to be $p < 0.05$.

All analysis and calculations were carried out in the statistical program Statistica 10.0 using standard spreadsheet functions of Microsoft Excel

RESULTS

Analysis Questionnaire SWLS

Demographic Data: Gender

Analysis by gender of doctors from both divisions revealed that males were a bigger group (60.0%). On the non-surgical wards there were more females (80.0%). In the surgical wards 100% of the participants were male. Given the level of $p < 0.05$ a significant statistical difference between the two groups of physicians by gender was observed. (Table 2).

A higher rate of high life satisfaction was recorded in the group of women - 41.7% at - 32.1% among men (Figure 2, Table 3). Slightly higher level of life satisfaction was recorded in the group of women.

Table 2. Physicians by gender

Ward	Non-Surgical		Surgical		Total		p Level
Gender	Number	%	Number	%	Number	%	
Female	16	80,0	0	0,0	16	40,0	p<0,05
Male	4	20,0	20	100,0	24	60,0	
Total	20	100,0	20	100,0	40	100,0	

Table 3. Results SWLS based on sex

Sex	Female		Male	
Results	Number	%	Number	%
Low	2	16,7	6	21,4
average	5	41,7	13	46,4
high	5	41,7	9	32,1
total	12	100,0	28	100,0

Figure 2. Distribution of the results of the average life satisfaction by gender

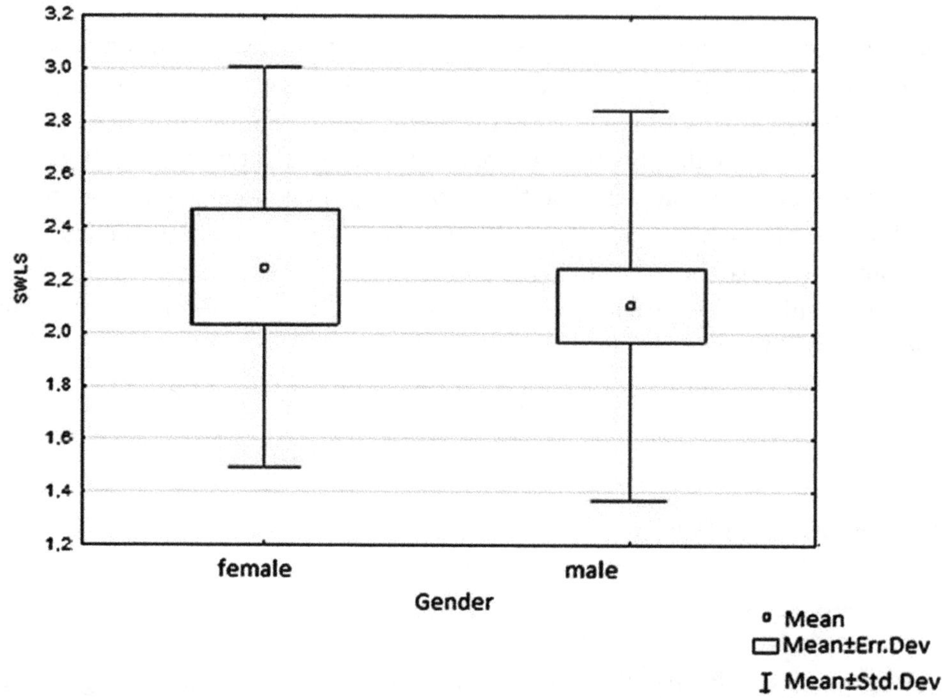

A higher rate of high level life satisfaction was observed in the group of doctors from non-surgical wards- 50.0%. In the group of doctors from the surgical wards this rate was 20%. Higher life satisfaction was recorded in the group of doctors from non-surgical wards (Figure 3, Table 4).

Age

Age group, which did not remain in a statistically significant correlation with the results of any position and the result of general life satisfaction (p> 0.05). The highest rate of high level life satisfaction was recorded in the age group 31-40 years - 45.5%. The lowest in over 60 years old - 27.8% (Figure 4).

Table 4. The results of SWLS in studied groups

Ward	Non-Surgical		Surgical	
Results	Number	%	Number	%
low	4	20,0	4	20,0
average	6	30,0	12	60,0
high	10	50,0	4	20,0
total	20	100,0	20	100,0

Figure 3. Distribution of the results of the average life satisfaction due to the ward

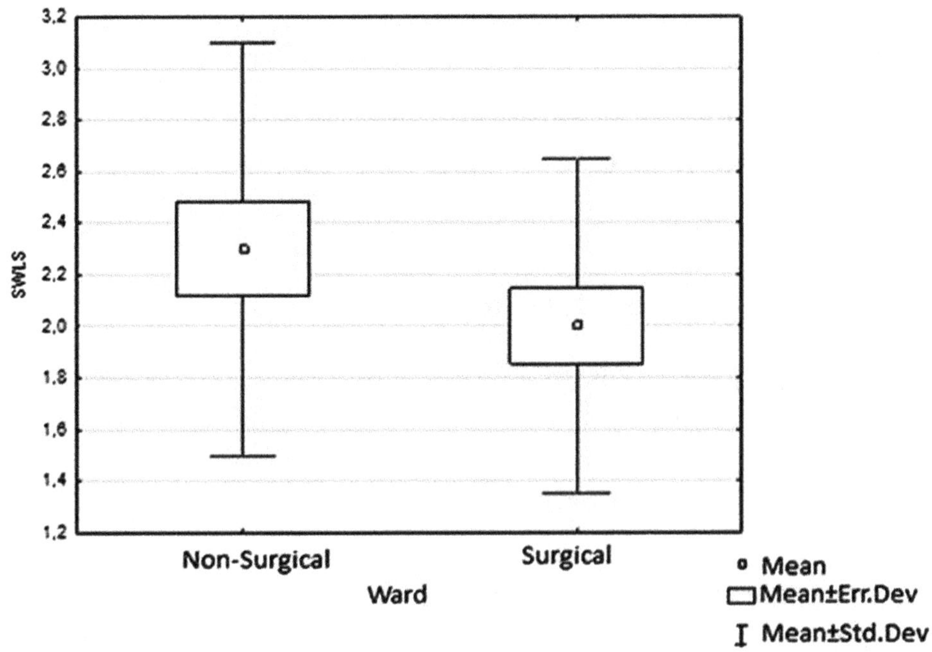

Figure 4. Distribution of the results of the average life satisfaction due to age

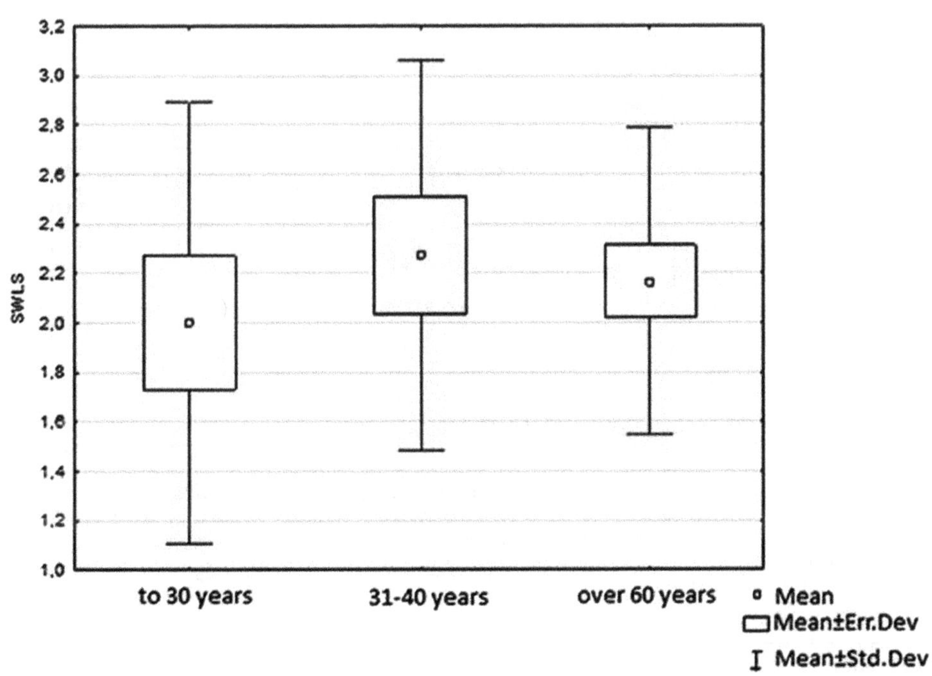

Satisfaction With Life: Sten and Point Value

Doctors as a group are people with an average level of life satisfaction, on the border of the high level. Both the average point result - 21.80 points, and the average sten result- 5.98 points (Table 5)

The highest rated statement was: "I am happy with my life" - average 5.20 point, and "I have achieved the most important things in life I wanted" - average 4.85 point. While the lowest position: "my life conditions are excellent" - average 3.90 points and "in many ways my life is close to perfect - average 3.70 point (Figure 5, Table 7, Table 8).

Differences in Life Satisfaction Between the Two Groups

Due to the level of significance ($p < 0.05$), there was a statistically significant difference between the groups regarding the position: in life I have achieved the most important things that I wanted. The "I am happy with my life, was" position on the border of significance (Table 8).

Table 5. The average value of the results of life satisfaction

Position	N	Average	Standard Deviation	Confidentiality -95,0%	Confidentiality +95,0%	Minimum	Maximum	Q25	Median	Q75
Points	40	21,80	4,558	20,34	23,26	12,0	32,0	19,0	21,5	25,0
Sten	40	5,98	1,687	5,44	6,51	3,0	10,0	5,0	6,0	7,0

Table 6. Results of satisfaction with life

Results	Number	%
Low level of satisfaction	8	20,0
medium level of satisfaction	18	45,0
high level of satisfaction	14	35,0
Total	40	100,0

Table 7. The averaged results of the position of life satisfaction

Position	$\overline{x}$	SD	Confidentiality -95,0%	Confidentiality +95,0%	Median	Min	Max
1. in many ways my life is close to perfect	3,70	1,620	3,18	4,22	4,0	1,0	7,0
2. my life conditions are excellent	3,90	1,446	3,44	4,36	4,0	1,0	7,0
3. I am quite happy with my life	5,20	0,723	4,97	5,43	5,0	4,0	7,0
4. I have achieved the most important things in life I wanted	4,85	1,001	4,53	5,17	5,0	2,0	7,0
5. I would not change a thing if I could live my life once again	4,15	1,460	3,68	4,62	4,0	1,0	7,0

Figure 5. Distribution of the average results of SWLS statements

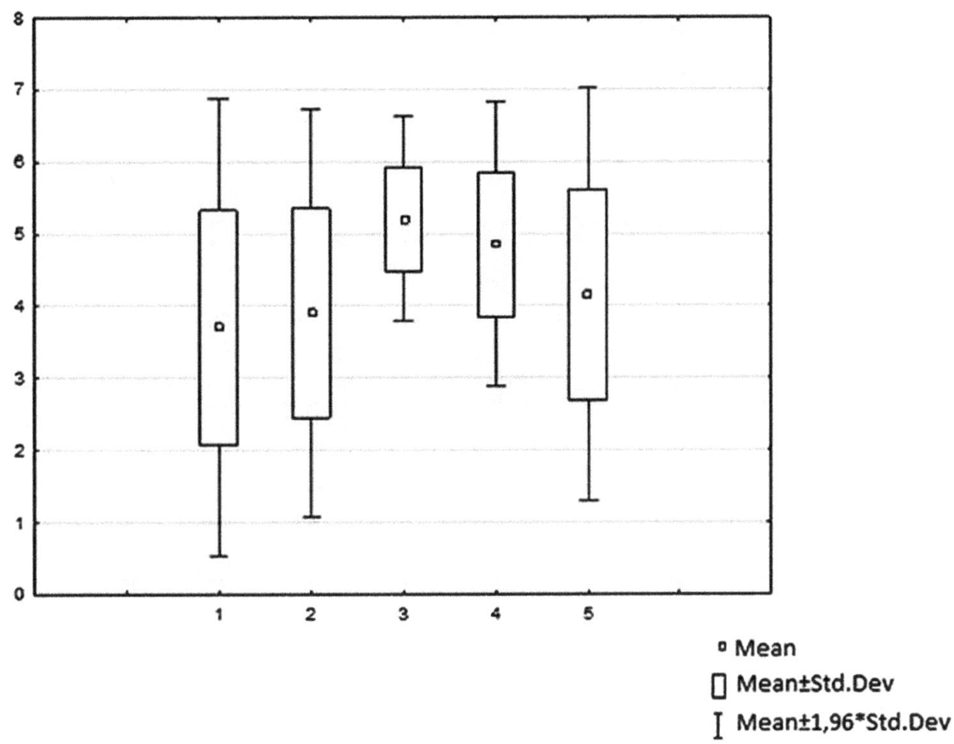

Table 8. Differences in life satisfaction between those two groups

Position	Sum. Rang Non-Surgical	Sum. Rang Surgical	U	Z	P Level	Z Popraw	P Level	N Ważn. Non-Surgical	N Ważn. Surgical	2*1str. Dokł. p
1	430,5	389,5	179,5	0,541	0,589	0,554	0,579	20	20	0,583
2	406,5	413,5	196,5	-0,081	0,935	-0,084	0,933	20	20	0,925
3	468,0	352,0	142,0	1,555	0,120	1,875	0,061	20	20	0,121
4	392,5	427,5	182,5	-0,460	0,646	-0,493	0,622	20	20	0,640
5	509,5	310,5	100,5	2,678	0,007	2,743	0,006	20	20	0,006
SWLS	458,0	362,0	152,0	1,285	0,199	1,387	0,166	20	20	0,201

The results of life satisfaction of surveyed physicians were statistically significant, average correlation with the results of aspects: In the time of need, how would you rate your availability for the patient, the biggest communication barrier between the doctor and the patient is, if you ask the patient before the end of the consultation to repeat instructions that the patient received during the visit and whether you think each medical consultation ends understandable to the patient instructions ($p < 0.05$). Results for position: "are you satisfied with the conversation with the patient", What methods do you use to reach an agreement with a "difficult patient" ?, "do you give the patient full information on the procedure in case of deterioration or lack of improvement in health", "in the course of medical consultation do you

Table 9. The average point results of SWLS positions in studied groups

Ward	Non-Surgical		Surgical	
Position	**Average**	**SD**	**AVERAGE**	**SD**
in many ways my life is close to perfect	3,85	1,79	3,55	1,47
my life conditions are excellent	3,85	1,57	3,95	1,36
I am quite happy with my life	5,40	0,68	5,00	0,73
I have achieved the most important things in life I wanted	4,85	0,75	4,85	1,23
I would not change a thing if I could live my life once again	4,80	1,20	3,50	1,43
SWLS	22,75	5,14	20,85	3,79

Table 10. Correlation between SWLS results and doctor's professional activities

No.	Occupational Activities	N	R	t(N-2)	Level p
1	Do you look at the medical records of a patient before the visit ?	40	0,143	0,892	0,378
2	Do you encourage your patient to discuss all ailments and health issues during medical consultation?	40	0,053	0,329	0,744
3	Do you think that the amount of time that you devote to a patient is sufficient ?	40	0,087	0,537	0,594
4	How would you rate your doctor-patient communication skills ?	40	0,075	0,466	0,644
5	Are you satisfied with the conversations with your patients ?	40	-0,290	-1,866	0,070
6	In the time of need, how would you rate your availability for the patient ?	40	0,337	2,208	0,033
7	In your opinion, do you clearly and in an understandable way describe the treatment and any side effects of prescribed drugs ?	40	0,149	0,928	0,359
8	do you always inform the patient about any complications that may occur during treatment ?	40	0,079	0,486	0,629
9	Are you always satisfied with the medical consultation you conducted ?	40	0,123	0,763	0,450
10	The biggest communication barrier between you and your patient is…	40	-0,403	-2,712	0,010
11	What are the best ways of overcoming the communication barrier ?	40	-0,140	-0,869	0,390
12	Is the time you devote to a patient sufficient enough to take the medical interview ?	40	-0,075	-0,462	0,647
13	What is the most common thing, that impede the relationship between doctor and patient ?	40	0,283	1,821	0,076
14	What is important in a doctor-patient relationship ?	40	-0,087	-0,540	0,592
15a	do you fully explain the health condition to the patient ?	40	0,043	0,263	0,794
15b	do you fully explain the method of treatment ?	40	0,090	0,556	0,581
15c	do you fully explain all information about any planed surgeries ?	40	-0,042	-0,258	0,798
15d	do you give you patient a comprehensive information on the procedure in case of deterioration or lack of health improvement ?	40	-0,306	-1,979	0,055
16	While talking with the patient do you take notice (point out) …	40	-0,230	-1,458	0,153
17	when the patient does not agree with the proposed therapy (diagnosis) are you able to persuade him/her to it ?	40	-0,063	-0,388	0,700
18	What methods do you use to reach an agreement with a "difficult patient" ?	40	0,006	0,036	0,972
19	During a medical consultation do you ask the patient if the treatment method is fully understandable and acceptable ?	40	-0,285	-1,832	0,075
20	during medical consultation do you ask your patient about any other, unrelated daily symptoms ?	40	-0,136	-0,847	0,402
21	do you write a note from the consultation for the patient and write down any essential information in the medical records ?	40	-0,134	-0,833	0,410
22	Do you ask the patient to repeat the recommendations at the end of the consultation ?	40	-0,363	-2,405	0,021
23	In your opinion, does every consultation ends with clear and understandable recommendations ?	40	-0,354	-2,333	0,025
24	Are you always satisfied with the consultation you have conducted?	40	0,018	0,113	0,911

Table 11. The results between the groups and aspects of life satisfaction

SWLS		Low		Medium		High	
Question	Answer	No.	%	No.	%	No.	%
In the time of need, how would you rate your availability for the patient	I am always available when the patient needs help or information	6	75,0	9	50,0	3	21,4
	When I am busy at the moment I will arrive the next free time I have	2	25,0	8	44,4	11	78,6
	Rather unavailable	0	0,0	1	5,6	0	0,0
The biggest communication barrier between you and your patient is…	Lack of trust	0	0,0	1	5,6	0	0,0
	Disease connected emotions	2	25,0	6	33,3	10	71,4
	Not understandable for patient usage of medical language	2	25,0	6	33,3	3	21,4
	I do not feel any barriers	4	50,0	5	27,8	1	7,1
Do you ask the patient to repeat the recommendations at the end of the consultation ?	Yes	0	0,0	0	0,0	2	14,3
	Rather yes	1	12,5	6	33,3	6	42,9
	Rather no	7	87,5	12	66,7	6	42,9
In your opinion, does every consultation ends with clear and understandable recommendations ?	Yes	1	12,5	5	27,8	5	35,7
	Rather yes	3	37,5	9	50,0	9	64,3
	Rather no	4	50,0	2	11,1	0	0,0
	I have no opinion	0	0,0	2	11,1	0	0,0

ask the patient whether the proposed method of treatment is understandable and fully accepted" were on the border of significance (Table 10).

Doctors with high SWLS results before the end of the consultation asking the patient to the greatest extent to repeat recommendations that the patient received during the visit - 14.3% for "yes" and 42.9% for "rather yes". Doctors with lower SWLS results rarely ask patients to repeat the recommendations - 87.5% declared rather not this. Medical consultation ends in understandable instructions for the patient, according to doctors with high SWLS. Answer yes - 35.7%. If the doctor's life satisfaction is low there is 12.5% chance that the patient did not fully understand the instructions (Table 11).

DISCUSSION

Literature, as well as numerous reports from ongoing studies indicate that there is a relationship between the level of life satisfaction of a doctor and socio-demographic factors (age, sex, marital status, place of residence, owned specialization, work experience in the profession), and environmental factors of work (e.g. The conditions and time of work, income) (Olatunji, 2014; Suresh, 2015; Bajcar, 2011; Katerndahl, 2009). The conducted study also confirms that satisfaction with doctor life, is related to the socio-demographic factors. The gender of the doctor was an important factor affecting the level of satisfaction with life. Women performing the medical profession have higher life satisfaction than men. In the case of male, life satisfaction increased with age and was associated with the choice of suitable specialization.

The highest rate of high life satisfaction was observed in the group of doctors in the age of 31-40 (45.5%), as well as in the group of doctors from non-surgical wards (50%). The conducted study are compatible with the findings of other researchers (Barak Y.,2011). Work satisfaction results among physicians (conducted in the US) showed that in non-surgical wards more doctors are satisfied with their life than in surgical wards (Kravitz, 2002). Satisfaction with the medical profession is associated with the perception of the employee of his professional role, particularly their place in the healthcare system (Tobiasz-Adamczyk, 2002; Lewtak, 2012; Sundquist, 2000; Lepnurm, 2006). It should be noted that satisfaction with the work may include assessment of overall satisfaction, like satisfaction with the current situation, as well as the satisfaction associated with a particular aspect of the work (interpersonal relationships with patients and colleagues, income) (Miles, 2010; Smith, 2001; Alemshet, 2011; Eckert, 2003). Health professionals can be satisfied with one aspect of the work and at the same time unhappy with another. Important factors influencing the satisfaction of a doctor turned out to be the ability to diagnose diseases easily as well as the ability to predict the results of treatment, which allows for an increase in its qualifications, and thus building proper doctor-patient relationships (Leigh, 2009). Establishing proper communication with the patient was therefore identified as a cornerstone in the process of hospital treatment as a prerequisite for proper diagnosis, management and quality of healthcare, which has a positive impact on doctor overall satisfaction with life and patient satisfaction with treatment (Tsou, 2013; Wu, 2015; Kenny, 2010; Cliff, 2012; Daaleman, 2014).

Analysis of the results of life satisfaction in both medical departments, revealed that doctors are an occupational group, with average and a high degree of life satisfaction. Doctors life satisfaction is in direct relation to its ability to communicate with the patient. This however was not yet confirmed by other studies (Kenny, 2010).

Among the non-surgical ward doctors reported a higher average score of the (22.75). This means that physicians in this group have a higher level of satisfaction with life, and thus better communicate with the patient. The results indicate a higher interpersonal skills of non-surgical ward doctors. Thus, they are able to diagnose the health problems faster, and provide better support to the patient.

Doctors characterized by a high level of life satisfaction have more patience for the patient, often ask the patient to repeat the medical recommendations and finish medical consultation with understandable messages for the patient. The study has revealed that doctors with a higher level of satisfaction with life have higher interpersonal skills. Thus, they are able to quickly diagnose the health problems of the patient and provide him with better support. In addition, a doctor with high level of satisfaction with life is more likely to make the patient cooperate and willingly participates as a partner in the healing process. This trend is confirmed by other researchers, who showed that in addition to support for the patient, doctors with a high degree of satisfaction with life are able to meet the emotional needs of the patient and engage them to cooperate actively in the process of healing (Clack, 2004; Brink-Muinen, 2002; Fong, 2010). Satisfaction with life influence the professional attitude, empathy for the patient, allows effective communication with the patient, and allows to effectively prevent undesired medical events (Moczydłowska, 2014). Therefore, medical institutions should pay attention to the overall improvement of life satisfaction of employees, because it is linked to better quality of services and better interpersonal communication (Iannuzi, 2015; Scholl, 2011; Otani, 2004).

Analyzing the problem of clinical communication in patient-doctor relationship we can conclude that this area needs improvement, especially in the case of doctors working with surgical patients. Emerging problems with doctor-patient communication are mainly the result of reduced life satisfaction in this group of doctors.

The results clearly show that at the surgical wards the preferred treatment activities are surgeries and preparing the patients for diagnostic tests, while doctors from non-surgical wards focus mainly on improving the life and educating the patients. Also, doctors form non-surgical wards have a higher level of satisfaction with life, and better contact with the patient.

Therefore, in order to improve the image of healthcare institutions and improve the quality of medical services hospital managers should aim not only to raise the qualifications of doctors in terms of proper communication with the patient, but also should take care to improve their satisfaction with life. For this purpose, it seems reasonable to employ additional staff in order to eliminate excessive bureaucracy, and educator in the field of clinical communication, which, together with the medical staff will take care of the high quality of the services and the proper doctor-patient communication. Moreover, the desire to improve physician satisfaction with life, especially in surgical wards contributes to better communication, which leads to a higher quality of services.

LIMITATION

The group of people, who took part in this study was restricted to doctors working in University hospitals, in Poland. Caution should be exercised in generalizing these findings to all hospital in the world. Although, the authors are not aware of any reasons to believe that doctors working in Poland are different from other doctors working in other country. Limitations of the study also include these elements as limitations associated with a doctors self-reported, cross-sectional, co-relational design and limitations associated with the simplicity of utilized statistics. Respondents' interpretations of the questions may be individual, but still there is some potential in collecting data about doctor behavior and life satisfaction

CONCLUSION

For a doctor satisfaction with life has a special place among the conditions significantly influencing the process of communication with the patient. Higher life satisfaction grants higher interpersonal skills. The results of life satisfaction of surveyed physicians were in statistically significant, average correlation with the results of aspects relating to the process of communicating with the patient. Doctors from non-surgical wards have higher levels of life satisfaction, which provide the patient with better support in the fight against the disease, have better contact with the patient and the medical consultation ends understandable instructions for the patient.

REFERENCES

Alemshet, Y., Leja, H., & Alima, H. (2014). Job Satisfaction and Its Determinants Among Health Workers in Jimma University. Expectations of patients towards medical staff. *Hygeia Public Health*, *49*(1), 142–151.

Bajcar, B. et al.. (2011). *Satysfakcja z pracy w zawodach z misją społeczną*. Gdańsk: GWP.

Barak, Y., Tishler, M., & Aizenberg, D. (2011). Satisfaction with life amongst psychiatrists and general physicians: Demographic and career variables. *Open Journal of Psychiatry*, *1*(03), 122–125. doi:10.4236/ojpsych.2011.13018

Bhatnagar, K., & Srivastava, K. (2012, January-June). Job satisfaction in health-care organizations. *Industrial Psychiatry Journal*, *21*(1), 75–78. doi:10.4103/0972-6748.110959 PMID:23766585

Brink-Muinen, A., van Dulmen, S., Messerli-Rohrbach, V., & Bensing, J. (2002). Do gender-dyads have different communication patterns? A comparative study in Western-European general practices. *Patient Education and Counseling*, *48*(3), 253–264. doi:10.1016/S0738-3991(02)00178-7 PMID:12477610

Cacioppo, J. T., Rourke, P. A., Marshall-Goodell, B. S., Tassinary, L. G., & Baron, R. S. (1990). Rudimentary physiological effects of mere observation. *Psychophysiology*, *27*(2), 177–186. doi:10.1111/j.1469-8986.1990.tb00368.x PMID:2247548

Clack, G. B., Allen, J., Cooper, D., & Head, J. O. (2004). Personality differences between doctors and their patients: Implications for the teaching of communication skills. *Medical Education*, *38*(2), 177–186. doi:10.1111/j.1365-2923.2004.01752.x PMID:14871388

Cliff, B. (2012). Excellence In patient satisfaction within a patient-centered culture. *Journal of Healthcare Management*, *57*, 157–159. PMID:22724373

Coomber, B., & Barriball, K. L. (2007). Impact of job satisfaction components on intent to leave and turnover for hospital based nurses: A review of the research literature. *International Journal of Nursing Studies*, *44*(2), 297–314. doi:10.1016/j.ijnurstu.2006.02.004 PMID:16631760

Daaleman, T. P., Shea, C. M., Halladay, J., & Reed, D. (2014). A method to determine the impact of patient-centered care interventions in primary care. *Patient Education and Counseling*, *97*(3), 327–331. doi:10.1016/j.pec.2014.09.009 PMID:25269410

DeMeester, R. H., Lopez, F. Y., Moore, J. E., Cook, S. C., & Chin, M. H. (2016, March 17). A Model of Organizational Context and Shared Decision Making: Application to LGBT Racial and Ethnic Minority Patients. *Journal of General Internal Medicine*, *31*(6), 651–662. doi:10.1007/s11606-016-3608-3 PMID:26988980

Di Blasi, Z., Harkness, E., Ernst, E., Georgiou, A., & Klejinen, J. (2001). Influence of context effects on health outcomes: A systematic review. *Lancet*, *357*(9258), 757–762. doi:10.1016/S0140-6736(00)04169-6 PMID:11253970

Surman, G., Lambert, T. W., & Goldacre, M. (2016). Doctors' enjoyment of their work and satisfaction with time available for leisure: UK time trend questionnaire-based study. *Postgraduate Medical Journal*. doi:10.1136/postgradmedj-2015-133743

Duffy, F. D., Gordon, G. H., Whelan, G., Cole-Kelly, K., Frankel, R., & Buffone, N. et al.. (2004). Assessing competence in communication and interpersonal skills: The Kalamazoo II report. *Academic Medicine*, *79*(6), 495–507. doi:10.1097/00001888-200406000-00002 PMID:15165967

Eckert, H., & Resch, K. L. (2003). Quality management –quo vadis? Perspectives for quality management in hospitals. *Zeitschrift fur Arztliche Fortbildung und Qualitatssicherung*, *97*(3), 219–226. PMID:12856550

Fong Ha, J., & Longnecker, N. (2010, Spring). Doctor Patient Communication A Review. *The Ochsner Journal, 10*(1), 38–43. PMID:21603354

Gordon Moore, L., & Wasson, J. H. (2007). The Ideal Medical Practice Model: Improving Efficiency, Quality and the Doctor-Patient Relationship. *Family Practice Management, 14*(8), 20–24. PMID:17912818

Iannuzi, J. C., Kahn, S. A., Zhang, L., Gestring, M. L., Noyes, K., & Monson, J. R. T. (2015). Getting satisfaction: Drivers of surgical Hospital Consumer Assessment of Health care Providers and Systems survey scores. *The Journal of Surgical Research, 197*(1), 155–161. doi:10.1016/j.jss.2015.03.045 PMID:25908102

Jopkiewicz S. (2011). Funkcja wizerunku i tożsamości placówki w komunikacji marketingowej, Studia i Materiały. *Miscellanea Oeconomicae, 2*.

Juczyński, Z. (2009). *Measurement Tools in the Promotion and Psychology Health*. Warsaw: Laboratory of Psychological Tests.

Katerndahl, D., Parchman, M., & Wood, R. (2009). Perceived complexity of care, perceived autonomy, and career satisfaction among primary care physicians. *Journal of the American Board of Family Medicine, 22*(1), 24–3. doi:10.3122/jabfm.2009.01.080027 PMID:19124630

Kenny, D. A., Valdhuijzen, W., van der Weijden, T., LeBlanc, A., Lockyer, J., Legare, F., & Campbell, C. (2010). Interpersonal perception in the context of doctor-patient relationships: A dyadic analysis of doctor-patient communication. *Social Science & Medicine, 70*(5), 763–768. doi:10.1016/j.socscimed.2009.10.065 PMID:20005618

Kenny, D. A., Veldhuijzen, W., van der Weijden, T., LeBlanc, A., Lockyer, J., Legare, F., & Campbell, C. (2010). Interpersonal perceptron in the context of doctor-patient relationships: A dyadic analysis of doctor-patient communication. *Social Science & Medicine, 70*(5), 763–768. doi:10.1016/j.socscimed.2009.10.065 PMID:20005618

Kissane, D. W., Bylund, C. L., Banerjee, S. C., Bialer, P. A., Levin, T. T., Maloney, E. K., & D'Agostino, T. A. (2012). Communication skills training for oncology professionals. *Journal of Clinical Oncology, 30*(11), 1242–1247. doi:10.1200/JCO.2011.39.6184 PMID:22412145

Klakovich, M. D., & Dela Cruz, F. A. (2006, January-February). Validating the Interpersonal Communication Assessment Scale. *Journal of Professional Nursing, 22*(1), 60–67. doi:10.1016/j.profnurs.2005.12.005 PMID:16459290

Leigh J.P, Tancredi D.J., Kravitz R.L. (2009). Physician career satisfaction within specialties *BMC Health Serv Res., 16*(9), 166.

Lepnurm, R., Dobson, R., Backman, A., & Keegan, D. (2006). Factors explaining career satisfaction among psy-chiatrists and surgeons in Canada. *Canadian Journal of Psychiatry, 51*(4), 243–255. doi:10.1177/070674370605100406 PMID:16629349

Lewtak, K., Poznańska, A., & Mirosław, J. (2012). Wysocki, Predyktory satysfakcji zawodowej lekarzy podstawowej opieki zdrowotnej. *Probl. Hig. Epidemiol., 93*(3), 558–567.

Maciąg, A. 2004. Rola informacji w procesie tworzenia jakości usług medycznych. *Zdrowie i Zarządzanie*, *6*(6).

Miles, S., & Leinster, S. J. (2010). Identifying Professional characteristics of the ideal medical doctor: The laddering technique. *Medical Teacher*, *32*(2), 136–140. doi:10.3109/01421590903196987 PMID:20163229

Olatunji, S.O. & Mokuolu, B.O. (2014). The Influence of Sex, Marital Status, and Tenure of Service on Job Stress, and Job Satisfaction of Health Workers in a Nigerian Federal Health Institution. An International Multidisciplinary Journal, 8(1), 126-133.

Otani, K., & Kurz, R. S. (2004, May). The impact of nursing care and other healthcare attributes on hospitalized patient satisfaction and behavioral intentions. *Journal of Healthcare Management*, *49*(3), 181–196. PMID:15190860

Paul, J. (2002). PhD; Kravitz R.L., MD, MSPH, Physician Career Satisfaction Across Specialties. *Archives of Internal Medicine*, *162*(14), 1577–1584. doi:10.1001/archinte.162.14.1577 PMID:12123400

Rider, E. A., & Keefer, C. H. (2006). Communication skills competencies: Definitions and a teaching toolbox. *Medical Education*, *40*(7), 624–629. doi:10.1111/j.1365-2929.2006.02500.x PMID:16836534

Scholl, J. C., Wilson, J. B., & Hughs, P. C. (2011). Expression of patients' and providers' identities during the medical interview. *Qualitative Health Research*, *21*(8), 1022–1032. doi:10.1177/1049732310393748 PMID:21263064

Smith, R. (2001). Why are doctors so unhappy? *British Medical Journal*, *322*(7294), 1073–1074. doi:10.1136/bmj.322.7294.1073 PMID:11337419

Street, R. L. Jr, Makoul, G., Arora, N. K., & Epstein, R. M. (2009). How does communication heal? Pathways linking clinician–patient communication to health outcomes. *Patient Education and Counseling*, *74*(3), 295–301. doi:10.1016/j.pec.2008.11.015 PMID:19150199

Sundquist, J., & Johannsson, S. E. (2000). High demand, low control, and impaired general health: Working conditions in a sample of Swedish general practitioners. *Scandinavian Journal of Public Health*, *28*(2), 123–131. doi:10.1177/140349480002800208 PMID:10954139

Suresh, S., Kodikal, R., & Kar, S. (2015). Measuring job satisfaction and impact of demographic characteristics among Doctors of Teaching Hospitals. *International Multispecialty Journal of Health*, *1*(9). Retrieved from http://www.imjhealth.org/admin/issues_detail/gallery/IMJH-NOV-2015-5.pdf

Teutsch, C. (2003, September). Patient-doctor communication. *The Medical Clinics of North America*, *87*(5), 1115–1145. doi:10.1016/S0025-7125(03)00066-X PMID:14621334

Tobiasz-Adamczyk, B. (2002). Relacje lekarz-pacjent w perspektywie socjologii medycyny, Wyd. *UJ Kraków*, *19*, 81–85.

Tsou, A. Y., Creutzfeldt, C. J., & Gordon, J. M. (2013). Chapter 9- The good doctor: Professionalism In the 21 st century. *Handbook of Clinical Neurology*, *118*, 119–132. doi:10.1016/B978-0-444-53501-6.00009-3 PMID:24182371 van Woerkum, C. M. (2003). The Internet and primary care physicians: Coping with different expectations. *The American Journal of Clinical Nutrition*, *77*(4 Suppl.), 1016S–1018S. PMID:12663310

Weiner, J. S., & Cole, S. A. (2004). Three principles to improve clinician communication for advance care planning: Overcoming emotional, cognitive, and skill barriers. *Journal of Palliative Medicine*, *7*(6), 817–829. doi:10.1089/jpm.2004.7.817 PMID:15684849

Williams, S. L., Haskard, K. B., & DiMatteo, M. R. (2007). The therapeutic effects of the physician-older patient relationship: Effective communication with vulnerable older patients. *Clinical Interventions in Aging*, *2*(3), 453. PMID:18044195

Wu, H., Zhao, X., Fritzsche, K., Leonhart, R., Schaefert, R., Sun, X., & Larisch, A. (2015). Quality of doctor-patient relationship in patient with high somatic symptom severity in China. *Complementary Therapies in Medicine*, *23*(1), 23–31. doi:10.1016/j.ctim.2014.12.006 PMID:25637149

Yagil, D., Biron, M., Pat, D., Mirzahi-Reuveni, M., & Zoller, L. (2015). Accurate diagnosis of patient's distress levels: The effect of family physicians' ability to take the patient's perspective. *Patient Education and Counseling*, *98*(12), 1631–1635. doi:10.1016/j.pec.2015.07.008 PMID:26215572

Yami, A., Hamza, L., Hassen, A., Jira, C., & Sudhakar, M. (2011). Job satisfaction and its determinants among health workers in Jimma University specialized hospital, southwest Ethiopia. Ethiopian journal of health sciences, 21(3). PMID:22435005

Yoshiaki, N. S. K., Onoda, K., Hamano, T., & Kimura, K. (2015). Job and life satisfaction and preference of future practice locations of physicians on remote islands in Japan. *Human Resources for Health*, *13*(1), 39. doi:10.1186/s12960-015-0029-z PMID:26008624

Chapter 14
The Physiotherapist as a Health Educator

Łukasz Sielski
Nicolaus Copernicus University, Poland

Julita Soczywko
Nicolaus Copernicus University, Poland

ABSTRACT

This chapter is devoted to the work of physiotherapists, who must be able to recognize a variety of limitations and contraindications. It presents physiotherapy as a profession and the physical therapist as a professional, a man perfectly prepared to work with the sick and needy and a member of the rehabilitation team (therapeutic) who is therapist-humanist ensuring his patients are treated properly and ethically.

INTRODUCTION

Exercise of trades involving, among other things, close physical relationship with another human being requires a certain predisposition. Important is the ease of contact with the patient, as well as discretion, tact, but especially good knowledge of the needs of others. In addition, knowledge of the principles of ethics has a significant impact on both the proper and improper conduct in the professional role. When this turns out to be a factor in the integration of these principles with the models adopted in practice with patients (Gabard 2003). Respect for human rights in health requires appropriate approach based on the principles of Justice and non-discrimination. The patient should be treated humanely, so that it can be an active, not just passive participant in the process of protection, whether restoring full fitness or health. Declaration adopted by the World Health Organization indicates three ethical principles: respect for human life, focus health services on health, and not primarily on the disease and new ethical perspective (Hebda 2004). And here is the question, as the background of these important moral values creates a profession of physiotherapist?

A physical therapist in a simple definition, is a specialist, which, thanks to the acquired knowledge and your manual skills and technical measures eliminates some disease processes in the body, prevents relapses and progression of diseases and ailments. Performs health massage, helps take care of the

DOI: 10.4018/978-1-5225-3946-9.ch014

health and well-being of patients. Helps in returning to the- physical fitness. Deals with the planning and conduct of physical activities and physical therapy treatments. To reliably perform their profession, physical therapists should have a vast knowledge of medicine, especially anatomy. The necessary are also high dexterity and resilience, and physical fitness. Important to physical therapist had to establish good interpersonal relationships, the desire to help and a high personal culture that rely on knowledge of the ethical requirements related to the exercise of the profession of physiotherapist (Kiebzak 2009). Its appropriate professional conduct stems from knowledge of ethics. This is probably a very important aspect, since the practice of physical therapy is deeply embedded in the multidimensional relationships with patients and their families or careers. Briefly summarize the role of the physiotherapist in society comes down not only to have the instrumental expertise, that is, high personal culture, but also require him to conduct humanitarian and ethical (Kenrick 2002). Physiotherapy is interdisciplinary, and therefore requires close interaction of medical specialists physical medicine and physical therapists. That's why education and shaping the nature of future physical therapist is difficult, which are influenced by academics, older experienced physiotherapists, as well as patients. A physical therapist must have a special sense of responsibility for the health of patients, keeping in mind that not only from the doctor, but also from his conscience duties depends on a faster return to health and life of the patient (Gabard 2003). Physical therapist, taking part in the rehabilitation of the patient should keep in mind that its work guided by the main rule: service health and human life. Appropriate therapeutic action by him should be subject to constant analysis and assessment in the context of the ideas of humanism, ethics and cultural achievements of society. In the good of culture contains a berth structure of its creator. Ethical and psychologically the correct behavior of the doctor and physiotherapist is revealed when they value of cultural goods in accordance with the intention of establishing an effective strategy treated (Wojciszke 2004).

The Responsibility of Higher Education for Shaping Appropriate Attitudes

The complexity of the tasks facing the universities requires excellence in management. The development and effective implementation of the processes described in General in the mission, and in more detail in the strategy requires knowledge, experience, but most of all the knowledge of the expectations, both academic, and environment of each University. Modern organized the University is not only a grouping of scholars and researchers. It is primarily the United and open academic community, whose aim is the development of science and education students based on the principles of moral and ethical, with the highest possible quality. The education of students, or future intellectual elites, is tremendously responsible. Of course, this applies to all colleges and all fields of study, however, these specialties, which are directly linked to human health, deserve special attention (Hejwosz 2008). The role of the University is not only ethically appropriate to the training of students. The essence of things is instilling the appropriate attitudes in such a way as to be forwarded. In this chain of ethics the University is the actual health educator to promote not only a healthy lifestyle, but also the training of ethical and responsible professionals of physiotherapy. The person preparing the health educators are required to show them respect, treat them as other students and to offer high-quality education that benefits professional and society (Kenrick 2002). Education of the competent ethical action is not an easy task. The results of many studies show that there is a clear link between the ability of students to resolve conflicts and their ability to deal with practical problems in complicated ambiguous areas of practice. In addition, the ethical issues are included in the perception of students on further than issues related to knowledge about the process of treatment or rehabilitation. Keep in mind that the quality of the relationship the physiotherapist with the patient dictate how. This causes the implications for education and physical therapists. Receipt of social knowledge or presented is as important as the other elements of the profession (Kenrick 2002). In broad terms, a physical therapist is responsible primarily for the patient. This is possible only when he knows value system. This knowledge is the complement of the knowledge possessed by a physical therapist, but without it, it is not possible to create a sufficiently close contact with the patient.

It is therefore important that in the process of education of future physical therapists more emphasis placed on the development of skills in interpersonal communication and conflict resolution (Woynarowska 2010).

Future Physical Therapist as a Graduate of the University and Social Expectations

The discovery of the relationship between health and lifestyle resulted in the need for society to promote a healthy lifestyle. Health is an area in which the individual or group is able, on the one hand, meet their aspirations and needs, and, on the other hand, change your surroundings, affecting the surrounding environment. Health is seen as one of the resources that we have in everyday life. The concept of health stresses both the social and the individual's resources and physical capabilities. On the other hand, higher education institutions, recognizing this need, should effectively respond to active participation in this process. Modification of the system of values or behavior requires knowledge and potential. The strength of this may serve as the University and its graduates, who, in fact, further transmission of knowledge. Awareness of the need for a healthy lifestyle causes an increase in liability for health (Hejwosz 2008). The availability of multiple sources of knowledge ensures that patients have the opportunity to acquire information to the extent many times wider than ever. This leads to an increase in health awareness, but growth expectations of patients, both in quality, informative, and ethical.

The answer to these expectations may be patient-oriented approach as opposed to the authoritarian approach. It is worth to keep in mind that the increasing commercialization of health carries serious dangers in the area. This includes the rise of profit, which defers the relationships related to the protection of health of non or to health purposes. Keep in mind that the most important thing is the welfare of the patient and that it must not become a means of increasing the profit (Karski 2011). Human health should be considered inclusive: protect-thanks to prevention, improve – through health promotion, restore, when disease-with the treatment and rehabilitation of Perfect physical therapist is not only very good practices, it is above all a good man who does not hesitate to take responsibility for joint education generations of valuable citizens (Pezdek 2001).

Ethical Attitude of Physiotherapist

Ethical attitude, an attitude which is characterized by a certain regularity. Is subject to sanctions, passed down from generation to generation, and its volatility is coincident with a society or culture. Such an attitude sets usually dynamic layout of three components: behavioral, emotional and intellectual. Ethical attitude of physiotherapist, is his relationship to the patient and the team. Characterized by the constancy, is a component of his personality and affects his disposition. Creation of theoretical types of moral attitudes is undoubtedly the procedure, in which you must walk to the idealization of the ethical assumptions and empirical situation (Michalin 2003). This team of physiotherapist behavior in relation to the patient, is formed in the process of meeting the needs of specific social conditions modulated,.

As was mentioned earlier, shaping the attitudes of ethical physiotherapists should be initiated during the learning process during their studies. It should be noted that the main message of the medical profession is helping others through the use of the acquired knowledge and skills. Physical therapist learns that, by imitating teachers, who provide knowledge and teach its practical use. These people should be of great intellect and integrity, propriety, justice, and that the moral sense. Teachers should shape the correct hierarchy of values, attitudes and opinions of young people open to learning. Should therefore be aware of the huge impact on the atmosphere and the relationship between master and pupil in the didactic process (Jemielniak 2005).

The attitude of the physiotherapist in relation to the patient is his subjective reference to it. Describe it attitude to life, death, health, people with disabilities and the elderly. These attitudes, including attitudes toward values derive from the human processes of socialization and play a significant role in the development of the relationship between the therapist and the patient. The attitude of social discipline – this awareness by physiotherapist standards, principles and rules that make up its disciplined conduct and abide by them, it is also a sensitivity the readiness to self-discipline. A physical therapist that I present this type of attitude is a man willing to comply with the rules, to the readiness of being useful. The attitude of social utility – physical therapist expresses this attitude in how to prepare for work, activities to the creative activities (Rusin 2013). The attitude of the social economy – physical therapist should recognize your and people's welfare, should also possess the ability to assess the situation, the trouble necessary to receive positive results. It is also the ability to management because of their ability to save. The attitude of social involvement-a physical therapist should enable as far as their capabilities in social activities.

Social attitude of openness is a social attitude of openness of physiotherapist in the fair judgements, assistance, cooperation with various specialists in therapeutic team, equal treatment of their charges (Litwiejko 2010). Attitude encourages interaction-is the ability of a physical therapist to work, life, loyalty, solidarity team. The meaning of these attitudes is apparent from the need to care for the welfare of others, positive and effective cooperation in the team is building a conducive atmosphere to life in the group. Another group of attitudes that are the basic form of the consideration of the silhouette of the physiotherapist is interpersonal attitudes or attitudes that are based on kindness, understanding, responsibility for his actions, or lack thereof. They meet three significant features: predispose to the evaluation itself, trigger a sense of responsibility for themselves and run the specific aspirations of perfection. To the needs, which are possible to meet people-to-people contacts, include: respect for human dignity, respect for life, tolerance, caregiving, respect for property, the reliability of the observation and respect for individuals, autonomy's empathizing with this result the following attitude: the attitude of respect for human dignity-a physical therapist working with your patient should keep in mind that a man crippled, helpless, that it is not for this reason treated worse than other patients with its surroundings (Pezdek 2001). An attitude of respect for life is an attitude of the medical profession. The patient should live in the sense that a physical therapist will do everything to ensure the optimum return to health both physical and mental. The attitude of tolerance – do not let to the arguments of religious, ethnic, racial, political or class can affect the performance of the obligation to the patient. The attitude of caring-a physical therapist should assist, cheer, is devoted to his work (Rusin 2013).

An attitude of respect for property – refers to the human right to have their own name, and reviews. The attitude of integrity of information – physical therapist by passing the knowledge the patient with a sense of responsibility for his word. The attitude of empathy – a good physiotherapist will be the one that is a good person, who understands the plight of the patient, which is demonstrated empathy. In addition, the physiotherapist are also between the staff attitudes, that derive from the attitudes of a sense of personal dignity, self-control, perfection, responsibility, optimism, self-reliance, personal courage and bravery (Makowska 2001).

Shaping the Attitudes of Physiotherapists

Moral development is a long-term process. The progressive a variety of directional changes allow a man to achieve ever higher levels of maturity. Shaping the attitudes of future physical therapists in the academic process is difficult and prolonged. The University's role is primarily to provide students with the educational and scientific staff prepared, respectively, access to specialized literature, ethics, demonstrating concern for the observance of ethical standards among employees (Michalin 2003). In the course of education, towards the shaping of attitudes, uses at least three methods: imitation, a forced commitment and humanistic education.

LIMITATION

Formation of attitudes in the relationship the master-pupil during the academic probably is the strongest component of the imitation, whose job is to present in a clear way the hierarchy of values and motivate to comply with them. In a relationship the master-student, the first must be, first and foremost, the right man, and in the second place, a professional teacher. Of course it is important he knows what he can, but at the same time, what is, what is committed and how, through your behavior, your personality shapes the attitude of ethical student. This process proceeds by patterns, word of mouth, the discussion, the relevant requirements, observation and active listening, providing feedback or motivating. Lecturer becomes a role model for his students when it is benevolent and treats their the entity, is a diligent and punctual, reliably fulfils its obligations, is prepared in substance, and by passing a knowledge and skills is responsible for the presented content. When you verify the knowledge students applies the principle of Justice, is forgiving. It is extremely important to the mistakes and verify the given message. Among the students are shown a variety of correct behavior, positive, negative, or even reprehensible. The role of educators is to respond to deviations from the academic ethos, not respect for fundamental ethical principles in relation to the leading classes, students and other staff. The role of educational and scientific worker is also to encourage the development of knowledge by research activities within the framework of scientific circles, enabling students to research projects and encourage participation in student scientific conferences (Rusin 2012).

Another factor in the shaping of attitudes is word of mouth and putting the requirements. This task is most often implemented in the classroom with the ethics and psychology. It is not enough to possess the theoretical knowledge with the science, which is why it seems to be teaching by lecturer-physical therapist with professional experience and knowledge of ethical issues. By presenting ethical issues should encourage reflection on the ethical aspects in physiotherapy and universal values of the medical profession. Each student of physiotherapy should know the rules for the conduct of studies and diagnoses-it takes place in the classroom and during student practice. On the subjective test and the material and perform the treatments the student must obtain the consent of the patient. Should sensitize the students for need of professional secrecy (Wojciszke 2004). In shaping the attitudes of students a large role of observation, active listening and giving feedback. Guardian of the students in the classroom or clinical practices should closely observe the attitude especially when dealing with patients, listen carefully to the relationship of students with diagnostic and therapeutic tests and respond to them. Constructive conversation physiotherapist with the students after the completed course is the perfect moment to exchange insights and a proper evaluation of (Straburzyńska – Lupa 2007).

ENFORCED COMMITMENT

Enforced commitment is an attempt to encourage students to the activities of for the public. Education should not focus on knowledge and skills and career planning, but primarily on education and strengthening the involvement of ethics (Hejwosz 2008). Among the medical profession in the first place, you should replace the high ethics and specifically in the sense of social responsibility, commitment to developing ethical sensitivity, the application of fundamental moral principles, in the sense of the dignity of the patient and of his own. The evolution of ethical attitudes during the involvement of students in the selfless actions. The correct motivation on the part of faculty, co-organizing charitable exercise the care of volunteer work in hospices, orphanages is of great importance in building a variety of attitudes, responsibility, tolerance and respect for human dignity (Pezdek 2001).

Humanistic Education

A third method which forms the attitude of students of physiotherapy is the so-called education of humanistic or humanistic reflection. Work with man and for man is not enough having medical expertise and instrumental values, typical for professional education, not enough in building positive relationships, physical therapist-patient. The threat of the ideology may appear when the young man does not find the alternatives in the form of other value systems (Woynarowska 2010).

Shaping an Ethical Posture at Work

After graduating from the ethical stance of physiotherapist are affected above all the type of work performed, the situation and employee relations that allow a man to liberate instilled rules and moral views. The environment is also active on the attitudes of people, perpetuates them or modifies the transforms. The attitude of the Physiotherapist should be such as to positively worked on the patient, as well as to ensure as soon as possible-better and how to perform them to the solemn veneration of all tasks arising from the obligation to a professional physiotherapist. It should respect their patients, and the strength to do good and to help her students (Rusin 2013).

Physical Therapist and Professional Culture

The culture of the profession is a derived culture of personal and collective, but also spiritual and material. It's a culture shared by people belonging to a given profession, associated with the nature of their work and the role that in society. The culture of the profession is in under the influence of vocational education, training, courses, specialization. It includes rules of conduct relating to the manufacture of goods or the provision of services and the same behaviors and the effects of that reflected in the results of the work unit (Jemielniak 2005).

Factors conducive to the formation of professional cultures include the frequent meetings of the representatives of the profession, in the framework of the activities of the organization. To be able to talk about the presence of the culture of professional physiotherapists, an attempt of analysis, whether the representatives of this profession notice referred to bond with other representatives of the same profession. That is why it is so important to each physical therapist was affiliated to the organization representing all its members. Professional culture allows you to specify the stereotypical roles in both broad and narrow sense. Professional culture is shaped in order to facilitate the interpretation of internal emotions, taming and translations. In addition, the professional culture responds to the needs of contractors, individual works-creates symbols and rituals needed specific profession. The broadcast of the identity in the eyes of their own units, assigning gender stereotypes in the eyes of others, satisfying emotional needs related to the job – are part of the particular culture (Jemielniak 2005).

The Pattern of Personal Physical Therapist

To deliberations of aspects of ethical physiotherapies defining the personality model of the physiotherapist which is supposed to become an indicator is included of aim of action edifying and aiming at the internalization of bent features in the personality of the physiotherapist. Strengthened personality traits in the teaching process expected are becoming a guarantor of meeting determined norms of professional duties. The physiotherapist can gain the name of the compliant career in the situation, when it is possible aptly to trust his care and won't disappoint as well as he will do everything, as for it belongs. In this place such universal attributes are meriting attention, like aspiration of the perfection, the openness of the mind, the self-discipline, the tolerance, the activity, the moral courage, the intellectual honesty, the criticism and the responsibility for the word (Pezdek 2001).

Warning by him ethical general and detailed norms should guarantee the presence of the personality model to which the physiotherapist can aspire, of him multilevel professional competence.

Rules for the Implementation of the Profession of Physiotherapist

The occupational group of physiotherapists is third in terms of the size with community amongst medical professions and feints of the public trust. Physiotherapists fly's to have high professional qualifications resulting from guidelines concerning educating on the higher education. They are providing health services, therefore in Poland last works on d with conclusive legal record concerning qualifications for taking this occupational activity.

Propriety of the Physiotherapist

A propriety of the man is an entirety of the modus operandi, the thought, notions and views which is purchasing as a result of the permanent work on oneself through the entire private life itself and professional, it is certain stood with property which determines keeping the man irrespective of the time, the place and circumstances. Being a man about the high propriety they are perceived positively in the surrounding environment. Taking into consideration defining the notion, one should perceive the culture as the degree of excellence, fitness in mastering diverse specialization, ability and the highest level of the intellectual development, whereas a cultured man is a man distinguishing himself big with culture, educated and very well brought up. Apart from ethical code, role model, theory of the profession, a peculiar culture of the occupational group and a propriety of every her member are one of characteristics of the profession (Rusin 2012). To elements shaping the culture personal to count the physiotherapist it is possible: intellectual advantages, the intelligence of emotions and the intelligence emotional, directional features, the manner and behaviors oneself towards other people, the efficiency of action and effects of this activity, the general rule of ethics and professional ethics, care of the health, hygiene personal and care of the appearance, openness to contacts with other people, the ability of the harmonious cooperation and co-existing, and the ability of the rule over its emotions and the temperament, as well as senses of humor. Such abilities of the man like the way and the efficiency to think, comprehending notions and the intelligence include intellectual advantages.

Physiotherapist having high professional competence and above abilities, efficiently he is taking the right decisions and is focusing on the relevant problem. Efficiency of the thinking the processing of information enables him which are encrypted in observations, ideas and notions, thanks to which he is getting to know reality in which he lives and is working (Makowska 2001). Having abilities of analysing, synthesis, generalizing, crystallizing, the physiotherapist well deals with diverse problem situations concerning manners and the selection of methods and centers in the rehabilitation process. Thanks to these abilities easily he is establishing contact with partners forming a rehabilitation team, is able from the easiness to create announcements and without unnecessary information and to hand them over with exploiting the appropriate form to the statement. An intelligent physiotherapist is the one which is demonstrating the adaptability, of the learning, the problem solving and the processing of information. With successive factor shaping the culture personal of man there are an intelligence of emotions and an emotional intelligence.

The one first is manifesting itself with abilities of sympathy, the intuition, understanding and the ability of the insight into oneself. To a considerable degree a success or a defeat depend on it in the family life and professional. The physiotherapist is learning the emotional intelligence from the moment of the birthday throughout the period of the education, and then during the career. Thanks to these abilities the physiotherapist easily is establishing contact with patients, often with people suffering and incurable, being in terminal states. In the development of the personality of every man marking soils directional features among which we can rank interests, emotions, thoughts and an attention concentrated for some phenomenon or the thing, as well as instructions for the performance of activities with them are playing tied. It is essential for the development of the personality so that the man has extensive interests, however too extensive can influence the downgrade of the knowledge and the ability and social competence.

In case of medical professions specializing is a general occurrence. The physiotherapist has detailed knowledges physiological and pathophysiology and general about all illnesses and the complaint, and detailed in one's specialization. He knows the sequence of healing factors physical and of therapeutic methods. He can take specializations, but so that his abilities aren't superficial, often chooses the specific group of healing problems.

With further factor shaping the culture is personal the manner and behaviors oneself towards other people which contains observing good manners and pretentious habits, using the appropriate tongue and expressions, showing the respect and the interest, desire for bringing help and of applying the principle of being just.

The physiotherapist should always behave tactfully towards patients and partners of the rehabilitation team. Using the appropriate tongue is a base of the efficient transport. Addressing patients indirectly is inadmissible or grandfather, grandmother and into the incomprehensible way using the transmission of information specialist vocabulary. The physiotherapist should demonstrate also a particular interest with every patient, to show the respect him, understanding and to be ready to bring help (De Walden-Gałuszko 2000).

With successive factor building the culture up an efficiency of action and her effect are personal. Physiotherapist beginning one's should carefully plan the work one's diagnostic and therapeutic procedures in order to work effectively. To effects frequently he must very much long await the work, because in many disease entities the therapeutic process is long-term, and with times in spite of employing from both sides - of the physiotherapist and the patient - one can't see the effect. Therefore in this profession ruthlessly a patience and a huge humility are demanded.

Physiotherapist with the high propriety it is an acting man according to principles of general ethics and professional ethics. Until recently physiotherapists in Poland referred to code of the ethical doctor, but a created Ethical Code of the Physiotherapist stayed in 2008 in order to help physiotherapists develop own sensitivity and of individual responsibility for one's action.

Ethical advantages, that is internal norms and rules of conduct social are unusually essential in the relation with the second man, particularly an ill man and the needy of the special care and the support. Ethical principles are helping every occupational group efficiently to solve peculiar professional problems, as well as influence it elevating.

A care of the health is a next factor influencing the propriety, hygiene personal and care of the external appearance. The physiotherapist should have an avocation for the adherence to the principles of the healthier living, neatly to be dressed, always in the clean uniform and caring about hygiene. It a polite, clean and neat person should be. The appearance of the man is delivering a lot of interesting information to the recipient, he is an indicator of character, the personality, as well as the upbringing. Based on the external appearance it is possible to predict behaving of given person. To character of the relation physiotherapist the patient, apart from verbal announcements, is playing the great significance body language which is a team of non-verbal announcements, sent and get back by all people (visual, hearing instrument, taste and tactile and olfactory) with channel sensory simultaneously (Makowska H. 2001).

The physiotherapist about the high propriety is open to contacts with other people, should possess a skill of the harmonious cooperation and having intercourse with partners, with patients and from family of the sick person.

With the last determinant propriety an ability of the rule over emotions and the temperament, as well as having a sense of humor are. The physiotherapist incessantly is exposed to conflictual situations of different kind in which the physiotherapist but the patient, the physiotherapist but the family of the patient, the physiotherapist but the team member are participating. Every man has other temperament, otherwise is responding to the stress, but the medical personnel peculiarly should have control of emotions, to be calm and taken control in every circumstances. As regards a sense of humor, of course the smiling man is perceived through other as very kind, clear, patients more willingly are cooperating with him. It is important so that a sense of humor is exploited in the appropriate situation what is marking not everywhere and not always. It is also element of therapy, influences for motivating the patient to the work, encouraging it for the active participation in the treatment.

Psychological Factors Being Significant in the Relation Patient: Medical Staff

Observing the history of medicine, without hesitation it is possible to state that dynamically he is developing, and hence for her the effectiveness is growing. However a changing lifestyle of people and world which is surrounding us, are putting new challenges still. Looking at all latest medical achievements so as development of the molecular biology, or genetics, we cannot permit the entity of influences of these achievements disappear from view. For this reason in the process of curing psychological influencing factors are an important component to relations between the patient, but the medical staff (Ostrowska 2001).

n order to understand how, in the process of curing psychological influencing factors are an important component to relations between the patient, but the medical staff one should acquaint it oneself with different models of the relation the medical staff but the patient, to distinguish positive and negative factors, as well as to learn, what relations are occurring between individual team members interdisciplinary and for sick persons.

The given aspect is important in medicine, in it with reference to physiotherapy, since to the health of the patient an approach of the medical staff towards his person, as well as an attitude of the patient towards the staff are enjoying considerable influence what results from a psychological point of view (Karski 2011).

Models of the Relation the Patient but the Medical Staff

The Model of the Relation of the Patient but the Medical Staff Classified Based on Interests of the Physiotherapist

The given model is divided into two fundamental models. First, which the climb concentrated on illness is standing out in is called the somatic sense of direction. Here not a patient is the main character as person, but bad organ or disease entity. The whole process of the treatment has a biological aspect both in terms of the possibility of the treatment as well as signs and causes of illness. The other model is putting the climb concentrated on the patient on and it is general sense of direction (Karski 2011). Here up to the attention they are overcome factors of the biological, psychological and social nature of patient. An aspiration to establishing the correct contact and bonds with the sick person and a look at his illness are also a main sign of the general sense of direction in the psychosocial aspect as the main cause of the appearance of illness.

Theory of Conflict

In previous models the patient but the medical staff as the main purpose are laying the report behind, both one as well as for the other party, health of the sick person. Now a situation will be presented, when it can fade away. According to many theories of conflict the behavior of the medical staff towards the patient results from different relations. Other purposes of achieving the benefit are motivating every side, on the part of the staff it is for financial benefits, as the deciding individual, but the sick person about regaining health. With consequence of it for example favoring wealthy patients can be. Appearing of such negative reports is inducing immediately to reflection which is obvious towards due ethical proceedings.

Ideology Associated With Being a So-Called Consultant

The given ideology is presenting the contact of the physiotherapist with the patient, as relations of the type consultant - customer. To her determined influence a development is aware of a society, simpler access to the information by the Internet and television. With consequence of it there is a change of the posture of the patient on more active. The sick person not only wants recommendations are heard doctor, but also to participate in the decision making, what at one time was booked only for the person pursuing a medical profession (Hebda 2004). In this relation the physiotherapist is acting as the adviser and the partner which has a professional authority, but there is no power. Both sides in this case are aware of an own relation what is a new element in relations.

Elements of Correct Reports the Patient but the Medical Staff

Empathy

Empathy constitutes empathizing with the role of the second man. One should distinguish empathy from sympathy, since this getting to know the more widely psychological situation, i.e. understanding the state are. Empathy will depend on many biological factors and social. A person which has is able to demonstrate greater empathy similar situations, is under the influence of the similar environment.

With one of important factors of the forming oneself for relation of the medical staff with the sick person there is empathy. For them higher abilities empathy all the better contact with the patient which is being displayed both for verbal as well as non-verbal sphere. Empathy is protecting from certain patterns of behaviors and the routine alert with patients.

To main factors empathy, essential for the physiotherapist, it is possible to rank:

- To rebel against in the situation of the patient
- Will stay along with him in the same place and time
- Setting oneself a question which he will put for you
- Trying to experience the same emotions, of which if it is possible to think, a sick person is experiencing
- Telling him, what in this situation alone the physiotherapist would make
- The same as very physiotherapist would like the procedure for the patient so that they act towards him.

Ability of the Transmission of Information for Patients by the Physiotherapist

The scope of information a patient should receive which is different. Therefore the physiotherapist should be guided by a manner of the receipt. He considers himself, that interest patient with the own health and progress of the treatment, as well as the impact of measures pharmacological to his state it is natural, and should be a primary source of this information person pursuing a medical profession.

In Poland conducted examinations stayed about an interest of patients in the condition of its health. It results from them that the 75% is demonstrating will of obtaining such information even in the event that they are disadvantageous.

Effects uninformed are as a rule very negative for the health of the patient. The sick person is feeling insecure then as well as doesn't have confidence in an interdisciplinary team, feels threatening, of what not-applying to recommendations, for example is resulting not performing exercises recommended by the physiotherapist. The unaware patient is starting seeking information about own illness, what it often becomes an incorrect image of his coincidence.

Benefits sailing out from informing the patient are huge. For example sick persons informed of the possible appearance of pain complaints after physiotherapy treatment far more easily they endured pain, as well as didn't use from yes of lot of painkillers like patients which weren't informed of it. In informing patients adapting amounts handed over to information is a next element depending on the person. Individual expectations patient constitute the risk, that both too vague, as well as specific information can arouse the market intense anxiety. Generally it is possible to divide the receipt of information in two separate styles:

- Vigilant observing which relies on turning inattention to the source of the threat, search, accumulation and for using information,
- Explaining warnings, which on avoiding specific information about the threat, as well as on so manipulating them so that subjectively the stress is picked up less intensively.

The communication is of special importance, when information is regarding unfavourable negotiations. In this situation one should be guided by a principle of the gradual transmission of information, that is not everything for the time. The physiotherapist which is informing patients must however pay attention, what demand of the patient for information is, since if asked questions stay, it belongs on not to answer and not to leave in the uncertainty. That's all guarantees adaptations of the sick person to the situation. Unfortunately, always many problems will cause the aspect, how to recognize the quantity of the information, which patient, given for it is possible to hand over. In literature he is meeting with the notion called the determined notion: with warning shot. He relies on it, around one should signal his state to the patient, with for example saying: I am afraid that the situation is graver than I supposed. Next depending on the reaction of the patient one should fit replies.

One should urgently observe the patient in order in every moment to know, whether provided information isn't outgrowing him. After this fact, it is necessary also to see to it .. so that don't leave the patient to one's own devices, and provide the contact with somebody close with whom he will be able to talk about it for him.

Psychological Factors in the Profession of the Being Physiotherapist Educator Medical

Psychological factors which influence relations the physiotherapist but the patient are very much wide and of May significant effect to effects of the treatment. Bad applying methods in relations very much quickly can cause the degeneration of the morbidity of the patient. Presenting above is indicating types of models explicitly for depicting the diversity of issues and multitudes of factors having a deciding influence on the patient and relations between the sick person and the physiotherapist are determining (Ostrowska 2001).

A communication and an amount of provided information and their quality are playing the key role. Described various aspects which they have stayed in the text or can affect relations between the physiotherapist and the patient. Above it appears from shown descriptions that psychological factors in the disease process are playing the very important role both for the patient, for example awareness of what with it is happening, and because of that faster recuperation, as well as of medical staff what influences for example to satisfaction from effects of the performed work.

Analysing all above characteristics, lets for expressing conclusions with reference to the profession of the physiotherapist:

- Having the theory of the profession, the role model, the ethical code, principles of the practicing a profession and the peculiar personal culture, is speaking for professional proceedings of the occupational group of physiotherapists and regarding her unquestionably as the medical profession.
- Is essential regulation of qualifications for the practicing a profession
- Competence of the physiotherapist and recognizing them by the patient are source of trusting towards the professional, of which observing norms is a purpose and a task and of high professional standards.
- The humanistic attitude of physiotherapists is covering treating the patient always as persons with, of subject of one's influence.
- To the professionalism of the entire occupational group units are working, therefore is so essential so that act in concert as part of professional organisations to build the culture up professional, to fortify it so that everyone notice the bond with other representatives of its profession since the automatic identification is a necessary and essential requirement for due action.

REFERENCES

De Walden–Gałuszko, K. (2000). *Problems of communication, Avid (red. K. De Walden-Gałuszko).* Kraków: Psychiatry Library.

Gabard, D., & Martin, M. (2003). *Physical therapy ethics.* Philadelphia: F.A. Davis.

Hebda, P., & Madejski, J. (2004). *A profession with passion.* Bielsko-Biała: At the Metropolitan Museum. Park.

Hejwosz, D. A. (2008). Patient-oriented approach in the process of education. In Health education. The possibilities, problems, restrictions with regard. Polish Scientific Medical University.

Jemielniak, D. (2005). Culture: trades and professions. In Zbytniewska k. Works and material. ISM Publishing House.

Karski, J.B. (2011). *Practice and theory of health promotion.* CeDeWu.

Kenrick, P. T., Neuberg, S. L., & Cialdini, R. B. (2002). *Social psychology.* Gdańsk: GWP.

Kiebzak W., Giermek K., Florczyk M., & Kiljański M. (2009). Code of conduct Physiotherapist of the Republic of Poland. *Physiotherapy Poland, 9*(3), 266-272.

Litwiejko, A. (2010). *The basics of public health in terms of legal and social Publishing House.* Wroclaw.

Makowska, H. (2001). Informing the patient by a doctor. Whether people ill want to know everything threatens? In The basics of Health Psychology. Publishing House of the University of Wrocław.

Michalin, M. (2003). From ethics to business ethics. Foundation for Innovation, Higher Socio-Economic School.

Ostrowska, A. (2001). The relationship patient doctor-new quality. Health promotion. *Social Science & Medicine*, *21*, 109–121.

Pezdek, K. (2010). Responsibility as a value in the work of physiotherapist. *Physiotherapy*, *18*(1), 72–77. doi:10.2478/v10109-010-0047-2

Rusin, M. (2013). *Attitude and ethical principles of physiotherapist*. Bielsko-Biała: WSA.

Rusin, M. (2012). Model bed modern physiotherapist. *Medical Rehabilitation, 16*(2), 34-46.

Straburzyńska-Lupa,A.Straburzyński,G. (2007). *Physiotherapy*. PZWL.

Chapter 15
Cross-Cultural Decision-Making in Healthcare:
Theory and Practical Application in Real Clinical Conditions

Tomasz Komendziński
Nocolaus Copernicus University, Poland

Emilia Mikołajewska
Nocolaus Copernicus University, Poland

Dariusz Mikołajewski
Nicolaus Copernicus University, Poland

ABSTRACT

This chapter describes how people are connected to each other through a common system of encoding and decoding messages. Opening the European gate has made intercultural communication omnipresent, and this includes health care. Internationally-based tasks need new, culture-aware medical practitioners. The challenges, barriers, and solutions in the aforementioned area based on the personal experiences of the authors. The chapter concludes that in spite of personal experience, intercultural tension continues to be a major hinderance to patient healthcare services.

INTRODUCTION

Culture constitutes a complex structure that includes habitual ways of thinking, acting, and interacting. This built-in set of procedures is "the software of the mind" and can be shared, learned, and updated, but is also subject to typically gradual change. Many attempts at defining culture describe it as a non-monolythic, overlapping set of internal "scripts" defining the functioning of social norms and values: "culture involves the ideas, beliefs, values, and assumptions about life that are widely shared among a group of people and guide much of their behavior" (Brislin, 1993). Assuming this perspective allows us to realize that people are equipped with various cultural "tools", and some of them may overlap or

DOI: 10.4018/978-1-5225-3946-9.ch015

even cut across different cultures (national, regional, organizational, professional, etc.). It can be also shaped by many factors: family, religion, political and educational systems, art and other activities. Culture also influences our vision of the world and interactions with other people: cognition (behaviors, information) and recognition and interpretation of emotions (both our own as well as those of others). Within a particular culture, people are connected to each other through a common system of encoding and decoding messages. Messages are sent, received and confirmed through verbal and nonverbal behaviors (Kim, 1988).

The multiculturalism of the European society is deep due to the migration of people and extensive tourism. There is no doubt that opening the European gates made social interaction and mutual understanding between representatives of different cultures much easier. Intercultural communication helps us become more familiar with foreign countries, organizations, and cultures and affords new opportunities for intercultural communication (Hornakova, 2006).

Figure 1. Cultural categories and their relations to health and compensation
Côté, 2013.

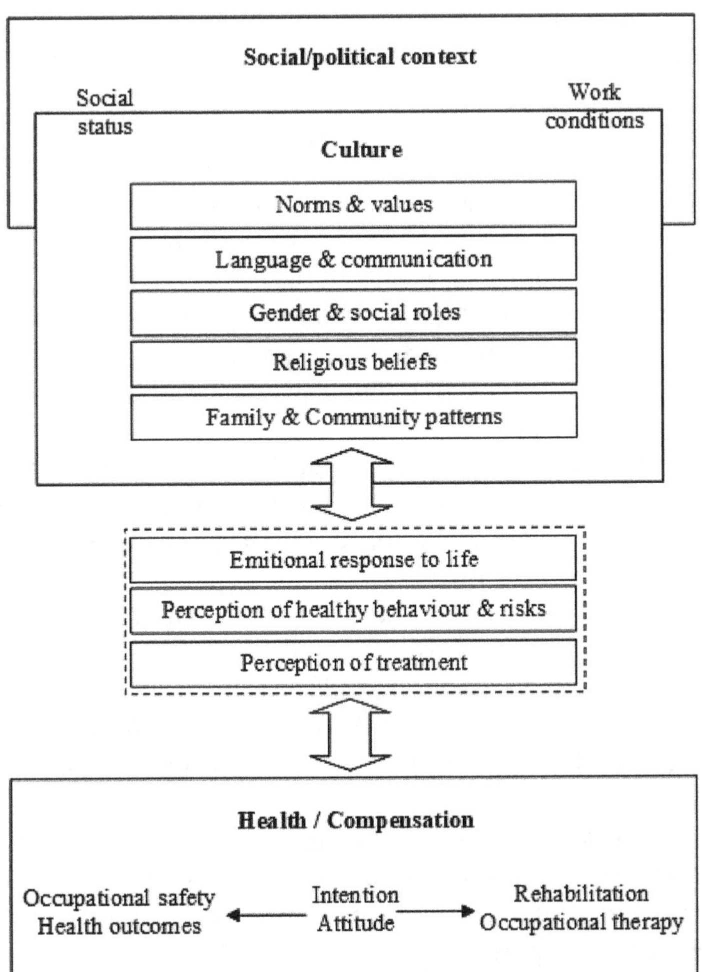

Current approaches to understanding other cultures are divided into a dissecting (superficial) model and a classifying (quantifying) one. Both these approaches have their strengths and weaknesses, but there is a clear need to develop, implement, and evaluate high-quality semi-automated education and training programs that focus on human perception and deeper understanding of other cultures without stereotyping. This way every culture can be recognized and "decoded" thanks to the cultural intelligence, even though the cultural mindset of a typical Polish person might be very different from that of a Japanese, which results in different interpretations of the same behaviour. Our aim is to think how to predict and avoid failing in inter-cultural interactions within a working health care system.

This issue is important for organizations operating in both national and international environments. The specific organizations in question are health care units and their everyday clinical practice. In times of hardship, full of social tensions and unrest, there might arise sudden and drastic cultural shifts, which often make the biases and limits of the existing models of culture more visible. They may provide only a partial view of culture and significantly influence the effects of clinical practice. Taking into consideration various perspectives and interpretation of own behavior may be thus critical. Cross-cultural decision making, culturally-aware education systems and highly-developed information gathering and analysing capabilities have become a foundational part of health care systems, which allows for implementing effective forms of treatments (higher quality of life for the patient in terms of health condition). Even those organisations that are described as most conservative and reflexively opposed to changes in the health care system are aware that medical knowledge and clinical experience are not enough to assure recovery and respect the patients' free will and choice. The ultimate therapeutic success is now measured by different standards than before, namely, by the patients' capacity to return to education/work, participation in everyday life of their family and community, and finally by the general patient satisfaction. Such a success may be achieved despite the impossibility of complete recovery.

The challenges that international medicine poses call for a new breed of culture-aware medical practitioners. We do not know if transcultural orientation is the best possible solution, but we have to take it into consideration. There is often the need for new solutions, joint research, health care or educational activities. This instigates adaptive reformulations of the progressive health care guidelines, standards, and procedures. Moreover, we do not know if institutional health care culture really can pose significant obstacles to organizational adaptation.

The phenomenon of non-native or foreign patients and health care staff is not limited to one country or even one continent. What is more, the percentage of non-native physicians in selected countries may in the future increase up to 30% - understanding dialects, colloquial speech, and body language may be difficult for them.

Even the most homogenous society is not a society without differences. Demographic shifts make cultural diversity an important factor in the workplace of the medical staff. Due to the diversity of patients' backgrounds, clinical specialties, approaches and diagnostic/therapeutic methods, understanding the importance of communication in health care delivery becomes the key issue. The same patients communicate with physicians, therapists, doctors, and other health care professionals from differing cultural backgrounds.

The term "health care provider" encompasses the organization and its workers, i.e. not only medical specialists, but also pharmacists, medical secretaries, medical IT specialists, the administrative personnel and others. These people may get in touch with patients (even accidentally) and influence the public relations of a particular health care provider. Thus, the term "delivery of health care" encompasses all services offered by a health care provider (not only treatment, rehabilitation and care). We should be aware that the aforementioned terms and definitions, as far as some strict regulations and procedures, may be perceived by patients as an attempt at dehumanization of the health care and a lack of an individual approach to each particular patient.

BACKGROUND: INTERCULTURAL COMMUNICATION IN HEALTH CARE AND ITS CHALLENGES

Health care workers have to learn how to communicate effectively with people from other cultures (Collier, 1989). Effective intercultural communication in health care affects patients' physical and mental well-being (Voelker, 1995). Understanding and respecting the values, beliefs, and attitudes of the patients constitutes a key element of this process (Bronner, 1994; Moore, 1992).

Interactions within the health care system are intercultural, since patients do not share the terminology, assumptions, and norms of the health profession culture (Ulrey & Amason, 2001). Setting up an effective health care system requires recognizing the importance of communication: faster and more precise diagnosis. Shortcomings in communication may lead to shortcomings in health care. Strict health care procedures are not the same as communication between two parties: the medical team and its patients. The medical jargon and lack of time make patients feel as if they were communicating with a machine (internet bot): quick procedural questions, lack of confirmation, poor understanding, weak patient-therapist co-operation.

A better ability to communicate across cultures may provide a significant market advantage, since improved communication may influence public relations and produce credentials as a patient-friendly and effective brand.

Miscommunication may, at the very least, cause dissatisfaction and stress for both providers and patients, but it can also lead to misunderstandings and costly mistakes, including misdiagnoses and violations of patients' ethical beliefs (Ulrey & Amason, 2001). A common example of this is when patients from different cultures report pain in various ways (Lee et al., 1992), and even informed consent (full information enabling them to freely make decisions about their own health care) may be culture-sensitive (Gostin, 1995).

The medical staff should learn to decode non-verbal expressions characteristic of patients from different cultures, they should study their traditions, customs, religions and lifestyles as well (Hornakova, 2006). The traditional, monocultural health care organizations contribute to the exclusion of certain social groups (Stone, 2009).

Health care is not typically a competitive market, but it nonetheless needs to advance and prove successful in its endeavours. Market decisions that are confusing or difficult to understand to the society bring infamy and may influence the reputation of the health care unit. Intercultural issues in health care may take away the attention from work-related factors and emphasize the attitude, expressions of feelings, perceptions, therapist-patient relationships and modalities of intervention in intercultural settings (Côté, 2013).

INTERCULTURAL COMMUNICATION IN HEALTH CARE: BARRIERS

We can consciously, though not always directly, assess the effectiveness of our communication with others.

There may be defined four primary cultural dimensions:

- **Patterns of Thought:** Common ways of thinking, beliefs, values, norms, and emotional attitudes,
- **Patterns of Behavior:** Common ways of behaving, speaking, etc., with intentional/unintentional, unconscious/subconscious or individual/interactive behaviour,
- **Patterns of Artifact Utilisation:** Common ways of manufacturing and using things, dwellings, tools, machines, and media,
- **Imprints in Nature:** The long-lasting imprints left by a group in the natural surroundings, (agriculture, trash, roads, etc.).

The most important factors influencing health care communication are as follows:

- Sensitivity to cultural differences where cultural sensitivity is defined as "willingness to use cultural knowledge while interacting with patients and considering culture during discussions and recommendations for treatment" (Brislin, 1993; Dennis & Giangreco, 1996; Jackson & Haynes, 1992))
- Language barriers (not only in clinical assessment, but also in translating prescriptions, etc.), including night shifts in hospital, where the number of bi- or multi-lingual personnel is limited
- Religious or spiritual beliefs, taboos, sex-role differences
- Patients' assumptions and beliefs concerning health care
- Prejudicial attitudes (sets of ideas based on stereotypes) influencing health care delivery, which is defined as "different ways that some cultural groups are treated in the health care system"
- Tensions between the patient and his/her family and the medical staff
- Disabilities, disorders, pain, stress, depression (including non-disclosed aliments and deficiencies, e.g. driver who resist diagnosing and healing eyes failure because he fears that he will lose his job
- Power differences (imbalances of power) – built into the health care structure
- Health care as a business (e.g. limitation of health care services)
- Intercultural vision of medical ethics
- Some controversial subjects: mental illness, AIDS, sexually transmitted diseases, vaccines, impotence, abortion, euthanasia, and in-vitro fertilisation
- Medical miscommunication - cultural misunderstanding resulting in medical mistakes, problems with patient use of medication, etc.

Physicians can give information about the patient's health within four general frameworks:

- **Strict Paternalism:** Reflects a physician's decision to provide misinformation to the patient when the physician believes it is in the best interest of the patient (e.g. in the case of a patient with terminal cancer)
- **Benevolent Deception:** When the physician chooses to communicate only a part of a patient's diagnosis (e.g. in the case of patients with poor prognosis)
- **Contractual Honesty:** Telling the patient only what she or he wants/wishes to hear or to know
- **Unmitigated Honesty:** When a physician chooses to communicate the entire diagnosis to a patient

Cultural sensitivity and effective intercultural communication undoubtedly benefit the health care providers personally by reducing their stress levels. Patients are often too scared and sick to focus on communication, whereas the providers are pressed for time or too focused on technology (Kreps & Kunimoto, 1994). Medical staff should endeavor to reduce the effects of lapses in communication whenever possible.

INTERCULTURAL COMMUNICATION IN HEALTH CARE: SOLUTIONS

Even though both sides – the patient and the medical specialist - are responsible for effective communication, it is the latter on whom the greater share of said responsibility lies, since it is them who is expected to use their training and communicative competence to develop positive relationships that facilitate an accurate diagnosing and effective treatment of patients (Ulrey & Amason, 2001). The trust on part of the patient and his/her family significantly influences the efficacy of the health-promoting strategies that are at the doctors' disposal.

Three dimensions of intervention in the context of cultural pluralism are highlighted by authors:

- Therapist-patient relationship
- Organisational structure
- Cultural competence, i.e. set of attitudes, practices and policies needed to develop culturally responsive caring (Côté, 2013)

Lots of attention should be focused on preventing and solving issues related to intercultural communication. If hospital staff understands cultural differences, it might help avoid many conflicts that might ensue from said differences.

Cultural sensitivity in health care settings includes:

- Avoiding routine
- Using culturally appropriate language
- Having knowledge of other cultures
- Understanding culture-specific value
- Considering culture in assessment of patients
- Adapting treatment according to the cultural knowledge they have regarding a patient (Bernal et al., 1995; Dennis & Giangreco, 1996)

Intercultural communication training programs for health care providers covers cultural accommodation of the medical staff. One of possible solutions is the LEARN model:

L: Listen to the patient's perception of the problem
E: Explain your point of view
A: Acknowledge and discuss the differences and disparities in perceptions of the problem,
R: Recommend treatment
N: Negotiate treatment (Edlin 2012)

Key issues are also: family involvement, community involvement: social support and feedback, chaplain involvement (where possible), and combating myths thanks to EBM-based therapy (but see also for role of alternative therapies as complementary medicine).

Study by Hornakova on Czech health care system showed that understanding the professional foreign terminology used in clinical practice is important for the majority of health care specialists. It is rarely possible to implement it in everyday clinical practice, and the most common way to maintain it are internet, professional literature, radio and television. Moreover, better financial prospects were much more important than higher qualifications or career development (Hornakova, 2006). Recommendations for effective intercultural communication in health care profession are as follows:

- Have enough time for each client from different culture
- Find a language for communication
- Use simple words and expressions which the patients from other cultures will understand
- Avoid medical terminology as much as you can
- Speak slowly and clearly, repeat words more often and require the same from different-culture patients
- Health care professionals should learn words for basic communication in the language of the Different-culture client and use them adequately
- Suppose possible prejudices and check the meaning of understanding
- Take your time to express yourself, do not be in a hurry
- To facilitate better understanding, smile and use gestures and visual aids in form of pictures
- Notice the non-verbal expressions of different-culture clients
- Find solutions that are a compromise, tolerate cultural varieties and ethics
- Help your clients express their feelings, ideas, opinions and needs
- Add schemes, drawings, communication cards, etc.
- Be patient and tolerant to all non-verbal expressions of different culture clients
- Verify whether the client understands the basic information you are trying to convey
- Provide the date(s) in numbers rather than words
- Listen carefully
- Encourage a client from the different culture to express their feelings, ideas, opinions and needs
- Use foreign language dictionaries and an interpreter if necessary (Hornakova, 2006)

COMMUNICATION WITH PATIENTS WITH NEUROLOGICAL DISORDERS

Stroke therapy focuses on reducing mortality, decreasing functional impairment, and increasing the patient's quality of life. Stroke may affect various levels of the nervous system and can lead to complex reception and/or perception deficits. Communication in post-stroke patients is impaired by aphasia, dysarthria, and many other syndromes. Patients with communicative disorders and special needs typically require further diagnosis and therapy aided by the speech pathologist. Medical staff and family/caregivers need obey rules related to the deficit areas, and certain possible psychological reactions and their influence on patient and his/her environment should be discussed (Pimentel, 1986). Although patient-staff communication is regarded as important, Laghorne et al. put little emphasis on it in their study in the section where they describe stroke patient care. They enumerate the following elements:

- Assessment procedures: medical, nursing and therapy assessments
- Early management policies: early mobilization, avoidance of urinary catheterization, treatment of hypoxia, hyperglycaemia, and suspected infection
- Ongoing rehabilitation policies: coordinated multidisciplinary team care, early assessment for discharge (Langhorne et al., 2002)

Most of stroke units offer both acute medical treatment and rehabilitation. A stroke unit is characterized by the following features:

- Is geographically defined with dedicated beds
- Has multidisciplinary and specially trained personnel
- Has standardised protocol for diagnostic evaluation, observation, acute treatment and rehabilitation (Indredavik, 2007)

Study by Pound & Ebrahim showed that on the stroke unit, teamwork was divided between doctors and therapists on the one hand and nurses on the other, while on the general medical ward, team working was not observed (Pound & Ebrahim, 2000).

Study conducted by Pound & Ebrahim showed that tasks at the stroke unit were divided between doctors and therapists on the one hand, and nurses on the other. No such tendency was observed at the general ward.

Following figure shows adaptation of the traditional Shannon-Weaver's communication model to communication taking into consideration patient's deficit. It may be modified individually for each patient.

Sudden hearing loss in post-stroke patients (both on brain stem or cortical level) is regarded as common. It may severely impair the patient's ability to communicate (Bamiou, 2015).

In the case of neurological rehabilitation services, multidisciplinary team approach is advocated. Coordinated work of various specialists better stimulates patients with neurological disorders, which also improves therapy outcomes. Despite general guidelines, lack of detailed procedures makes therapists'

Figure 2. Shannon-Weaver's communication model which takes into consideration patients' deficits
Own project based on original Shannon-Weaver's model (Shannon 1948).

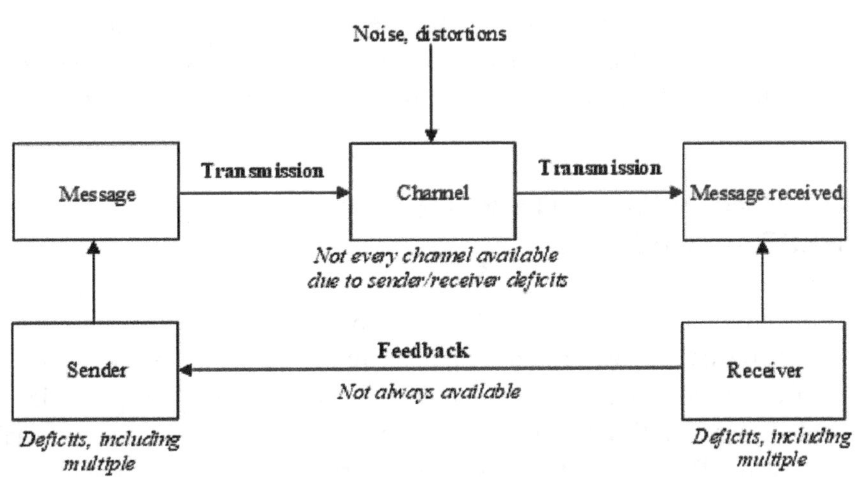

experiences and perceptions diverse, as far as structure and composition of the team are concerned (Suddick & De Souza, 2006).

Multidisciplinary team meetings are regarded as useful form of coordinating daily work and a form of institutionalised communication. However, to be effective, the meetings need to:

- Organise and communicate in the team adequately
- Achieve a consensus in a multidisciplinary discussion
- Offer consistency in the patient management standard
- Include a teaching element for junior team members
- Improve communication between different specialists
- Have a mature leadership
- Be democratic
- Entail constructive discussion. (Ruhstaller et al., 2006)

Now such meetings are regarded as a key component of a professional's routine. As opposed to the multidisciplinary team, integrated care methods may not reduce disability, institutionalisation, or duration of hospitalization. (Sulch et al., 2002).

Multidisciplinary team in stroke rehabilitation offers:

- Improved team working
- Better understanding of patients' needs
- Enhanced SMART (specific, measurable, achievable, realistic and time framed) goal-setting
- Greater patient involvement (Monaghan et al., 2005)

Nursing staff might be considered a weak point of post-stroke therapy and communication.

Nurses often talk with patients in a functional manner, use minimal social or affective communication, avoid patients with communication difficulties. They control conversation, its topic and flow. A certain asymmetry was observed: patients responded briefly to closed-ended questions, whereas the conversation focus should be on the patient's goals, hopes, worries and future expectations. Poor communication may impair the development of communication abilities and the potential to recovery. (Gordon et al., 2009).

The International Classification of Functioning, Disability and Health (ICF) may clarify team roles and clinical reasoning for rehabilitation planning purposes. It may also aid communication within multidisciplinary therapeutic team; moreover, it may structure service provision in the conditions of mixed skills, individuals' interests, and staffing levels within teams (Tempest & McIntyre, 2002).

COMMUNICATION WITH PATIENTS WITH AND POST-CONSCIOUSNESS DISORDERS

(Re)establishment of communication is one of the main goals in the assessment and therapy of patients with disorders of consciousness (DoC). Extensive motor impairment and lack of speech are challenges for further communication. What may also be apparent is the absence of external signs of consciousness. Patients are able to process stimuli of varying complexity even in cases of being unable to respond. Unfortunately, patients with DoC are the the most severely impaired; in effect, severe motor impairment, fatigue and attention disorders, may lead to severe communication deficits in this population. Little is known about the mental life of such patients, and it still needs further research. How can be sure, if certain person is conscious and aware. (One may ask how can we not be sure whether a certain person is conscious and aware or not) Current diagnoses and assessments, based mainly on behavioral measures, are unreliable and prone to errors. Disorders of communication similar to DoC may cause discerning the disorder and lead to false diagnoses. High rate of misdiagnosis (around 40%) is observed in assessment of awareness in patients in a vegetative state (VS, called also unresponsive wakefulness syndrome, UWS) and patients in a minimally conscious state (MCS).

Predicted response to external command constitutes reliable method which allows detecting awareness in patients with DoC. Answer may have various forms, usually measured using dedicated devices (EEG, fMRI, etc.). Action or intention reflected in the predicted pattern of activity observed in the brain (the so-called neural representation) can also constitute a response. Distinction between responsive and nonresponsive patients are still beyond our recognition, but it is fundamental for diagnosis, prognosis, clinical therapy, rehabilitation and care, and even medical ethics, legal rules, and decision-making process (Owen, 2013).

Attempts of communication with the aforementioned patients constitute a major challenge; however, the activity is not without a purpose. Certain percentage of such patients can respond to commands, but we have to help them in improving existing communication channels or providing a new one.

Some percentage of patients with DoC is able to respond to commands by willfully modulating their brain activity (e.g. by selectively paying attention, depending on the stimuli). A binary yes/no answer is much better than no response whatsoever. We hope patients with DoC can selectively maintain attention to certain events in their environment, process them and understand them thanks to coherent thought. We also anticipate that these patients can formulate answers, and wilfully manifest them thanks to a novel technical solution. Brain-based communication tests with the use of functional magnetic resonance imaging showed that all patients followed instructions from commands. Patients in these tests were able to answer either yes or no. As a result, behaviorally nonresponsive patients regained ability to communicate with environment (Naci & Owen, 2013).

Functional magnetic resonance imaging (fMRI) and electroencephalography (EEG)-cover areas of basic sensory, perceptual, language, and emotional processing assessment in patients with DoC. But a positive detection of conscious awareness and possibility for communication is much more difficult (Harrison & Connolly, 2013). Even patients in vegetative state (VS) who appear to be awake do not show any signs of awareness. Yet, they can respond to commands thanks to brain-computer interfaces: willfully modulating their brain activity according to instruction (Naci et al., 2012).

Discrimination between vegetative state and minimally conscious state are essential to subsequent rehabilitation and care. Some EEG procedures are developed to do it quasi-automatically (Mangia et al., 2014).

Binary response "yes/no" to the question may elicited by performing mental imagery tasks using fMRI. Such mental imagery process produces distinct activation patterns (compared to motor imagery in controls). 3 Tesla fMRI is required to provide an appropriate signal-to-noise ratio (Liang et al., 2014).

Variations of similar technical solutions are available for different DoC patients. UWS patients are regarded as having no awareness, while MCS patients are regarded as having their conscious awareness partially preserved. Lancioni et al. described two studies with various types of response:

- Willingly imaging of single- versus double-hand closure
- Increase engaging in leisure activities, and listen to audio-recordings of family members (Lancioni et al., 2014a)

Passive and isolated patients emerged (who recovered from?) from DoC have access to the broader repertoire of responses, despite speech and motor impairment constituting a huge difficulty. Thus, intervention programs relying on assistive technology are applied, including:

- Accessing brief periods of stimulation through one or two microswitches
- Combining a microswitch and a sensor connected to a speech generating device
- Controlling through computer or radio systems and a microswitch
- Communicating through modified messaging or telephone systems operated via microswitch
- Controlling and communicating options through computer systems operated via microswitch (Lancioni et al., 2014b; Lancioni et al., 2012)

What was also described were important brain markers detected in cognitive processes and awareness in the absence of behavioral manifestation; however, which of these are available for DoC patients remains unknown.

Various solutions based on distinct paradigms may be feasible to various DOC patients. Moreover, we should take into consideration clinical usefulness of each solution – e.g. limitations in fMRI due to its:

- Huge dimensions (lack of bedside version)
- Weight
- Complex procedure (both realizing and interpreting, hardly generalizable use in clinical routine)
- Weak temporal resolution
- Cost (Luauté et al., 2015)

Quasi-simultaneous fMRI-EEG measure, increases time resolution of the measurement, is available. But it seems current form of fMRI will not be individual equipment of the patient with DoC. Comtte et al. compared four fMRI-based methods correctly and accurately interpreting the communication task, but:

- None of them showed 100% correct detection during the communication
- 25% of participants did not provide the expected patterns of activations (Comte et al., 2015)

BCI paradigms are more feasible than individual equipment. Recent advances concerning studies on magnetoencephalography (MEG) may constitute another breakthrough in BCI technology. However, we still search for patient's bedside equipment. Several limitations of BCIs are important:

- Lack of awareness in itself
- Lack of spatial resolution (but computational solutions for EEG source localization still quickly develops)
- Atypical patterns of brain activity in brain damaged patients

Despite relatively quick progress – it may concern minority of DOC patients (Luauté et al., 2015).

Alternative diagnostic tools for asessment response to command are also developed. Detecting signs of consciousness in patients in vegetative state/unresponsive wakefulness syndrome (UWS/VS), minimally conscious state (MCS) is possible with the use of a breathing-controlled communication device. One of them achieves accuracy 84%. Patients with locked-in syndrome (LIS) were unable to use it (Charland-Verville et al., 2014).

Despite needs and reported efficacy, the development of the aforementioned systems is limited by many technical and clinical challenges. Such communication mode is difficult, and it also requires trained personnel. Inter-cultural communication using BCI is difficult but not impossible. It requires deep adaptation of the therapeutic team to the needs, knowledge, and previous experience of the DoC patient. Patient's family assistance seems to be very valuable.

COMMUNICATION WITH GERIATRIC PATIENTS

Caring for elderly people (especially: elderly parents) is common in many cultures, not only in the Western culture. Despite various co-occurring physical and/or mental diseases, the elderly is no different from other patients. Communication is crucial for them. Activities and interactions of elderly patients are useful for measurement of their cognitive and behavioural functioning. Study by Armstron-Esther et al. reported rather low levels of staff-patient interaction beyond expected routine of patient care. Staff did not engage patients in social activities or informal conversations while elderly patients require enjoyable and rewarding conversation (Armstron-Esther et al., 1994).

Optimal performance of medical procedures in the elderly needs adequate clinical communication with patients. Importantly, the traditional paternalistic relationship between the patient and the therapist is no longer appropriate. The optimal performance can be achieved by:

- Accuracy
- Empathy
- Efficacy
- Shared decision-making and setting common goals
- Informed consent process
- Adaptation to patient understanding (including level of education, personality, etc.)
- Adaptation to possible cognitive impairment (Giampieri, 2012)

Pain is regarded as a vital factor which influences the course of communication. The following issues were identified in pain-influenced communication:

- Nurse-to-nurse communication
- Nurse-to-patient communication
- Pain management strategies
- Environmental and organisational issues related to care
- Complex nature of pain (Manias, 2012)

Best practice for the management of pain in elderly patients is not fully covered within guidances, partly due to inconsistences and differences in the patients' profile, methods and definitions used. The problem is also influenced by attitudes and beliefs of older people influence all aspects of their pain experience (stoicism is prevalent). Therapies must be individualised and carefully monitored, and certain psychological approaches seem be useful in older population (Abdulla et al., 2013).

Conversational strategies in nurse-to-patient communication should fit the demands of elderly patients suffering, for example, from dementia. The aforementioned can be further divided into two sides of communication:

- **Nurse Conversational Strategies:** Moderating, clarifying, exploring, validating, rescuing, and general discourse markers,
- **Patients' Conversational Strategies:** Discourse markers, limited engagement, expanded responses, personalized response, self-initiated participation, disconnected or fragmented participation.

Even patients with dementia are able to participate in such adaptive conversation (Perry et al., 2005).

Patients with dementia are a special group of elderly patients. The language used by medical staff should match the comprehension abilities of residents. In effect, they become agitated (which is displayed by restlessness, strange noises, or negativism) if this language is too complex for them (Hart & Wells, 1997).

COMMUNICATION WITH PAEDIATRIC PATIENTS

Communication with paediatric patients and their caretakers is extremely difficult and requires not only sophisticated tools but also extraordinary abilities of the general practitioner. The concept of child-physician communication is based on mutual trust, knowledge and experience of the GP. It constitutes developmental intervention itself and shapes new intervention strategy in each patient.

The objective assessment of functional achievements in both healthy and ill children (including children with developmental disabilities) may change significantly due to such factors as: boredom, fear, hunger, thirst, etc. An easier diagnosis or even development of motor, cognitive, or social skills in young patients may be facilitated by the new generation of interactive toys. However, the use of toys as peacemakers is not always enough. The new findings on infant development are key to recent research: they allow to assess both physiological and pathological development and potential retardation, mainly through careful observation. Diagnosis and communication through gestures and toy usage is possible in 8- to 16-month-old infants, but their interpretation is not easy (Dimitrova et al., 2015). There is a need for classification of a whole range of gestures used by a particular infant. Play position, grasping, reaching, handedness, and object manipulation require knowledge shared between children and their caretakers, which would enable a proper interpretation (Miller & Gros-Louis, 2013; Olson & Masur, 2015). On the other hand, poor mobility of the upper limbs, asymmetrical performance, weak reactions to stimulus, poor coordination, or varied motor skills and general recurrent problems in adaptation of posture to the whole repertoire of various movements may characterise developing disorders. Videotaping may be useful for measurement and analysis of such behaviours.

Early detection and diagnosis is essential as it enables the implementation of preventive measures and therapy of pathological elements at a very early stage – every day makes a significant difference in further therapy. Effectiveness of the treatment seems to be closely connected with the proper diagnosis, communication and trust, as well as with the advanced methods, techniques and tools applied in a particular case.

The development of healthy children can be shaped by the toys used. The selection of such toys may influence the sensory, motor and cognitive development and facilitate new achievements. Toys may be useful for monitoring and measuring infants' behaviours but cannot be taken as the only determinant; therefore, more clinical tests are needed.

We present some individual and group toy-associated behaviours which are relatively easy to observe and assess:

- **Searching Behaviour for a Disappearing Toy:** In 5- to 6-month-old infants
- **Pushing a Button to Turn on a Distant Light or to Get a Toy:** In 7-month-old infants
- **Imitating Object Manipulation:** In 10- to 12- month-old infants
- **Performing the Aforementioned Actions Faster Using Various Grasp, a Variety of Objects, and Creative Thinking:** In toddlers
- **Simple Group Behaviours:** Imitating, repeating, passing a toy between children, group toy using, and cooperating during a game: in toddlers
- **Replicating Actions to Achieve Preestablished Effects:** In 19-month-old toddlers
- **Fighting Over a Single Attractive Toy:** Begins in much older children
- **Use of Musical Toys:** Can cause increased responsiveness in toddlers and children of all ages

Many of the aforementioned behaviours may be easily observed by the caretakers, but such an observation made by a stranger (new therapist, new physician) is not easy and needs to be stimulated by a person who is familiar to them.

Some toy-associated behaviours may also relate to the increased probability that a developmental disorder will occur. These include:

- Throwing blocks in 18-month-olds can be a predictor of *attention-deficit hyperactivity disorder* (ADHD) (Yoshikawa, 1997)
- Difficulties in hand-eye coordination
- Lack of manual dexterity
- Lack of recognition of causal relationships

Generally available, low-cost, fun, and functional toys facilitate diagnosis and treatment provided that they are chosen carefully. Moreover, technologically advanced solutions (games, virtual reality) are widely accepted by children.

Most of the studies concern children living in relatively wealthy Western or similar countries, and analyse intercultural factors which may change some of the observed behaviours entirely. We should be aware of the fact that there are still many threats and limitations concerning e.g. stimulation of children with epilepsy (if recognized). Diagnosis and therapy of children with developmental disorders in selected countries is still scarcely accepted. We do not know exactly how will the TV or computer games influence children's behaviours in the future. Their attention span becomes shorter, hence, toys must be more and more attractive. Intra-gender comparisons are not always possible due to social roles stereotypes and task division. On the other hand, hyper-stimulation of a child should be avoided.

The recovery from the paediatric developmental disorders is still limited. Thus, it may significantly influence the health-related quality of life of both the children and their families. In selected cultures such a child may be difficult to accept – we should take it into consideration while shaping the patient-physician communication.

Communication, diagnosis, therapy and care in case of infants should be shaped through play: the execution of the requested behaviours should be covert and therefore natural. Moreover, the same toy can play an important role in exercises performed by the infant – if the therapist or the caretaker provide the children with the same communicative-therapeutic activities at home.

A variety of developmental disorders, patients' and parents' profiles or factors influencing therapy outcomes make the whole intervention patient-oriented. This kind of approach, even NDT-Bobath derived, is often called eclectic or mixed.

It is difficult to apply detailed schemas describing communication in the therapy of infants with developmental disorders. Various toys, games, and robots (even artificial animals) are used, but none particular toy guarantees therapeutic success. Instead, it is better to think about stimulators such as colour, shape, texture, movement, light or sound.

Toys may become a very useful communicative and therapeutic tool in the examination of infants, toddlers and children. The effective use of toys needs a thorough understanding of normal and pathological development of the group discussed. Appropriate stimulation may significantly enhance motor, cognitive, and social skills. It seems that neither medical specialist nor parents are trained for conscious and wise application of such knowledge in clinical practice and everyday life.

Generally, we can say that communication with young patients is far from communication with adult patients. Child therapy and end-of-life care in the paediatric intensive care units are crucial. Six domains are identified as critical to high-quality, family-centred care:

- Communication with the child and family – concerning treatment goals and plans
- Continuity of care
- Family support
- Ethics and shared decision-making
- Pain and other symptoms reduction
- Grief and bereavement support (Truog et al., 2006)

COMMUNICATION IN PALLIATIVE CARE

Relation to disease, suffering and death varies across cultures and influences the palliative care. Physician-patient communication is the central element of quality care and family satisfaction. Nonetheless, communication in palliative care seems to be a very difficult but a rather well recognized issue. There is a need for effective communication, identification of effective communication systems, and exploration of the influence and value of the contemporary communication theories, models, and frameworks in palliative care. Alleviating pain and anxiety, promoting patient's quality of life, encouraging patients and their families, as far as situational control should constitute general basement of patient-staff relationship (Wallace, 2001).

Terminal patients and their families usually look for better quality of life – establishing certain and adequate ways of communication may play key role in this process. The study by de Andrade et al. (2013), concerning patient-nurse communication in palliative care extracted the three basic categories:

- "Palliative care and communication - interpersonal relation between the nurse and the terminally ill patient";
- "Communication in palliative care as a strategy for strengthening the bond between the nurse and the terminally ill patient";
- "The importance of communication between the nurse and the family of the terminally ill patient under palliative care".

Communication plays a significant role in the individual assessment of the patient. Intensive care units and palliative care units are regarded as "high quality" based on various criteria. Study by Nelson et al. (2010: 809) extracted such factors as:

- Timely, clear, and careful communication
- Therapy focused on patients' preferences, goals, and values
- Care concerning comfort, dignity, and personhood of the patient
- Family care with open access and proximity to patients
- Interdisciplinary support in the intensive care unit
- Bereavement care for families of patients who died

According to the study by Seccareccia et al. (2015), key elements of communication in high-quality palliative care are:

- Building trust and kinship with patients and families
- Meeting the expectations and explaining goals of care
- Keeping patients and families informed about the patient's condition
- Validating patients' concerns and needs by means of careful listening
- Intruding the issue of death and dying in a careful and controlled manner

Despite vast research, there is still no central and widely accepted set of communication skills in palliative care. Some of them may best be described as:

- Respectful and friendly attitude towards the patients
- Initiative to discuss the end-of-life issues (Slort et al., 2011)

On the other hand, limitations stemming from the nature of treatment and physicians' work are reported as well:

- Difficulty in dealing with former doctors' delay
- Demands from patients' family
- Dealing with emotions and troublesome doctor-patient relations
- Insufficient clarification of patients' problems

- Promises that could not be kept
- Helplessness
- Too close involvement
- Insufficient anticipation of various scenarios (Slort et al., 2011)

Family meetings are regarded as a space for implementing shared decision-making and improving communication in the relation to the patient's family – medical staff, empathy, and open discussion concerning death and dying. It may improve patient's test results, reduce trauma, depression, and anxiety, improve patient's quality of death and dying (Levin et al., 2010).

DISCUSSION

Research and associated guidelines to contemporary and future clinical practice should cover at least the following issues:

- Biopsychosocial approach and holistic therapy and care gradually replace previous biomedical approach
- Differences between roles, tasks, and power of various health care professionals (physicians, nurses, physical therapists, occupational therapists, medical technicians, etc.) within a multidisciplinary therapeutic team
- Some specialist may participate in a multidisciplinary therapeutic team only temporarily, but they need a coherent view of the whole therapy
- Research, education, and clinical practice should cover not only current problems but also problems emerging in the near future
- Theory and practice may differ significantly
- Homogenous populations (including medical staff and patients – their caretakers and families) seem not to be prepared to intercultural society or approach within health care system

We described various issues that are relevant to intercultural communication within health care system. As the population becomes more culturally diversified, intercultural communication becomes more important. Communication is crucial for the functioning of health service, and is not limited to the communication between the patient and the physician.

LIMITATIONS OF CURRENT RESEARCH

- Results are often limited to physicians and nurses – we do not know their impact e.g. on long-term rehabilitation
- Results may not be universal to all health care providers
- Results for a particular population are valid for members of this population – it is difficult to compare the results for various populations
- An increasing number of international students, immigrants, and foreign tourists may influence the results for a popular city or even the whole region

Despite common awareness and cultural education, competence within health care system is far from ideal. Possibility of being exposed to multicultural clinical settings should be sufficient to prevent from stereotypes, generalizations, and reductionism (Côté, 2013).

DIRECTIONS FOR FURTHER RESEARCH

There is a one general direction for further research: identification of intervention modalities and conceptual framework proposed by the researchers, clinicians, and organizations (both governmental and non-governmental) targeted at improving the services and care directed to the patients from different cultural backgrounds. A coherent strategy allows for improvement of the efficacy of the whole action.

The described problems have been studied by various disciplines: anthropology, sociology, medicine, cognitive science, and linguistics. Nevertheless, they need a coherent view from the practical perspective.

The detailed short- and long-term goals are more complex – a set of goals depends on many factors, including local settings. It may encompass the following ideas:

- Ways in which communication influences the delivery of medical services can be foreseen
- How much our society or family trusts physicians (or generally medical staff)
- How patients understand the importance of communication in health care situations
- Whether a more serious illness may require much interaction with a physician (or generally medical staff)
- How can health care professionals encourage more open communication
- To what extent gender is a relevant issue in the context of intercultural encounters in the medical environment
- The influence of the media on the relations between the patients and the health care staff
- Which training programmes focused on improving physicians' and staff's intercultural communication need to be implemented
- Whether appropriate facilities are provided to promote healthy behaviours among ethnic minorities
- Whether we are equipped (theoretical frameworks, intervention tools and guidelines) to provide a culturally appropriate response to disability management, return to work or rehabilitation with regard to the diversity of the workforce

Evidence in this field is limited: many studies do not provide requirements on the selection criteria (inclusion/exclusion) or keywords. Moreover, the confusion between the racial and ethnocultural categories (mixed phenotypes, national and religious labels, natives and immigrants, and economic or political migrations) (Côté, 2013) are omnipresent.

It may be difficult to assess the situation without any general plan or external support. Some communities have long histories of integration in their host country, and have developed their own social and integration structures, but some communities still live in internal isolation (Côté, 2013).

A newly implemented research may constitute an important background for training programmes which can minimize the negative results stemming from cultural differences.

CONCLUSION

There is a discrepancy between scientific research, current knowledge, and clinical practice.

Intercultural issues concerning health care system are hardly a new topic. The population of the European Union nations becomes more diversified culturally, and there is an urgent need to develop intercultural communication skills (Hornakova, 2006). Development of intercultural therapeutic relationships seems to be the key element of the novel approach to the health care system. The growth of immigration is a real challenge to the delivery of health care services. Despite growing concerns in providing culturally appropriate heath care, intervention models, tools and training tools are still not enough in the current health care systems (Côté, 2013).

Health care specialists perceive themselves as culturally sensitive and experience less anxiety in intercultural situations. Further, reduced anxiety may lead to better quality of health care (Ulrey & Amason, 2001).

We need more evidence concerning long-term results (i.e. concerning post-graduate education of the medical staff) of such programmes. New goals need new and more precise tools, which can be the main challenge for scientists from the aforementioned areas. Certain psychological approaches may be helpful as well.

ACKNOWLEDGMENT

This work was conducted as a part of work within the InteRDoCTor project.

REFERENCES

Abdulla, A., Adams, N., Bone, M., Elliott, A. M., Gaffin, J., Jones, D., & Schofield, P. et al.British Geriatric Society. (2013). Guidance on the management of pain in older people. *Age and Ageing*, *42*(Suppl. 1), i1–i57. doi:10.1093/ageing/afs199 PMID:23420266

Armstron-Esther, C. A., Brown, K. D., & McAfee, J. G. (1994). Elderly patients: Still clean and sitting quietly. *Journal of Advanced Nursing*, *19*(2), 264–271. doi:10.1111/j.1365-2648.1994.tb01080.x PMID:8188957

Bamiou, D. E. (2015). Hearing disorders in stroke. *Handbook of Clinical Neurology*, *129*, 633–647. doi:10.1016/B978-0-444-62630-1.00035-4 PMID:25726294

Bernal, G., Bonilla, J., & Bellido, C. (1995). Ecological validity and cultural sensitivity for outcome research: Issues for the cultural adaptation and development of psychosocial treatments with Hispanics. *Journal of Abnormal Child Psychology*, *23*(1), 67–82. doi:10.1007/BF01447045 PMID:7759675

Brislin, R. (1993). *Understanding culture's influence on behavior*. Orlando, FL: Harcourt Brace.

Bronner, Y. (1994). Cultural sensitivity and nutrition counseling. *Topics in Clinical Nutrition*, *9*(2), 13–19. doi:10.1097/00008486-199403000-00004

Charland-Verville, V., Lesenfants, D., Sela, L., Noirhomme, Q., Ziegler, E., Chatelle, C., & Laureys, S. et al. (2014). Detection of response to command using voluntary control of breathing in disorders of consciousness. *Frontiers in Human Neuroscience*, *8*, 1020. doi:10.3389/fnhum.2014.01020 PMID:25566035

Collier, M. J. (1989). Cultural and intercultural communication competence: Current approaches and directions for future research. *International Journal of Intercultural Relations*, *13*(3), 287–302. doi:10.1016/0147-1767(89)90014-X

Comte, A., Gabriel, D., Pazart, L., Magnin, E., Cretin, E., Haffen, E., & Aubry, R. et al. (2015). On the difficulty to communicate with fMRI-based protocols used to identify covert awareness. *Neuroscience*, *300*, 448–459. doi:10.1016/j.neuroscience.2015.05.059 PMID:26033566

Côté, D. (2013). Intercultural communication in health care: challenges and solutions in work rehabilitation practices and training: a comprehensive review. *Disability and Rehabilitation*, *35*(2), 153–163. doi:10.3109/09638288.2012.687034 PMID:22616895

de Andrade, C. G., da Costa, S. F., & Lopes, M. E. (2013). Palliative care: Communication as a strategy of care for the terminal patient. *Ciencia & Saude Coletiva*, *18*(9), 2523–2530. PMID:23989558

Dennis, R. E., & Giangreco, M. F. (1996). Creating conversation: Reflections on cultural sensitivity in family interviewing. *Exceptional Children*, *63*(1), 103–116. doi:10.1177/001440299606300109

Dimitrova, N., Moro, C., & Mohr, C. (2015). Caregivers interpret infants' early gestures based on shared knowledge about referents. *Infant Behavior and Development*, *39*, 98–106. doi:10.1016/j.infbeh.2015.02.015 PMID:25827260

Edlin, M. (2012). Cultural competency means better patience service. *Drug Topics*, *156*(6), 18.

Giampieri, M. (2012). Communication and informed consent in elderly people. *Minerva Anestesiologica*, *78*(2), 236–242. PMID:22127308

Gordon, C., Ellis-Hill, C., & Ashburn, A. (2009). The use of conversational analysis: Nurse-patient interaction in communication disability after stroke. *Journal of Advanced Nursing*, *65*(3), 544–553. doi:10.1111/j.1365-2648.2008.04917.x PMID:19222652

Gostin, L. O. (1995). Informed consent, cultural sensitivity, and respect for persons. *Journal of the American Medical Association*, *274*(10), 844–845. doi:10.1001/jama.1995.03530100084039 PMID:7650810

Harrison, A. H., & Connolly, J. F. (2013). Finding a way in: A review and practical evaluation of fMRI and EEG for detection and assessment in disorders of consciousness. *Neuroscience and Biobehavioral Reviews*, *37*(8), 1403–1419. doi:10.1016/j.neubiorev.2013.05.004 PMID:23680699

Hart, B. D., & Wells, D. L. (1997). The effects of language used by caregivers on agitation in residents with dementia. *Clinical Nurse Specialist CNS*, *11*(1), 20–23. doi:10.1097/00002800-199701000-00015 PMID:9233134

Horňáková, A. (2006). Language implementation of future health care workers and using of professional medical terminology in foreign language. In *Trends in Nursing IV* (pp. 84–93). Ostrava: University of Ostrava.

Indredavik, B. (2007). What characterises an effective stroke unit? *Tidsskrift for Den Norske Lægeforening*, *127*(9), 1214–1218. PMID:17479142

Jackson, C., & Haynes, T. (1992). *Cultural sensitivity: Aworking model*. Atlanta, GA: Southern Council on Collegiate Education for Nursing.

Kim, Y. Y. (1988). *Communication and cross-cultural adaptation: An integrative theory*. Philadelphia: Multilingual Matters.

Komendziński, T., Komendziński, J., Mikołajewska, E., & Mikołajewski, D. (2016). Ethics in communication with patients in the state of disorders of consciousness. Natural situation and the use of modern technologies. *Advances in Psychiatry and Neurology*, *25*(2), 85–92.

Kreps, G. L., & Kunimoto, E. N. (1994). *Effective communication in multicultural health care settings*. Thousand Oaks, CA: Sage. doi:10.4135/9781483326344

Lancioni, G. E., Bosco, A., Olivetti Belardinelli, M., Singh, N. N., O'Reilly, M. F., Sigafoos, J., & Oliva, D. (2014b). Technology-based intervention programs to promote stimulation control and communication in post-coma persons with different levels of disability. *Frontiers in Human Neuroscience*, *8*, 48. doi:10.3389/fnhum.2014.00048 PMID:24574992

Lancioni, G. E., Singh, N. N., O'Reilly, M. F., Sigafoos, J., Buonocunto, F., D'Amico, F., & Megna, M. et al. (2014a). Occupation and communication programs for post-coma persons with or without consciousness disorders who show extensive motor impairment and lack of speech. *Research in Developmental Disabilities*, *35*(5), 1110–1118. doi:10.1016/j.ridd.2014.01.029 PMID:24582854

Lancioni, G. E., Singh, N. N., O'Reilly, M. F., Sigafoos, J., & Olivetti Belardinelli, M. (2012). Technology-based intervention to help persons with minimally conscious state and pervasive motor disabilities perform environmentally relevant adaptive behavior. *Cognitive Processing*, *13*(Suppl. 1), S219–S222. doi:10.1007/s10339-012-0485-5 PMID:22806668

Langhorne, P., & Pollock, A.Stroke Unit Trialists' Collaboration. (2002). What are the components of effective stroke unit care? *Age and Ageing*, *31*(5), 365–371. doi:10.1093/ageing/31.5.365 PMID:12242199

Lee, M. E., Matsumoto, D., Kobayashi, M., Krupp, D., Maniatis, E. F., & Roberts, W. (1992). Cultural influences on nonverbals in applied settings. In *Applications of nonverbal behavior theories and research* (pp. 239–261). Hillsdale, NJ: Lawrence Erlbaum Associates, Inc.

Levin, T. T., Moreno, B., Silvester, W., & Kissane, D. W. (2010). End-of-life communication in the intensive care unit. *General Hospital Psychiatry*, *32*(4), 433–442. doi:10.1016/j.genhosppsych.2010.04.007 PMID:20633749

Liang, X., Kuhlmann, L., Johnston, L. A., Grayden, D. B., Vogrin, S., Crossley, R., & Cook, M. J. et al. (2014). Extending communication for patients with disorders of consciousness. *Journal of Neuroimaging*, *24*(1), 31–38. doi:10.1111/j.1552-6569.2012.00744.x PMID:22928842

Luauté, J., Morlet, D., & Mattout, J. (2015). BCI in patients with disorders of consciousness: Clinical perspectives. *Annals of Physical and Rehabilitation Medicine*, *58*(1), 29–34. doi:10.1016/j.rehab.2014.09.015 PMID:25616606

Mangia, A. L., Pirini, M., Simoncini, L., & Cappello, A. (2014). A feasibility study of an improved procedure for using EEG to detect brain responses to imagery instruction in patients with disorders of consciousness. *PLoS One*, *9*(6), e99289. doi:10.1371/journal.pone.0099289 PMID:24915148

Manias, E. (2012). Complexities of pain assessment and management in hospitalised older people: A qualitative observation and interview study. *International Journal of Nursing Studies*, *49*(10), 1243–1254. doi:10.1016/j.ijnurstu.2012.05.002 PMID:22640777

Miller, J. L., & Gros-Louis, J. (2013). Socially guided attention influences infants' communicative behavior. *Infant Behavior and Development*, *36*(4), 627–634. doi:10.1016/j.infbeh.2013.06.010 PMID:23906941

Monaghan, J., Channell, K., McDowell, D., & Sharma, A. K. (2005). Improving patient and carer communication, multidisciplinary team working and goal-setting in stroke rehabilitation. *Clinical Rehabilitation*, *19*(2), 194–199. doi:10.1191/0269215505cr837oa PMID:15759535

Moore, S. E. (1992). Cultural sensitivity treatment and research issues with Black adolescent drug users. *Child & Adolescent Social Work Journal*, *9*(3), 249–260. doi:10.1007/BF00755864

Naci, L., Monti, M. M., Cruse, D., Kübler, A., Sorger, B., Goebel, R., & Owen, A. M. et al. (2012, September). Brain-computer interfaces for communication with nonresponsive patients. *Annals of Neurology*, *72*(3), 312–323. doi:10.1002/ana.23656 PMID:23034907

Naci, L., & Owen, A. M. (2013). Making every word count for nonresponsive patients. *JAMA Neurology*, *70*(10), 1235–1241. PMID:23939634

Nelson, J. E., Puntillo, K. A., Pronovost, P. J., Walker, A. S., McAdam, J. L., Ilaoa, D., & Penrod, J. (2010, March). In their own words: Patients and families define high-quality palliative care in the intensive care unit. *Critical Care Medicine*, *38*(3), 808–818. doi:10.1097/CCM.0b013e3181c5887c PMID:20198726

Olson, J., & Masur, E. F. (2015). Mothers' labeling responses to infants' gestures predict vocabulary outcomes. *Journal of Child Language*, *3*, 1–23. PMID:25643656

Owen, A. M. (2013). Detecting consciousness: A unique role for neuroimaging. *Annual Review of Psychology*, *64*(1), 109–133. doi:10.1146/annurev-psych-113011-143729 PMID:23043305

Perry, J., Galloway, S., Bottorff, J. L., & Nixon, S. (2005). Nurse-patient communication in dementia: Improving the odds. *Journal of Gerontological Nursing*, *31*(4), 43–52. doi:10.3928/0098-9134-20050401-10 PMID:15839524

Pimental, P. A. (1986). Alterations in communication. Biopsychosocial aspects of aphasia, dysarthria, and right hemisphere syndromes in the stroke patient. *The Nursing Clinics of North America*, *21*(2), 321–337. PMID:3517820

Pound, P., & Ebrahim, S. (2000). Rhetoric and reality in stroke patient care. *Social Science & Medicine*, *51*(10), 1437–1446. doi:10.1016/S0277-9536(00)00040-X PMID:11077948

Ruhstaller, T., Roe, H., Thürlimann, B., & Nicoll, J. J. (2006). The multidisciplinary meeting: An indispensable aid to communication between different specialities. *European Journal of Cancer (Oxford, England)*, *42*(15), 2459–2462. doi:10.1016/j.ejca.2006.03.034 PMID:16934974

Seccareccia, D., Wentlandt, K., Kevork, N., Workentin, K., Blacker, S., Gagliese, L., & Zimmermann, C. et al. (2015). Communication and Quality of Care on Palliative Care Units: A Qualitative Study. *Journal of Palliative Medicine*, *18*(9), 758–764. doi:10.1089/jpm.2014.0408 PMID:26069934

Shannon, C. (1948). A Mathematical Theory of Communication. *The Bell System Technical Journal*, *27*(3), 379–423, 623–656. doi:10.1002/j.1538-7305.1948.tb01338.x

Slort, W., Blankenstein, A. H., Deliens, L., & van der Horst, H. E. (2011). Facilitators and barriers for GP-patient communication in palliative care: A qualitative study among GPs, patients, and end-of-life consultants. *The British Journal of General Practice*, *61*(585), 167–172. doi:10.3399/bjgp11X567081 PMID:21439174

Stone, J. (2009). Cultural considerations in disability and rehabilitation. *Disability and Rehabilitation*, *31*(14), 1109–1110. doi:10.1080/09638280902773679 PMID:19479534

Suddick, K. M., & De Souza, L. (2006). Therapists' experiences and perceptions of teamwork in neurological rehabilitation: Reasoning behind the team approach, structure and composition of the team and teamworking processes. *Physiotherapy Research International*, *11*(2), 72–83. doi:10.1002/pri.325 PMID:16808088

Sulch, D., Melbourn, A., Perez, I., & Kalra, L. (2002). Integrated care pathways and quality of life on a stroke rehabilitation unit. *Stroke*, *33*(6), 1600–1604. doi:10.1161/01.STR.0000017144.04043.87 PMID:12052998

Tempest, S., & McIntyre, A. (2006). Using the ICF to clarify team roles and demonstrate clinical reasoning in stroke rehabilitation. *Disability and Rehabilitation*, *28*(10), 663–667. doi:10.1080/09638280500276992 PMID:16690581

Truog, R. D., Meyer, E. C., & Burns, J. P. (2006). Toward interventions to improve end-of-life care in the pediatric intensive care unit. *Critical Care Medicine*, *34*(11 Suppl.), S373–S379. doi:10.1097/01.CCM.0000237043.70264.87 PMID:17057601

Ulrey, K. L., & Amason, P. (2001). Intercultural communication between patients and health care providers: An exploration of intercultural communication effectiveness, cultural sensitivity, stress, and anxiety. *Health Communication*, *13*(4), 449–463. doi:10.1207/S15327027HC1304_06 PMID:11771806

Voelker, R. (1995). Speaking the languages of medicine and culture. *Journal of the American Medical Association*, *273*(21), 1639–1641. doi:10.1001/jama.1995.03520450007003 PMID:7752395

Wallace, P. (2001). Improving palliative care through effective communication. *International Journal of Palliative Nursing*, *7*(2), 86–90. doi:10.12968/ijpn.2001.7.2.8919 PMID:12271254

Yoshikawa, R. (1997). Hyperactivity at 18 months of age and attention-deficit hyperactivity disorder before entry to school - follow up study from 18 months to 6 years. *Seishin Shinkeigaku Zasshi. Psychiatria et Neurologia Japonica*, *99*(2), 47–67. PMID:9086845

Compilation of References

(1996). WHO determinant with participatory decision-making styles. *Annals of Internal Medicine, 124*(5), 497–504. doi:10.7326/0003-4819-124-5-199603010-00007 PMID:8602709

(2016). Rosiek A et all, Evaluation of stress intensity and anxiety level in preoperative period of cardiac patients. *Biomedical Research.*

Abdul-Hakim, R., Ismail, R., & Abdul-Razak, N. A. (2010) The relationship between social capital and quality of life among rural households in Terengganu, Malaysia, *International Journal of Sustainable Development,* 1(5). Retrieved 20 May 2014 from http://www.ssrn.com/link/OIDA-Intl-Journal-Sustainable-Dev.html

Abdulla, A., Adams, N., Bone, M., Elliott, A. M., Gaffin, J., Jones, D., & Schofield, P. et al.British Geriatric Society. (2013). Guidance on the management of pain in older people. *Age and Ageing, 42*(Suppl. 1), i1–i57. doi:10.1093/ageing/afs199 PMID:23420266

Academy of Medical Sciences. (2016, September). Improving the health of the public by 2040: optimising the research environment for a healthier, fairer future. Retrieved April 26, 2017 from https://acmedsci.ac.uk/policy/policy-projects/health-of-the-public-in-2040

Act of 27 August 2009 on Public Finance (Journal of Laws of 2016.1870 with later amendments).

Act of December 5, 1996 on the profession of doctor and dentist (Journal of Laws of 2015.464 amended).

Adamiec, M., & Kożusznik, B. (2000). *Zarządzanie zasobami ludzkimi: aktor-kreator-inspirator.* Katowice.

Agency for Healthcare Research and Quality. (n.d.). National Healthcare Quality Report, Rockville. Retrieved 3.02.2015 from http://www.ahrq. gov/qual/nhqr06/nhqr06.htm

Ahmed, B., Lischke, S., Straight, F., Gogo, P., Leffler, S., Kutler, M., & Dauerman, H. L. et al. (2009). Consistent door-to-balloon times of less than 90 minutes for STEMI patients transferred for primary PCI. *The Journal of Invasive Cardiology, 21*, 429–433. PMID:19726811

Ako-Nai, E. A. (2011). *Effect of Customer Service on Customer Satisfaction, a Case Study of Fidelity Bank* (p. 85). Kumasi: Adum.

Alemshet, Y., Leja, H., & Alima, H. (2014). Job Satisfaction and Its Determinants Among Health Workers in Jimma University. Expectations of patients towards medical staff. *Hygeia Public Health, 49*(1), 142–151.

Ammo, M. A., Abu-shaheen, A. K., Kobrosly, S., & Al-tannir, M. A. (2014). Determinants of Patient Satisfaction at Tertiary Care Centers in Lebanon. *Open Journal of Nursing, 4*(December), 939–946. doi:10.4236/ojn.2014.413100

Amoozegar, J. B., Rupert, D. J., Sullivan, H. W., & O'Donoghue, A. C. (2017). Consumer confusion between prescription drug precautions and side effects. *Patient Education and Counseling.*

Anczewska, M., Switaj, P., & Roszczyńska, J. (2005). *Professional burnout.* In Phases of Psychiatry and Neurology.

Anderson, L. M., Oliver, S. R., Michie, S., Rehfuess, E., Noyes, J., & Shemilt, I. (2013). Investigating complexity in systematic reviews of interventions by using a spectrum of methods. *Journal of Clinical Epidemiology, 66*(11), 1223–1229. doi:10.1016/j.jclinepi.2013.06.014 PMID:23953087

Aniszewska, G. (2007). *Kultura organizacyjna w zarządzaniu* (p. 23). Warszawa: Polskie Wydawnictwo Ekonomiczne.

Anita, F. (2012). The Movement to Improve Care: The Institute of Medicine Quality Reports and Implications for the Advanced Practice Registered Nurse. *The Nursing Clinics of North America, 47*(2), 251–260. doi:10.1016/j.cnur.2012.02.006 PMID:22579060

Anne, A., Wu, A. W., Angela, L., Peter, N., Kumar, A. N., Bates, D. W., & Itziar, L. (2013, December). Patient Safety Research Training and Education Expert Working Group of WHO Patient Safety. Case Studies of Patient Safety Research Classics to Build Research Capacity in Low- and Middle-Income Countries. *Joint Commission Journal on Quality and Patient Safety, 39*(12), 553–560. doi:10.1016/S1553-7250(13)39071-0 PMID:24416946

Antonovsky, A. (1987). *Unraveling The Mystery of Health. How People Manage Stress and Stay Well.* San Francisco: Jossey-Bass Publishers.

Argyle, M. (1987). *The psychology of happiness.* London: Methuen.

Armstron-Esther, C. A., Brown, K. D., & McAfee, J. G. (1994). Elderly patients: Still clean and sitting quietly. *Journal of Advanced Nursing, 19*(2), 264–271. doi:10.1111/j.1365-2648.1994.tb01080.x PMID:8188957

Arystoteles. (2008) *Retoryka. Reotoryka dla Aleksanda. Poetyka.* Warsaw: PWN.

Atłachowicz, J. (2013). Historia ubezpieczeń zdrowotnych w Polsce [History of health insurance in Poland]. Retrieved from http://wartowiedziec.org/index.php/zdrowie/aktualnosci-i-ekonomia/14708-historia-ubezpiecze-w-polsce

Aujoulat, A., d'Hoore, W., & Deccache, A. (2007). Patient empowerment in theory and practice: Polysemy or cacophony? *Patient Education and Counseling, 66*(1), 13–20. doi:10.1016/j.pec.2006.09.008 PMID:17084059

Babska K., Tkaczyk M., & Nowicki M. (2008). Współpraca w zespole terapeutycznym – Podstawowa zasada profesjonalnej opieki nad chorym dializowanym otrzewnowo – założenia a rzeczywistość. *Pol Merk Lek, 14*(12 Suppl. 4), 12-14.

Babu, T. S. and N. S. (2012). A STUDY ON PATIENT SATISFACTION IN HOSPITALS (A Study on Three Urban Hospitals in Guntur District, Andhra Pradesh) T. *International Journal of Management Research and Business Strategy, 1*(1), 100–118.

Bajcar, B. et al.. (2011). *Satysfakcja z pracy w zawodach z misją społeczną.* Gdańsk: GWP.

Baker, G. R., & Norton, P. G. (2004). The Canadian Adverse Events Study: The incidence of adverse eventsamong hospitalized patients in Canada. *Canadian Medical Association Journal, 170*(11), 1678–1686. doi:10.1503/cmaj.1040498 PMID:15159366

Baker, W. (2000). *Achieving Success Through Social Capital: Tapping the Hidden Resources in Your Personal and Business Networks.* Michigan: Jossey-Bass.

Bamiou, D. E. (2015). Hearing disorders in stroke. *Handbook of Clinical Neurology, 129*, 633–647. doi:10.1016/B978-0-444-62630-1.00035-4 PMID:25726294

Banaś, I., & Zając, M. (2016). Koordynowana opieka zdrowotna –cele i zasady organizacji [Coordinated healthcare - goals and principles of organization]. Retrieved from http://akademia.nfz.gov.pl/wp-content/uploads/2016/06/Koordynowana-opieka-zdrowotna-cele-i-zasady-organizacji.-Izabela-Bana%C5%9B-Magdalena-Zaj%C4%85c.pdf

Banaszak-Holl, J., Levitsky, S., & Zald, M. (2010). *Social movements and the transformation of American health care*. Oxford, CA: Oxford University Press. doi:10.1093/acprof:oso/9780195388299.001.0001

Bańka, A., & Derbis, R. (1994). *Psychologiczne i pedagogiczne wymiary jakości życia (The Psychological and Pedagogical Dimensions of Life)*. Poznan: Gemini.

Barak, Y., Tishler, M., & Aizenberg, D. (2011). Satisfaction with life amongst psychiatrists and general physicians: Demographic and career variables. *Open Journal of Psychiatry*, *1*(03), 122–125. doi:10.4236/ojpsych.2011.13018

Bartkowski, J. (2007). *Kapitał społeczny i jego oddziaływanie na rozwój w ujęciu socjologicznym* (*Social Capital and Its Impact on Developemnt: A Sociological Perspective*). In M. Herbst (Ed.), *Kapitał ludzki i kapitał społeczny a rozwój regionalny (Human and Social Capital versus Regional Development)*. Warsaw: SCHOLAR.

Basińska, M. (Ed.) (2016). Elastyczne radzenie sobie ze stresem w zdrowiu i chorobie [Coping flexibility with stress in health and in disease]. Bydgoszcz: Wydawnictwo Uniwersytetu Kazimierza Wielkiego.

Bellingrath, S., Rohleder, N., & Kudielka, B. (2010). Healthly working teachers with high effort-reward-imbalance and overcommitment show increased pro-inflammatory immune activity and a dampened innate immune defence. *Brain, Behavior, and Immunity*, *24*(8), 1332–1339. doi:10.1016/j.bbi.2010.06.011 PMID:20599495

Benien, K. (2005). *Jak prowadzić trudne rozmowy*. Kraków: Wydawnictwo WAM.

Berger-Schmitt, R. (2000) Social Cohesion as an Aspect of the Quality of Societies: Concept and Measurement (Working Paper 14). EU Reporting. Mannheim: ZUMA.

Berkman, L. F., & Syme, S. L. (1979). Social Networks, Host Resistance, and Mortality: A Nine-year Follow-up Study of Almeda County Residents. *American Journal of Epidemiology*, *109*(2), 186–204. doi:10.1093/oxfordjournals.aje.a112674 PMID:425958

Bernal, G., Bonilla, J., & Bellido, C. (1995). Ecological validity and cultural sensitivity for outcome research: Issues for the cultural adaptation and development of psychosocial treatments with Hispanics. *Journal of Abnormal Child Psychology*, *23*(1), 67–82. doi:10.1007/BF01447045 PMID:7759675

Besciu, C. (2015). Patient Satisfaction in the Hospital's Emergency Units in Bucharest. *Procedia Economics and Finance*, *32*, 870–877. doi:10.1016/S2212-5671(15)01534-8

Bhatnagar, K., & Srivastava, K. (2012, January-June). Job satisfaction in health-care organizations. *Industrial Psychiatry Journal*, *21*(1), 75–78. doi:10.4103/0972-6748.110959 PMID:23766585

Bjornskov, C. (2003). The happy few: Cross country evidence on social capital and life satisfaction. *Kyklos*, *56*(1), 3–16. doi:10.1111/1467-6435.00207

Blanchard, K., & Hodges, P. (2003). *Transforming Your Heart, Head, Hands & Habits*. Nashville, TN: Countryman.

Bodak, A. (2007). Skuteczność w komunikacji wewnętrznej we współczesnych zespołach pracowniczych. In S. Rudolf (Ed.), *Perspektywy rozwoju partycypacji pracowniczej w Polsce w warunkach Unii Europejskiej*. Wydawnictwo Uniwersytetu Łódzkiego.

Boland, P. (2001). *Making Managed Healthcare Work: A Practical Guide to Strategies and Solutions*. Jones & Bartlett Learning.

Bonenberger, M., Aikins, M., Akweongo, P., & Wyss, K. (2014). The effects of health worker motivation and job satisfaction on turnover intention in Ghana: A cross-sectional study. *Human Resources for Health*, *12*(43), 10–1186. PMID:25106497

Borkowski, G. (2012). *Zarządzanie ryzykiem*. Katowice, CA: Uniwersytet Ekonomiczny.

Bowling, A., Rowe, G., Lambert, N., Waddington, M., Mahtani, K. R., Kenten, C., & Francis, S. A. et al. (2012). The measurement of patients' expectations for health care: A review and psychometric testing of a measure of patients' expectations. *Health Technology Assessment, 16*(30), 1–509. doi:10.3310/hta16300 PMID:22747798

Boxman, E., De Graaf, P., & Flap, H. (1991). The impact of social and human capital on the income attainment of Dutch managers. *Social Networks, 13*(1), 51–73. doi:10.1016/0378-8733(91)90013-J

Boyd, W. D., Kodera, K., Stahl, K. D., & Rayman, R. (2002). Current status and future directions in computer-enhanced video- and robotic-assisted coronary bypass surgery. *Seminars in Thoracic and Cardiovascular Surgery, 14*(1), 101–109. doi:10.1053/stcs.2002.31893 PMID:11977023

Boylan, J. M., & Ryff, C. D. (2013). Varieties of anger and the inverse link between education and inflammation: Toward an integrated framework. *Psychosomatic Medicine, 75*(6), 566–574. doi:10.1097/PSY.0b013e31829683bd PMID:23766379

Brammer, L. M. (1985). *The helping relationship: process and skills*. Englewood Cliffs, N.J.: Prentice-Hall.

Brasaite, I., Kaunonen, M., Martinkenas, A., Mockiene, V., & Suominen, T. (2016). Health care professionals' skills regarding patient safety. *Medicina, 52*(4), 250–256. doi:10.1016/j.medici.2016.05.004 PMID:27697239

Bravo, P., Edwards, A., Barr, P. J., Scholl, I., Elwyn, G., & McAllister, M. (2015). Conceptualising patient empowerment: A mixed methods study. *BMC Health Services Research, 15*(1), 252. doi:10.1186/s12913-015-0907-z PMID:26126998

Brennan, J., & Krohmer, J. (Eds.). (2005). Principles of EMS Systems. Jones and Bartlett Publishers.

Bridges, J.F.P., Loukanova, S., & Carrera, P.M. (2017). Patient Empowerment in Health Care. Reference Module in Biomedical Sciences. In International Encyclopedia of Public Health (2nd ed., pp. 416-425).

Brink-Muinen, A., van Dulmen, S., Messerli-Rohrbach, V., & Bensing, J. (2002). Do gender-dyads have different communication patterns? A comparative study in Western-European general practices. *Patient Education and Counseling, 48*(3), 253–264. doi:10.1016/S0738-3991(02)00178-7 PMID:12477610

Brislin, R. (1993). *Understanding culture's influence on behavior*. Orlando, FL: Harcourt Brace.

Bronner, Y. (1994). Cultural sensitivity and nutrition counseling. *Topics in Clinical Nutrition, 9*(2), 13–19. doi:10.1097/00008486-199403000-00004

Brosschot, J. (2010). Markers of chronic stress: Prolonged physiological activation and (un)conscious perseverative cognition. *Neuroscience and Biobehavioral Reviews, 35*(1), 46–50. doi:10.1016/j.neubiorev.2010.01.004 PMID:20096302

Brudecka, B. (2007). Rozwój kształcenia pielęgniarek. *Magazyn Pielęgniarki i Położnej, 6*, 13–14.

Bukowska-Piestrzyńska, A. (2007). Marketing usług zdrowotnych. Warszawa, CA: CeDeWu.

Buła, P. (2015). *System zarządzania ryzykiem w przedsiębiorstwie, jako element nadzoru korporacyjnego*. Kraków, CA: Uniwersytet Jagielloński.

Buntin, M. B., Burke, M. F., Hoaglin, M. C., & Blumenthal, D. (2011). The benefits of health information technology: A review of the literature shows predominantly positive results. *Health Affairs (Project Hope), 30*(3), 464–471. doi:10.1377/hlthaff.2011.0178 PMID:21383365

Burt, R. S. (2005). *Brokerage & closure. An introduction to social capital*. New York, Oxford: Oxford University Press.

Burt, S. R. (1997). A note on social capital and network content. *Social Networks, 19*(4), 355–373. doi:10.1016/S0378-8733(97)00003-8

Bytnar, B. (2010). *Quality of life of instrumentalists working in shifts.* Rzeszów: Przegląd Medyczny Uniwersytetu Rzeszowskiego.

Cacioppo, J. T., Rourke, P. A., Marshall-Goodell, B. S., Tassinary, L. G., & Baron, R. S. (1990). Rudimentary physiological effects of mere observation. *Psychophysiology, 27*(2), 177–186. doi:10.1111/j.1469-8986.1990.tb00368.x PMID:2247548

Cadiere, G. B., Himpens, J., & Germay, O. et al.. (2001). Feasibility of robotic laparoscopic surgery: 146 cases. *World Journal of Surgery, 25*, 1467–1477. PMID:11760751

Campbell, A., Converse, P., & Rodgers, W. (1976). *The Quality of American Life: Perceptions, Evaluations, and Satisfactions*. New York: Russel Sage Foundation.

Caplan, G. (1961). *An approach to community mental health.* New York: Behavioral Publication.

Caplan, G. (1964). *Principles of preventive psychiatry.* New York: Basic Books.

Caplan, G. (1986). Caplan, G. (1986). Recent development in crisis intervention and in the promotion of support services. In M. Kessler & S. E. Goldston (Eds.), *A decade of progress in primary prevention* (pp. 235–260). Hanover, NH: University Press of New England.

Caplan, G., Caplan, R. B., & Erchul, W. P. (1994). Caplanian Mental Health Consultation: Historical Background and Current Status. *Consulting Psychology Journal: Practice and Research.* https://msrc.fsu.edu/system/files/Caplan%20G%20et%20al%201994%20Caplanian%20mental%20health%20consultation-20historical%20background%20and%20current%20status.pdf

Carter, S. M., Entwistle, V. A., & Littie, M. (2015, August). Relational conceptions of paternalism: A way to rebut nanny-state accusations and evaluate public health interventions. *Public Health, 129*(8), 1021–1029. doi:10.1016/j.puhe.2015.03.007 PMID:25917003

Cassella, C. (2011). Burnout and the relative value of dopamine. *Anesthesiology, 114*(1), 213–217. doi:10.1097/ALN.0b013e318201c8cd PMID:21169792

Castro, E. M., Van Regenmortel, T., Vanhaecht, K., Sermeus, W., & Van Hecke, A. (2016). Patient empowerment, patient participation and patient-centeredness in hospital care. A concept analysis based on a literature review. *Patient Education and Counseling, 99*(12), 1923–1939. doi:10.1016/j.pec.2016.07.026 PMID:27450481

Central Statistical Office. (2015). Population Project 2014–2015. Statistical Analyses and Studies, Warsaw 2014, Poland. Retrieved 6 August 2015 from http://www.stat.gov.pl/

Centrum Monitorowania Jakości w Ochronie Zdrowia. (2009). *Zestaw standardów akredytacyjnych.* Kraków: CMJ.

Chaiyakulsil, C., & Pandee, U. (2015, August). Validation of pediatric early warning score in pediatric emergency department. *Pediatrics International, 57*(4), 694–698. doi:10.1111/ped.12595 PMID:25639996

Chandola, T., Heraclides, A., & Kumari, M. (2010). Psychophysiological biomarkers of workplace stressors. *Neuroscience and Biobehavioral Reviews, 35*(1), 51–57. doi:10.1016/j.neubiorev.2009.11.005 PMID:19914288

Charland-Verville, V., Lesenfants, D., Sela, L., Noirhomme, Q., Ziegler, E., Chatelle, C., & Laureys, S. et al. (2014). Detection of response to command using voluntary control of breathing in disorders of consciousness. *Frontiers in Human Neuroscience, 8*, 1020. doi:10.3389/fnhum.2014.01020 PMID:25566035

Chase, A. (2000). Information to users. doi:10.16953/deusbed.74839

Chida, Y., & Steptoe, A. (2009). Cortisol awakening response and psychosocial factors: A systematic review and meta-analysis. *Biological Psychology, 80*(3), 265–278. doi:10.1016/j.biopsycho.2008.10.004 PMID:19022335

Choma, A. (2011). Zarządzanie ryzykiem. *Think*, *4*(8), 12.

Christakis, N. A., & Fowler, J. H. (2011). *W sieci. Jak sieci społeczne kształtują nasze życie* [On the Web. How social networks shape our lives]. Sopot: Smak Słowa.

Chrzan-Dętkoś, M., & Pietkiewicz, A. (2015). How can we cooperate better? The determinants of conflict solving competence in Polish pediatric nurses' relations with parents of hospitalized children. *Health Psychology Review*, *3*(4), 345–351. doi:10.5114/hpr.2015.51906

Cierpiałkowska, L., & Sęk, H. (red.) (2016). Psychologia kliniczna [Clinical psychology] Warszawa: Wydawnictwo Naukowe PWN.

Clack, G. B., Allen, J., Cooper, D., & Head, J. O. (2004). Personality differences between doctors and their patients: Implications for the teaching of communication skills. *Medical Education*, *38*(2), 177–186. doi:10.1111/j.1365-2923.2004.01752.x PMID:14871388

Cliff, B. (2012). Excellence In patient satisfaction within a patient-centered culture. *Journal of Healthcare Management*, *57*, 157–159. PMID:22724373

Clow, A., Hucklebridge, F., Stadler, T., Evans, P., & Thorn, L. (2010). The cortisol awakening response: More than a measure of HPA axis function. *Neuroscience and Biobehavioral Reviews*, *35*(1), 97–103. doi:10.1016/j.neubiorev.2009.12.011 PMID:20026350

Coleman, J. (1988). Social Capital in the Creation of Human Capital. *American Journal of Sociology*, *94*, 95–120. doi:10.1086/228943

Coleman, J. (1990). *The Foundations of Social Theory*. Cambridge: Harvard University Press.

Collier, M. J. (1989). Cultural and intercultural communication competence: Current approaches and directions for future research. *International Journal of Intercultural Relations*, *13*(3), 287–302. doi:10.1016/0147-1767(89)90014-X

Compas, B. E., Beckjord, E., Agocha, B., Sherman, M. L., Langrock, A., Grossman, C. I., & Luecken, L. et al. (2006). Measurement of coping and stress responses in women with breast cancer. *Psycho-Oncology*, *15*(12), 1038–1054. doi:10.1002/pon.999 PMID:17009343

Comte, A., Gabriel, D., Pazart, L., Magnin, E., Cretin, E., Haffen, E., & Aubry, R. et al. (2015). On the difficulty to communicate with fMRI-based protocols used to identify covert awareness. *Neuroscience*, *300*, 448–459. doi:10.1016/j.neuroscience.2015.05.059 PMID:26033566

Coomber, B., & Barriball, K. L. (2007). Impact of job satisfaction components on intent to leave and turnover for hospital based nurses: A review of the research literature. *International Journal of Nursing Studies*, *44*(2), 297–314. doi:10.1016/j.ijnurstu.2006.02.004 PMID:16631760

Côté, D. (2013). Intercultural communication in health care: challenges and solutions in work rehabilitation practices and training: a comprehensive review. *Disability and Rehabilitation*, *35*(2), 153–163. doi:10.3109/09638288.2012.687034 PMID:22616895

Csikszentmihalyi, M. (1990). *Flow: The Psychology of Optimal Experience*. New York: Harper Collins.

Cummins Fred, A. (2017). *Agile Enterprise Leadership. In Building the Agile Enterprise* (2nd ed., pp. 333–368). doi:10.1016/B978-0-12-805160-3.00011-9

Cunningham, L. (1991). *The Quality Connection in Health Care: Integrating Patient Satisfaction and Risk Management*. San Francisco: Jossey-Bass Publishers.

Curry, E., Li, X., Nguyen, J., & Matzkin, E. (2014). Prevalence of Internet and social media usage in orthopedic surgery. *Orthopaedic Review*, *6*(3). PMID:25317312

Cutler, D. M. (2004). *Your money or your life: strong medicine for America's health care system.* Oxford, CA: Oxford University Press.

Ćwiąkała-Małys, A., & Łagowski, P. (2013). Ewolucyjny obraz przekształceń systemu ochrony zdrowia w Polsce [The evolutionary picture of the transformation of the healthcare system in Poland]. *Przegląd Prawa i Administracji*, *93*, 90–101.

Cydulka, R. K., & Korte, R. (2008). Career satisfaction in EM: The ABEM longitudinal study of Emergency Physicians. *Annals of Emergency Medicine*, *51*(6), 714–722. doi:10.1016/j.annemergmed.2008.01.005 PMID:18395936

Czapiński, J. (2007). Indywidualna jakość życia (Individual Quality of Life). In J. Czapiński, & T. Panek (Eds.), Diagnoza społeczna [Social Diagnosis]. Warsaw: VizjaPress@IT.

Czapiński, J. (2004). *Ekonomiczne przesłanki i efekty dobrostanu psychicznego* (*Economic determinants and effects of mental well-being*). In T. Tyszka (Ed.), *Psychologia ekonomiczna (Economic psychology)* (pp. 192–242). Gdansk: GWP.

Czekaj, J. (2012). *Podstawy zarządzania informacją*. Kraków: Wydawnictwo Uniwersytetu Ekonomicznego w Krakowie.

Czerniak, J. (2012). Accidental bumps. *Magazyn Pielęgniarki i Położnej*, 7-8.

Czerw, A., Religioni, U., Matuszna, A., Lesiak, K., Olejnik, A., & Śniadała, D. (2012). Principles of effective communication in medical entities. *Hygeia Public Health*, *47*(3), 247–253.

Daaleman, T. P., Shea, C. M., Halladay, J., & Reed, D. (2014). A method to determine the impact of patient-centered care interventions in primary care. *Patient Education and Counseling*, *97*(3), 327–331. doi:10.1016/j.pec.2014.09.009 PMID:25269410

de Andrade, C. G., da Costa, S. F., & Lopes, M. E. (2013). Palliative care: Communication as a strategy of care for the terminal patient. *Ciencia & Saude Coletiva*, *18*(9), 2523–2530. PMID:23989558

de la Billiere, S. P. (2007). Przywodztwo, [w:] Biznes – Zarządzanie firmą cz. 2, praca zbior. Wyd. PWN, Warszawa.

De Walden–Gałuszko, K. (2000). *Problems of communication, Avid (red. K. De Walden-Gałuszko)*. Kraków: Psychiatry Library.

Debrand-Passard, A., & Luce-Wunderle, G. (2010). *Operational nursing*. Wroclaw: Urban & Partner.

Dębska, G., Pasek, M., & Wilczek-Rużyczka, E. (2014). *Psychological burden and professional burnout among nurses working in various occupational specializations*. Poland: Hygeia Public Healt.

Deckard, G., Hicks, L., & Hamory, B. (1992). The occurrence and distribution of burnout among infectious diseases physicians. *The Journal of Infectious Diseases*, *165*(2), 224–228. doi:10.1093/infdis/165.2.224 PMID:1730889

Degni, F., Suominen, S., Essen, B., El, A. W., & Vehvilainen-Julkunen, K. (2012). Communication and cultural issues in providing reproductive health care to immigrant women: health care providers' experiences in meeting the needs of Somali women living in Finland. *Journal of Immigrant and Minority Health*, *14*(2), 330–343. doi:10.1007/s10903-011-9465-6 PMID:21465142

DeMeester, R. H., Lopez, F. Y., Moore, J. E., Cook, S. C., & Chin, M. H. (2016, March 17). A Model of Organizational Context and Shared Decision Making: Application to LGBT Racial and Ethnic Minority Patients. *Journal of General Internal Medicine*, *31*(6), 651–662. doi:10.1007/s11606-016-3608-3 PMID:26988980

Den Brink-Muinen, V., Van Dulmen, S. M., De Haes, H. C., Visser, A. P., Schellevis, F. G., & Bensing, J. M. (2006). Has patients' involvement in the decision-making process changed over time? *Health Expectations*, *9*(4), 333–342.

Denecke, K., Bamidis, P., Bond, C., Gabarron, E., Househ, M., Lau, A. Y., & Hansen, M. (2015). Ethical Issues of Social Media Usage in Healthcare. *Yearbook of Medical Informatics*, *10*(1), 137–147. doi:10.15265/IY-2015-001 PMID:26293861

Denis, C., & Robert, S. (2007). Taking Steps Toward Integration. *Health Affairs*, *26*, 69–71. PMID:17148492

Dennis, R. E., & Giangreco, M. F. (1996). Creating conversation: Reflections on cultural sensitivity in family interviewing. *Exceptional Children*, *63*(1), 103–116. doi:10.1177/001440299606300109

Deussom, R., Jaskiewicz, W., Dwyer, S., & Tulenko, K. (2012). Holding Health Workers Accountable: Governance Approaches to Reducing Absenteeism (Technical Brief 3).

Di Blasi, Z., Harkness, E., Ernst, E., Georgiou, A., & Klejinen, J. (2001). Influence of context effects on health outcomes: A systematic review. *Lancet*, *357*(9258), 757–762. doi:10.1016/S0140-6736(00)04169-6 PMID:11253970

Diener, E. (1984). Subjective Well-being. *Psychological Bulletin*, *95*(3), 542–575. doi:10.1037/0033-2909.95.3.542 PMID:6399758

Diez Roux, A. (2011). Complex systems thinking and current impasses in health disparities research. *American Journal of Public Health*, *101*(9), 1627–1634. doi:10.2105/AJPH.2011.300149 PMID:21778505

Dimitrova, N., Moro, C., & Mohr, C. (2015). Caregivers interpret infants' early gestures based on shared knowledge about referents. *Infant Behavior and Development*, *39*, 98–106. doi:10.1016/j.infbeh.2015.02.015 PMID:25827260

Dimsdale, J. (2008). Psychological stress and cardiovascular disease. *Journal of the American College of Cardiology*, *51*(13), 1237–1246. doi:10.1016/j.jacc.2007.12.024 PMID:18371552

Dłużewska, M. (2012). Exploration of conditions in the formation of the burnout process - analysis based on own research. *Pielęgniarstwo Polskie*, *2*(44), 63–72.

Dobek-Ostrowska, B. (1999). *Podstawy komunikowania społecznego*. Wrocław: Wyd. Astrum.

Dobranzkil, S., Hammond, I., Khan, G., & Holdsworth, H. (2002). The nature of hospital prescribing errors. *Br. J. Clin. Govern.*, *7*(3), 187–193. doi:10.1108/14664100210438271

Doligalski, T. (2013). *Internet w zarządzaniu wartością klienta* (p. 222). Warszawa: Oficyna Wydawnicza SGH.

Dougherty, D., Mistry, K. B., LLanos, K., Lillie-Blanton, M., & Chesley, F. (2014, September–October). An AHRQ and CMS Perspective on the Pediatric Quality Measures Program. *Academic Pediatrics*, *14*(5 Suppl.), S17–S18. doi:10.1016/j.acap.2014.06.017 PMID:25169452

Drat-Ruszczak, K. (2000). Teorie osobowości – podejście psychodynamiczne I humanistyczne. [Theories of personality - psychodynamic and humanistic approach] In J. Strelau (Ed.), *Psychologia* [Psychology. Academic manual] (Vol. 1, pp. 601–652). Gdańsk: Gdańskie Wydawnictwo Psycholgiczne.

Dudek, B., Waszkowska, M., Merecz, D., & Hanke, W. (2004). Protection of workers' health from the effects of occupational stress. Institute of Occupational Medicine, Łódź.

Duffey, K. J., & Popkin, B. M. (2011). Energy density, portion size, and eating occasions: Contributions to increased energy intake in the United States, 1977–2006. *PLoS Medicine*, *8*(6). doi:10.1371/journal.pmed.1001050 PMID:21738451

Duffy, F. D., Gordon, G. H., Whelan, G., Cole-Kelly, K., Frankel, R., & Buffone, N. et al.. (2004). Assessing competence in communication and interpersonal skills: The Kalamazoo II report. *Academic Medicine, 79*(6), 495–507. doi:10.1097/00001888-200406000-00002 PMID:15165967

Działek, J. (2011). *Kapitał społeczny jako czynnik rozwoju gospodarczego w skali regionalnej i lokalnej w Polsce (Social capital as the determinant of economic growth in Poland in regional and local perspective).* Krakow: Jagiellonian University Press.

Eastwood, J. B., Conroy, R. E., Naicker, S., West, P. A., Tutt, R. C., & Plange-Rhule, J. (2005). Loss of health professionals from sub-Saharan Africa: The pivotal role of the UK. *Lancet, 365*(9474), 1893–1900. doi:10.1016/S0140-6736(05)66623-8 PMID:15924988

EC. (2009) Retrieved 20.02.2017 from: http://ec.europa.eu/health//sites/health/files/patient_safety/docs/council_2009_pl

Eckert, H., & Resch, K. L. (2003). Quality management –quo vadis? Perspectives for quality management in hospitals. *Zeitschrift fur Arztliche Fortbildung und Qualitatssicherung, 97*(3), 219–226. PMID:12856550

Economist Intelligence Unit. (2011). The future of healthcare in Europe [cited 2015 Mar 18]. Retrieved from http://www.janssen.pt/sites/default/files/The- Future-Of-Healthcare-In-Europe.pdf

Edlin, M. (2012). Cultural competency means better patience service. *Drug Topics, 156*(6), 18.

Elissen, A., Hertroijs, D., Shaper, N., Vrijhoef, H., & Ruwaard, D. (2016). Profiling Patients' Healthcare Needs to Support Integrated, Person-Centered Models for Long-Term Disease Management (Profile): Research Design. *International Journal of Integrated Care, 16*(2), 1. doi:10.5334/ijic.2208 PMID:27616957

Emanuel Ezakiel, J., & Emanuel Linda, L. (1992). Four models of the physician-patient relationship. *Journal of the American Medical Association, 267*(16), 2221–2226. doi:10.1001/jama.1992.03480160079038 PMID:1556799

Encyclopedia Britannica. (n.d.). Information system. Retrieved 09.04.2017 from http://www.britannica.com/EBchecked/topic/287895/information-system

Encyclopedia of Mathematics. (n.d.). Set. Retrieved 25.04.2017 from https://www.encyclopediaofmath.org/index.php/Set

Environment, V. (n.d.). *The Rising Importance of Patient Satisfaction in a Value-Based Environment.*

Erenkfeit, K., Dudzińska, L. & Indyk, A. (2012). The impact of the working environment on the emergence of professional burnout. *Medycyna Środowiskowa* [Enviromental Medicine], *15*(3), 121-128.

Eriksson, M., & Lindstöm, B. (2005). Validity of Antonovsky's sense of coherence scale: A systematic review. *Journal of Epidemiology and Community Health, 59*(6), 460–466. doi:10.1136/jech.2003.018085 PMID:15911640

European Commission. (2015). DG Health & Consumers. European Core Health Indicators (ECHI). Self-reported chronic morbidity. Proportion of people aged 65+ reporting any long-standing chronic illness or longstanding health problem. Retrieved March 18, 2015 from http://ec.europa.eu/health/indicators/echi/list/

European Union. (n.d.). Recommendation of the Council of the European Union of 9 June 2009 on security The patient and the prevention and combating of infections related to health, 2009 / C 151/01. Technical Report (2008) Improving Patient Safety in the EU developed for Commissioned by the European Commission, the RAND Corporation. Retrieved 09.03.2017 from https://pl.wikipedia.org/wiki/Kodeks_Hammurabiego

Farnicka, M., Liberska, H., & Niewiedział, D. (2016). *Psychologia agresji* [Psychology of aggression]. Warszawa: Wydawnictwo Naukowe PWN.

Fedorowski, J. J. (2017). Definition of KOZ. Retrieved from http://ptkoz.org/definicja-koz

Feinglass, S. (2002). The Toll of Chronic Illness. *Health Affairs*, *21*(5), 297–298. doi:10.1377/hlthaff.21.5.297

Fejfer-Wirbał, E., Gładczuk, J., & Marcinowicz, L. (2013). Relacje lekarz-pielęgniarka w polskiej literaturze medycznej. *Medycyna Rodzinna*, *1*, 19–22.

Felcenloben, M. (2007). Samokształcenie pielęgniarek i położnych. *Magazyn Pielęgniarki i Położnej*, *4*, 13–14.

Felton, J. (1998). Burnout as a clinical entity – its importance in health care workers; occupational. *Medicine*, *48*(4), 237–250. PMID:9800422

Fengler, J. (2000). *Helping to tire-burn in work*. Gdansk: Gdańskie Wydawnictwo Psychologiczne.

Ferlie, S. (2001). *Improving the Quality of Health Care in the United Kingdom and the United States: A Framework for Change. University of London*. Berkeley: University of California.

Fernandez, I., Hayan, S., Winters, P., & Liang, H. (2010). Association of workplace chronic and acute stressors with employee weight status: Data from worksites in turmoil. *Journal of Occupational and Environmental Medicine*, *52*(Suppl. 1), s34–s41. doi:10.1097/JOM.0b013e3181c88525 PMID:20061885

Finegood, D. T. (2011). The complex systems science of obesity. In J. Cawley (Ed.), *The Oxford handbook of the social science of obesity* (pp. 208–236). New York: Oxford University Press.

Florkowski, M. (2009). *Working nights. Work and Health*. Warszawa: Unimedia.

Foley, P., & Kirschbaum, C. (2010). Human hypothalamus-pituitary-adrenal axis responses to acute psychosocial stress in laboratory settings. *Neuroscience and Biobehavioral Reviews*, *35*(1), 91–96. doi:10.1016/j.neubiorev.2010.01.010 PMID:20109491

Fong Ha, J., & Longnecker, N. (2010, Spring). Doctor Patient Communication A Review. *The Ochsner Journal*, *10*(1), 38–43. PMID:21603354

Forgas, J. P. (2012). Belief and affect: On the mental pre-cursors of health-related cognition and behaviour. *Journal of Health Psychology*, *18*(1), 3–9. doi:10.1177/1359105312448869 PMID:22850972

Forgas, J. P. (Ed.). (2006). *Affect in Social Cognition and Behavior*. New York: Psychology Press.

Forgas, J. P., & Moylan, S. J. (2002). Affective influences on self-perception and self-disclosure. In J. P. Forgas & K. D. Williams (Eds.), *The social self: Individual, interpersonal and intergroup perspectives* (pp. 73–96). New York: Psychology Press.

Forster, A. J., Clark, H. D., Menard, A., Dupuis, N., & Chernish, R. et al.. (2004). Adverse events among medical patients after discharge from hospital. *Canadian Medical Association Journal*, *170*(3), 345–349. PMID:14757670

Frączkiewicz-Wronka, A., & Austen-Tynda, A. (Eds.) (2009). Przywództwo w ochronie zdrowia.

Frączkiewicz-Wronka, A. (2012). *Wykorzystanie analizy interesariuszy w zarządzaniu organizacją zdrowotną*. Katowice, CA: Śląsk.

French, S. A. (2005). Public health strategies for dietary change: Schools and worksites. *The Journal of Nutrition*, *135*, 910–912. PMID:15795458

Freud, S. (1995). Wykłady ze wstępu do psychoanalizy. Nowy cykl [Lectures from the introduction to psychoanalysis. New cycle]. Warszawa: KR.

Freudenberger, H. J. (1974). Staff burn-out. *The Journal of Social Issues*, *30*(1), 159–165. doi:10.1111/j.1540-4560.1974.tb00706.x

Freudenberger, H. J. (1983). *Burnout: Contemporary issues, trends and concerns. Stress and burnout in the human service professions*. New York: Pergamon.

Friedman, E. M., & Ryff, C. D. (2012). Living well with medical co-morbidities: A biopsychosocial perspective. *The Journals of Gerontology. Series B, Psychological Sciences and Social Sciences*, *67*(5), 535–544. doi:10.1093/geronb/gbr152 PMID:22377799

Frydrychowicz, S. (2009). Komunikacja interpersonalna w zarządzaniu, *Wydawnictwo Forum Naukowe Poznań*, 17.

Gabard, D., & Martin, M. (2003). *Physical therapy ethics*. Philadelphia: F.A. Davis.

Gabryś, E. (2009). Zarządzanie ryzykiem w szpitalach publicznych w Polsce. In R. Holly & J. Suchecka (Eds.), *Szpital Publiczny w polskim systemie ochrony zdrowia. Zarządzanie i gospodarka finansowa* (pp. 93-115). Łódź-Warszawa, CA: Agencja Wydawnicza Sowa.

Gallant, M. P. (2003). The influence of social support on chronic illness self-management: A review and directions for research. *Health Education & Behavior*, *30*(2), 170–195. doi:10.1177/1090198102251030 PMID:12693522

George, W. (2014). *Chronic disease in Twentieth Century. A history*. JHU Press.

Giampieri, M. (2012). Communication and informed consent in elderly people. *Minerva Anestesiologica*, *78*(2), 236–242. PMID:22127308

Gierszewska, G. (2016). Male i średnie przedsiębiorstwa, innowacyjność, konkurencyjność- głos w dyskusji [w:] Grzeszczyk T.A.: Wybrane problemy wzrostu innowacyjności i konkurencyjności przedsiębiorstw. Oficyna Wydawnicza Politechniki Warszawskiej, Warszawa.

Giza-Poleszczuk, A., Marody, M., & Rychard, A. (2000). *Strategie i system. Polacy w obliczu zmiany społecznej [Strategies and the System. Polish People against a Social Change]*. Warsaw: Institute of Philosophy and Sociology at the Polish Academy of Sciences.

Głębocka, A., & Lisowska, E. (2007). Professional burnout and stress among Polish physicians explained by the Hobfoll resources theory. *Journal of Physiology and Pharmacology*, *58*(Suppl. 5), 243–252. PMID:18204134

Glińska, J., & Lewandowska, M. (2007). Autonomiczność zawodu pielęgniarskiego w świadomości pielęgniarek z uwzględnieniem pełnionych funkcji zawodowych. *Problemy Pielęgniarstwa*, *15*(4), 249–253.

Glossmann, J.P., Schliebusch, O., Diehl, V., Walshe, R. *Lean management in hospitals: potentials and limitations*. Munich, CA: Med Klin.

Gold, D. L., Mihalov, L. K., & Cohen, D. M. (2014, November). Evaluating the Pediatric Early Warning Score (PEWS) system for admitted patients tn the pediatric emergency department. *Academic Emergency Medicine*, *21*(11), 1249–1256. doi:10.1111/acem.12514 PMID:25377402

Golembiewski, R. T., Boudreau, R. A., Sun, B. C., & Luo, H. (1998). *Estimates of burnout in public agencies*. Public Administr Rev.

Gordon Moore, L., & Wasson, J. H. (2007). The Ideal Medical Practice Model: Improving Efficiency, Quality and the Doctor-Patient Relationship. *Family Practice Management*, *14*(8), 20–24. PMID:17912818

Gordon, C., Ellis-Hill, C., & Ashburn, A. (2009). The use of conversational analysis: Nurse-patient interaction in communication disability after stroke. *Journal of Advanced Nursing*, *65*(3), 544–553. doi:10.1111/j.1365-2648.2008.04917.x PMID:19222652

Gordon, T. (1998). *Wychowanie bez porażek w praktyce*. Warszawa: Instytut Wydawniczy PAX.

Gostin, L. O. (1995). Informed consent, cultural sensitivity, and respect for persons. *Journal of the American Medical Association*, *274*(10), 844–845. doi:10.1001/jama.1995.03530100084039 PMID:7650810

Gottman, J. M., & Silver, N. (2000). *The Seven Principles for Making Marriage Work*. New York: Crown.

Graban, M. (2011). *Lean Hospitals. Improving Quality, Patient Safety, and Employee Satisfaction*. Wrocław, CA: Prod-Publishing.

Granovetter, M. S. (1973). The Strength of Weak Ties. *American Journal of Sociology*, *78*(6), 1360–1380. doi:10.1086/225469

Grant, J. (2010, January). What does it take to make integrated care work? *The McKinsey Quarterly*.

Greenhalgh, L. (1986). Managing conflict. *Sloan Management Review*, *27*(4), 45–51.

Grontved, A., & Hu, F. B. (2011). Television viewing and risk of type 2 diabetes, cardiovascular disease, and all-cause mortality: A meta-analysis. *Journal of the American Medical Association*, *305*(23), 2448–2455. doi:10.1001/jama.2011.812 PMID:21673296

Grootaert, C., *Narayan, D.,* Nyhan Jones, V. and Woolcock, M. (2003) *Integrated Questionnaire for the Measurement of Social Capital*. he World Bank.

Grootaert, C., & Van Bastelaer, T. (2002). *Understanding and Measuring Social Capital. A Multidisciplinary Tool for Practicioners*. Washington, DC: The World Bank. doi:10.1596/0-8213-5068-4

Grzesiuk, L. (2001). *Umiejętności menedżera. Psychologia stosowana dla menedżerów, Wydawnictwo Wyższej Szkoły Handlu i Prawa im*. Warszawa: Ryszarda Łazarskiego.

Halpern, D. (2005). *Social capital*. Cambridge: Polity Press.

Hamrol, A., & Mantura, W. (2011). *Zarządzanie jakością Teoria i praktyka*. Warszawa, CA: PWN.

Hänsel, A., Hong, S., Cámara, R., & von Känel, R. (2010). Inflammation as a psychophysiological biomarker in chronic psychosocial stress. *Neuroscience and Biobehavioral Reviews*, *35*(1), 115–121. doi:10.1016/j.neubiorev.2009.12.012 PMID:20026349

Hansen, A., Larsen, A., Ragulies, R., Garde, A., & Knudsen, L. (2009). A review of the effect of the psychosocial working environment on physiological changes in blood and urine. *Basis & Clincal Pharmacolgy & Toxicology*, *105*, 73–83. PMID:19563453

Hardin, L., Kilian, A., & Spykerman, K. (2017). Competing health care systems and complex patients: An inter-professional collaboration to improve outcomes and reduce health care costs. *Journal of Interprofessional Education & Practice*, *7*(June), 5–10. doi:10.1016/j.xjep.2017.01.002

Harrison, A. H., & Connolly, J. F. (2013). Finding a way in: A review and practical evaluation of fMRI and EEG for detection and assessment in disorders of consciousness. *Neuroscience and Biobehavioral Reviews*, *37*(8), 1403–1419. doi:10.1016/j.neubiorev.2013.05.004 PMID:23680699

Hart, B. D., & Wells, D. L. (1997). The effects of language used by caregivers on agitation in residents with dementia. *Clinical Nurse Specialist CNS*, *11*(1), 20–23. doi:10.1097/00002800-199701000-00015 PMID:9233134

Hawley Sarah, T., & Morris Arden, M. (2017). Cultural challenges to engaging patients in shared decision making. *Patient Education and Counseling*, *100*(1), 18–24. doi:10.1016/j.pec.2016.07.008 PMID:27461943

Hebda, P., & Madejski, J. (2004). *A profession with passion*. Bielsko-Biała: At the Metropolitan Museum. Park.

Hejwosz, D. A. (2008). Patient-oriented approach in the process of education. In Health education. The possibilities, problems, restrictions with regard. Polish Scientific Medical University.

Heller, A. S., van Reekum, C. M., Schaefer, S. M., Lapate, R. C., Radler, B. T., Ryff, C. D., & Davidson, R. J. (2013). Sustained ventral striatal activity predicts eudaimonic well-being and cortisol output. *Psychological Science*, *24*(11), 2192–2000. doi:10.1177/0956797613490744 PMID:24058063

Helliwell, J. F. (2002). Social Capital, the Economy and Well-being. *The Review of Economic Performance and Social Progress*. In K. Banting, A. Sharpe, & F. St-Hilaire (Eds.), *The Review of Economic Performance and Social Progress* (pp. 43–60). Montreal, Ottawa: Institute for Research on Public Policy and Centre for the Study of Living Standards.

Henderson, L. N., & Tulloch, J. (2008). Incentives for retaining and motivating health workers in Pacific and Asian countries. *Human Resources for Health*, *6*(1), 18. doi:10.1186/1478-4491-6-18 PMID:18793436

Henderson, S. (2003). Power imbalance between nurses and patients: A potential inhibitor of partnership in care. *Journal of Clinical Nursing*, *12*(4), 501–508. doi:10.1046/j.1365-2702.2003.00757.x PMID:12790863

Heng, C. C. (2011). Customer's satisfaction towards service quality of private hospitals in Kuching.

Herron, P. D. (2015). Opportunities and ethical challenges for the practice of medicine in the digital era. *Current Reviews in Musculoskeletal Medicine*, *8*(2), 113–117. doi:10.1007/s12178-015-9264-0 PMID:25786848

Heszen, I., & Sęk, H. (2017). Psychologia zdrowia [Health psychology]. *Intervention (Amstelveen, Netherlands)*, *5*(4), 329–339. doi:10.1093/brief-treatment/mhi030

Hobfoll, S., Nadler, A., & Leiberman, J. (1986). Satisfaction with social support during crisis: Intimacy and self-esteem as critical determinants. *Journal of Personality and Social Psychology*, *51*(2), 296–304. doi:10.1037/0022-3514.51.2.296 PMID:3746613

Holanowski, R. (2016, 27 października).Ryzyko kliniczne, czyli uczmy się na błędach, aby było ich coraz mniej [wypowiedź zarejestrowana podczas XII Forum Rynku Zdrowia, Warszawa 26-27 października 2016 roku]. Obtained from http://rynekzdrowia.pl

Holmes, T. H., & Rahe, R. H. (1967). The social readjustment rating scale. *Journal of Psychosomatic Research*, *11*(2), 213–218. doi:10.1016/0022-3999(67)90010-4 PMID:6059863

Horňáková, A. (2006). Language implementation of future health care workers and using of professional medical terminology in foreign language. In *Trends in Nursing IV* (pp. 84–93). Ostrava: University of Ostrava.

House, J. S., Landis, K. R., & Umberson, D. (1988). Social Relationship and Health. *Science*, *241*(4865), 540–545. doi:10.1126/science.3399889 PMID:3399889

Huczynski, A., & Buchanan, D. A. (2007). *Organisational Behaviour* (6th ed.). Harlow, England: FT Prentice Hall.

Hu, F. B., Li, T. Y., Colditz, G. A., Willett, W. C., & Manson, J. E. (2003). Television watching and other sedentary behaviors in relation to risk of obesity and type 2 diabetes mellitus in women. *Journal of the American Medical Association*, *289*(14), 1785–1791. doi:10.1001/jama.289.14.1785 PMID:12684356

Hwang, B., Moser, D. K., & Dracup, K. (2014). Knowledge Is Insufficient for Self-Care Among Heart Failure Patients With Psychological Distress. *Health Psychology*, *33*(7), 588–596. doi:10.1037/a0033419 PMID:23815766

Iannuzi, J. C., Kahn, S. A., Zhang, L., Gestring, M. L., Noyes, K., & Monson, J. R. T. (2015). Getting satisfaction: Drivers of surgical Hospital Consumer Assessment of Health care Providers and Systems survey scores. *The Journal of Surgical Research*, *197*(1), 155–161. doi:10.1016/j.jss.2015.03.045 PMID:25908102

Indes, J., Gates, L., Mitchell, E., & Muhs, B. (2013). Social media in vascular surgery. *Journal of Vascular Surgery*, *57*(4), 1159–1162. doi:10.1016/j.jvs.2012.09.065 PMID:23321344

Indredavik, B. (2007). What characterises an effective stroke unit? *Tidsskrift for Den Norske Lægeforening*, *127*(9), 1214–1218. PMID:17479142

Inglehart, R. (1997). *Modernization and Postmodernization. Cultural, Economic and Political Change in 43 Societies*. Princeton: Princeton University Press.

Institute of Medicine. (2001). *Crossing the Quality Chasm*. Washington, DC: National Academy Press.

Inzucchi, S. E., Bergenstal, R. M., Buse, J. B., Diamant, M., Ferrannini, E., Nauck, M., & Matthews, D. R. et al. (2012). Management of hyperglycemia in type 2 diabetes: A patient-centered approach. *Diabetes Care*, *35*(6), 1364–1379. doi:10.2337/dc12-0413 PMID:22517736

ISO. (2012, March). ISO 31000: 2009 Risk Management. Rules and Guidelines - Polish edition PN ISO 31000.

Iwanowicz-Palus, G. (2005). *Valuing work. Management in nursing*. Lublin. Czelej, Iwanowicz- Palus, G. J. & Kicia, M. (2005). *To burn must be on fire - stress and professional burnout in nurses and midwives*. Poland. *Pielęgniarstwo*, *XXI*, 25–27.

Jackson, C., & Haynes, T. (1992). *Cultural sensitivity: Aworking model*. Atlanta, GA: Southern Council on Collegiate Education for Nursing.

Jahns, L., Siega-Riz, A. M., & Popkin, B. M. (2001). The increasing prevalence of snacking among U.S. children from 1977 to 1996. *Pediatrics*, *138*(4), 493–498. doi:10.1067/mpd.2001.112162 PMID:11295711

Jakubaszko, J. (2004). *Nauczanie pierwszej pomocy. Zalecenia metodyczne*. Wrocław: Biblioteka Polskiego Towarzystwa Medycyny Ratunkowej.

Jakubaszko, J. (2005). *Kwalifikowana pierwsza pomoc. Zalecenia metodyczne*. Wrocław: Biblioteka Polskiego Towarzystwa Medycyny Ratunkowej.

Jakubaszko, J. (2007). *Medical rescue. Undergraduate Course (BSc)*. Wroclaw: Library of Polish Society for Emergency Medicine.

James, S., Reddy, S. P., Ellahebokus, A., Sewpaul, R., & Naidoo, P. (2017). The association between adolescent risk behaviours and feelings of sadness or hopelessness: A cross-sectional survey of South African secondary school learners. *Psychology Health and Medicine*, *22*(7), 778–789. Published online14Mar2017. doi:10.1080/13548506.2017.1300669 PMID:28290218

Janicka, I., & Liberska, H. (red.) (2014). Psychologia rodziny [Psychology of family]. Warszawa: Wydawnictwo Naukowe PWN.

Jankowiak, B., & Bartoszewicz, A. (2003). Komunikowanie się w obrębie zespołu terapeutycznego In A. Kwiatkowska, E. Krajewska – Kułak, C. Czabała et al. (Eds.). Komunikowanie interpersonalne w pielęgniarstwie (pp. 117-126). Czelej, Lublin: Wyd.

Janowska, Z. (2014). The role of management in the adaptation of multicultural work teams. *Prace Naukowe Uniwersytetu Ekonomicznego we Wrocławiu*, *349*, 120-129.

Janowska, J. (2016). Cztery wymiary komunikowania się w organizacji. *Marketing i Rynek*, *3*, 252–262.

Januszek, H., & Sikora, J. (1997). *Podstawy socjologii* (p. 37). Poznań: Wyd. AE.

Jasiński, Z. (2016). Decisions made by organizer of an employees' teams making their functioning difficult. *Prace Naukowe Uniwersytetu Ekonomicznego we Wrocławiu, 421*, 199-204.

Jaworzyńska, M. (2014). Market equilibrium in the health market- the theoretical background. Annales Universitatis Mariae Curie-Skłodowska, XLVIII(2).

Jędralska, K. (2010). *Niepewność jako źródło paradoksów strategicznych. W: J. Lichtarski, H. Jagoda (red.) Kierunki i dylematy rozwoju nauki i praktyki zarządzania przedsiębiorstwem.* Wrocław, CA: Uniwersytet Ekonomiczny.

Jemielniak, D. (2005). Culture: trades and professions. In Zbytniewska k. Works and material. ISM Publishing House.

Joint Learning Initiative. (2004). *Human Resources for Health: Overcoming the Crisis*. Cambridge, MA: Harvard University Press.

Jopkiewicz S. (2011). Funkcja wizerunku i tożsamości placówki w komunikacji marketingowej, Studia i Materiały. *Miscellanea Oeconomicae, 2.*

Juczyński Z. (2001). Spostrzegana kontrola a strategie radzenia sobie z przewlekłym bólem [Perceived control and coping strategies for chronic pain]. *Sztuka Leczenia, 7*(2), 9-16.

Juczyński, Z. (2014). Pomiar wsparcia społecznego – polska adaptacja Skali Znaczenia Innych [Measurement of social support - Polish adaptation of the Scale of Meaning of Others]. In E. Zasępa & T. Gałkowski (Eds.), Oblicza psychologii klinicznej. Pamięci Profesora Janusza Kostrzewskiego [Faces of clinical psychology. The memory of Professor Janusz Kostrzewski] (pp. 437–461). Warszawa: PWN.

Juczyński, Z. (2009). *Measurement Tools in the Promotion and Psychology Health.* Warsaw: Laboratory of Psychological Tests.

Juczyński, Z. (2009). *Narzędzia pomiaru w promocji i psychologii zdrowia (wydanie drugie)* [Measurement tools in promotion and health psychology (2nd ed.)]. Warszawa: Pracownia Testów Psychologicznych PTP.

Judgment of the Supreme Court: July 5, 1967, I PR 74/67, OSN of 1968 No. 2, item. 26 and of 7 June 1969, II CR 165/69, OSPiKA of 1969, no. 7-8, pos. 155, dated June 13, 2000, V CKN 34/00, Lex No. 52689, 17 May 2007, III CSK 429/06, Lex no. 274129); Gloss to the judgment of M. Nesterowicz, Lex No. 1222168, OSP 2013/6/61.

Kabengele Mpinga, K., & Chastonay, P. *Patient Satisfaction Studies and the Monitoring of the Right to Health: Some Thoughts Based on a Review of the Literature*, Global Journal of Health Science, Vol. 3, No. 1; April 2011, Retrieved 08.05.2017 from http://www.ccsenet.org/journal/index.php/gjhs/article/viewFile/8093/7143

Kaczmarek, T. T. (2010). Filozofia ryzyka – nowe tendencje w gospodarce globalnej. W: T. Kaczmarek (red.), Zarządzanie ryzykiem-ujęcie interdyscyplinarne (s.:11-14,29-30). Warszawa, CA: Difin S.A.

Kaducakova, H., & Lehotska, M. (2010). *Factors influencing the work of nurses in social welfare centers* (pp. 176–183). Cracow: AFM.

Kamrowska, A. (2007). Wypalenie zawodowe. *Polski Merkuriusz Lekarski, 23*(136), 317–319. PMID:18293860

Kamrowska, A., & Kamrowski, C. (2010). Wypalenie zawodowe wśród lekarzy psychiatrów. *Polski Merkuriusz Lekarski, 28*(165), 242–243. PMID:20815178

Kanner, A. D., Coyne, J. C., Schaefer, C., & Lazarus, R. S. (1981). Comparison of two modes of stress measurement: Daily hassles and uplifts versus major life events. *Journal of Behavioral Medicine, 4*(1), 1–39. doi:10.1007/BF00844845 PMID:7288876

Kapała, W. (2007). Lekarze i pielęgniarki – w stronę aktywnego współdziałania. *Nowoczesne Pielęgniarstwo i Położnictwo*, *1*, 1–14.

Kaplan, S. H., Greenfield, S., Gandek, B., Rogers, W. H., & Ware, J. E. (1996). Characteristics of physicians with participatory decision-making styles. *Annals of Internal Medicine*, *124*(5), 497–504.

Karimzadeh, M. (2013). Impact of Social Capital on Quality of Life: Evidence from India. *International Journal of Economic Practices and Theories*, *3*(4), 264–270.

Karski, J.B. (2011). *Practice and theory of health promotion*. CeDeWu.

Kasiewicz, S. (2011). *Zintegrowane zarządzanie ryzykiem przedsiębiorstwa w Polsce*. Warszawa, CA: Wolter Kluwer.

Katerndahl, D., Parchman, M., & Wood, R. (2009). Perceived complexity of care, perceived autonomy, and career satisfaction among primary care physicians. *Journal of the American Board of Family Medicine*, *22*(1), 24–3. doi:10.3122/jabfm.2009.01.080027 PMID:19124630

Kathleen, C. (2006, February). JCAHO'S National Patient Safety Goals 2006. *Journal of Perianesthesia Nursing*, *21*(1), 6–11. doi:10.1016/j.jopan.2005.11.005 PMID:16446238

Kawula, S. (1997). Spirala życzliwości: od wsparcia do samodzielności (The Kindness Spiral: From Support to Self-Reliance). *Wsparcie Społeczne*, *1*, 13–21.

Keiffer Melanie, R. (2015, June). Utilization of Clinical Practice Guidelines: Barriers and Facilitators. *The Nursing Clinics of North America*, *50*(2), 327–345. doi:10.1016/j.cnur.2015.03.007 PMID:25999074

Keith, T. (2009, February). Paternalism, participation and partnership- The evolution of patient centeredness in the consultation. *Patient Education and Counseling*, *74*(2), 150–155. doi:10.1016/j.pec.2008.08.017 PMID:18930624

Kenny, D. A., Valdhuijzen, W., van der Weijden, T., LeBlanc, A., Lockyer, J., Legare, F., & Campbell, C. (2010). Interpersonal perception in the context of doctor-patient relationships: A dyadic analysis of doctor-patient communication. *Social Science & Medicine*, *70*(5), 763–768. doi:10.1016/j.socscimed.2009.10.065 PMID:20005618

Kenrick, P. T., Neuberg, S. L., & Cialdini, R. B. (2002). *Social psychology*. Gdańsk: GWP.

Kępiński, A. (2005). *Jak leczyć i poznawać człowieka*. Kraków: Wydawnictwo Literackie.

Kiebzak W., Giermek K., Florczyk M., & Kiljański M. (2009). Code of conduct Physiotherapist of the Republic of Poland. *Physiotherapy Poland, 9*(3), 266-272.

Kilmann, R., & Thomas, K. W. (1974). *Thomas-Kilmann Conflict Mode Instrument. Xicom*. Tuxedo.

Kim, Y. Y. (1988). *Communication and cross-cultural adaptation: An integrative theory*. Philadelphia: Multilingual Matters.

Kissane, D. W., Bylund, C. L., Banerjee, S. C., Bialer, P. A., Levin, T. T., Maloney, E. K., & D'Agostino, T. A. (2012). Communication skills training for oncology professionals. *Journal of Clinical Oncology*, *30*(11), 1242–1247. doi:10.1200/JCO.2011.39.6184 PMID:22412145

Kitaoka-Higashiguchi, K., Morikawa, Y., Miura, K., Sakaurai, M., Ishizaki, M., Kido, T., & Nakagawa, H. et al. (2009). Burnout risk factors for arteriosclerotic disease: Follow up study. *Journal of Occupational Health*, *51*(2), 123–131. doi:10.1539/joh.L8104 PMID:19212087

Klakovich, M. D., & Dela Cruz, F. A. (2006, January-February). Validating the Interpersonal Communication Assessment Scale. *Journal of Professional Nursing*, *22*(1), 60–67. doi:10.1016/j.profnurs.2005.12.005 PMID:16459290

Kliszcz, J. (2012). *Psychologia w ratownictwie*. Warszawa: Difin SA.

Knoll, N., & Schwarzer, R. (2004). "Prawdziwych przyjaciół" Wsparcie społeczne, stres, choroba i śmierć ["Real friends" Social suport, stress, ilness and death.] In H. Sęk & R. Cieślak (Eds.), Wsparcie społeczne, stres i zdrowie [Social Support, Stress, Health] (pp. 29-48).Warszawa: Wydawnictwo Naukowe PWN.

Kodeks Etyki Lekarskiej. (n.d.). Retrieved 09.03.2017 from http://www.nil.org.pl

Komendziński, T., Komendziński, J., Mikołajewska, E., & Mikołajewski, D. (2016). Ethics in communication with patients in the state of disorders of consciousness. Natural situation and the use of modern technologies. *Advances in Psychiatry and Neurology*, *25*(2), 85–92.

Kongstvedt, P. R. (2001). *The Managed Health Care Handbook*. Jones & Bartlett Learning.

Kongstvedt, P. R. (2012). *Essentials of Managed Health Care*. Jones & Bartlett Publishers.

Kotarbiński, K. (1985). *Wykłady z dziejów logiki* (2nd ed.). Warszawa: PWN.

Kotler, P. (2004). *Marketing od A do Z*. Warszawa: PWE.

Kotter. J. (2005). Co właściwie robią przywódcy? [What Do Leaders Do?]. *Harvard Business Review*.

Kouzes, J.M., & Posner, B.Z. (2012). The Leadership Challenge: How to Make Extraordinary Things Happen in Organizations.

Kowalik, S. (2007). *Psychologia rehabilitacji* [Psychology of Rehabilitation]. Warszawa: Wydawnictwa Akademickie i Profesjonalne.

Kratochvil, S. (2016). *Terapia małżeńska* (p. 123). Gdańsk: Via Medica.

Kravitz, R. (1998). Patient Satisfaction with Health Care. Critical Outcome or Trivial Pursuit? *Journal of General Internal Medicine*, *13*(4), 280–282, Retrieved 07.052017 from https://www.ncbi.nlm.nih.gov/pmc/articles/PMC1496942/

Kravitz, R. L., Bell, R. A., Azari, R., Kelly-Reif, S., Krupat, E., & Thom, D. H. (2003). Direct observation of requests for clinical services in office practice: What do patients want and do they get it? *Archives of Internal Medicine*, *163*(14), 1673–1681. doi:10.1001/archinte.163.14.1673 PMID:12885682

Kreps, G. L., & Kunimoto, E. N. (1994). *Effective communication in multicultural health care settings*. Thousand Oaks, CA: Sage. doi:10.4135/9781483326344

Kripalani, S., LeFevre, F., Phillips, C. O., Williams, M. V., Basaviah, P., & Baker, D. W. (2007). Deficits in communication and information transfer between hospital-based and primary care physicians: Implications for patient safety and continuity of care. *Journal of the American Medical Association*, *297*(8), 831–841. doi:10.1001/jama.297.8.831 PMID:17327525

Król, H., & Ludwiczyński, A. (2007). Zarządzanie zasobami ludzkimi. Tworzenie kapitału ludzkiego organizacji. Warszawa. *PWN*, *31*, 336.

Kruk-Kupiec, G. (2011) National Consultant in Nursing, Consultant's recommendations National nursing field for good nursing practice, Safe Hospital - Safe Patient, Risk Management of Adverse Events, Project Safe medical practice. Retrieved 21.08.2012 from http: // www.mz.gov.pl

Krzakiewicz, K. (2008). *Kognitywne podejście do zarządzania strategicznego. W: J. Rokita (red.), Ku nowym paradygmatom nauk o zarządzaniu*. Katowice, CA: GWSH.

Krzych, Ł. J., Pawlak, A., Woźnica, A., Skarysz, J., Eysymontt, Z., Krupka-Matuszczyk, I., & Cisowski, M. et al. (2009). Conditions of severity of anxiety and depression in the perioperative period in the economically active men undergoing coronary artery and cardiopulmonary bypass. *Cardio-Thoracic Surgery Poland*, *6*(3), 238–243.

Ksykiewicz-Dorota, A. (2005). *Ergonomic analysis of the work. Management in nursing*. Lublin: Czelej.

Ksynkiewicz-Dorota, A. (2005). *Zarządzanie w Pielęgniarstwie*. Lublin: Czelej.

Kuleta, M., & Trzópek, J. (2003). Zmiana stylu życia jako efekt przezwyciężenia kryzysu – szansa czy konieczność? [Change of lifestyle as a result of overcoming the crisis - chance or necessity?] In D. Kubacka-Jasiecka, & K. Mudyń (Eds.), Kryzys, interwencja i pomoc psychologiczna. Nowe ujęcia i możliwości [Crisis, intervention and psychological help. New shots and opportunities] (pp. 121- 144). Toruń: Wydawnictwo: Adam Marszałek.

Kuriata, E., Felińczak, A., Grzebieluch, J., & Szachniewicz, M. (2011). Detrimental factors and workload of nurses employed in the hospital. Part II. Nursing. *Public Health*, 269–273.

Kutryba, B., Kutaj-Wąsikowska, H., & Tombarkiwewicz, M. (2015). *Zdarzenia niepożądane. Analiza przyczyn źródłowych zdarzeń niepożądanych*. Kraków, CA: Centrum Monitorowania Jakości w Ochronie Zdrowia.

Labott, S. M., Ahleman, B. A., Wolever, M. E., & Martin, R. B. (2010). The Physiological and Psychological Effects of the Expression and Inhibition of Emotion. *Journal of Behavioral Medicine*, 16(4), 182–189. PMID:2271804

Labott, S. M., & Martin, R. B. (1990). Emotional coping, age, and physical disorder. *Behavioral Medicine (Washington, D.C.)*, *16*(2), 53–61. doi:10.1080/08964289.1990.9934592 PMID:2364177

Lancioni, G. E., Bosco, A., Olivetti Belardinelli, M., Singh, N. N., O'Reilly, M. F., Sigafoos, J., & Oliva, D. (2014b). Technology-based intervention programs to promote stimulation control and communication in post-coma persons with different levels of disability. *Frontiers in Human Neuroscience*, *8*, 48. doi:10.3389/fnhum.2014.00048 PMID:24574992

Lancioni, G. E., Singh, N. N., O'Reilly, M. F., Sigafoos, J., Buonocunto, F., D'Amico, F., & Megna, M. et al. (2014a). Occupation and communication programs for post-coma persons with or without consciousness disorders who show extensive motor impairment and lack of speech. *Research in Developmental Disabilities*, *35*(5), 1110–1118. doi:10.1016/j.ridd.2014.01.029 PMID:24582854

Lancioni, G. E., Singh, N. N., O'Reilly, M. F., Sigafoos, J., & Olivetti Belardinelli, M. (2012). Technology-based intervention to help persons with minimally conscious state and pervasive motor disabilities perform environmentally relevant adaptive behavior. *Cognitive Processing*, *13*(Suppl. 1), S219–S222. doi:10.1007/s10339-012-0485-5 PMID:22806668

Langhorne, P., & Pollock, A.Stroke Unit Trialists' Collaboration. (2002). What are the components of effective stroke unit care? *Age and Ageing*, *31*(5), 365–371. doi:10.1093/ageing/31.5.365 PMID:12242199

LaPietra, A., Grossi, E. A., Derivaux, C. C., Applebaum, R. M., Hanjis, C. D., Ribakove, G. H., & Colvin, S. B. et al. (2000). Robotic-assisted instruments enhance minimally invasive mitral valve surgery. *The Annals of Thoracic Surgery*, *70*(3), 835–838. doi:10.1016/S0003-4975(00)01610-6 PMID:11016319

Laviolette, P. (1981). *A system view of man*. Boulder, CO: Westview Press.

Lazarus, R. S. (1986). Paradygmat stresu i radzenia sobie [Paradigm of stress and doping]. *Nowiny Psychologiczne*, *3*, 2–39.

Lazarus, R. S., & Folkman, S. (1984). *Stress, appraisal, and coping*. Berlin, Heidelberg, New York: Springer.

Lee Ventola, C. (2014). Social Media and Health Care Professionals: Benefits, Risks, and Best Practices. *P&T*, *39*(7), 491–499, 520. PMID:25083128

Lee, K., Yoon, K., Ha, M., Park, J., Cho, S., & Kang, D. (2010). Heart rate variability and urinary catecholamines from job stress in Korean male manufacturing workers according to work seniority. *Industrial Health*, *48*, 331–338.

Lee, M. E., Matsumoto, D., Kobayashi, M., Krupp, D., Maniatis, E. F., & Roberts, W. (1992). Cultural influences on nonverbals in applied settings. In *Applications of nonverbal behavior theories and research* (pp. 239–261). Hillsdale, NJ: Lawrence Erlbaum Associates, Inc.

Leigh J.P, Tancredi D.J., Kravitz R.L. (2009). Physician career satisfaction within specialties *BMC Health Serv Res.*, *16*(9), 166.

Lepnurm, R., Dobson, R., Backman, A., & Keegan, D. (2006). Factors explaining career satisfaction among psy-chiatrists and surgeons in Canada. *Canadian Journal of Psychiatry*, *51*(4), 243–255. doi:10.1177/070674370605100406 PMID:16629349

Leslie, R. C. (1983). Management of Conflict. *Industrial Management & Data Systems*, *83*(1/2), 77. doi:10.1108/eb057300 PMID:6551214

Leung, A., Kier, C., Fung, T., Fung, L., & Sproule, R. (2011). Searching for Happiness: The Importance of Social Capital. *Journal of Happiness Studies*, *12*(3), 443–462. doi:10.1007/s10902-010-9208-8

Levenson, P. M., Morrow, J. R. Jr, & Pfefferbaum, B. J. (1984). Attitudes toward health and illness. A comparison of adolescent, physician, teacher, and school nurse views. *Journal of Adolescent Health Care*, *5*(4), 254–260. doi:10.1016/S0197-0070(84)80127-8 PMID:6490480

Levin, T. T., Moreno, B., Silvester, W., & Kissane, D. W. (2010). End-of-life communication in the intensive care unit. *General Hospital Psychiatry*, *32*(4), 433–442. doi:10.1016/j.genhosppsych.2010.04.007 PMID:20633749

Lewandowska, A., & Litwin, B. (2009). Professional burnout as a threat to nursing work. In Yearbook of the Pomeranian Medical Academy in Szczecin.

Lewicki, A. (1978). Niektóre problemy teorii zachowania [Some problems of the theory of behavior]. In A. Lewicki (Ed.), Psychologia kliniczna [Clinical psychology] (pp. 21 – 43). Warszawa: PWN.

Lewtak, K., Poznańska, A., & Mirosław, J. (2012). Wysocki, Predyktory satysfakcji zawodowej lekarzy podstawowej opieki zdrowotnej. *Probl. Hig. Epidemiol.*, *93*(3), 558–567.

Liang, X., Kuhlmann, L., Johnston, L. A., Grayden, D. B., Vogrin, S., Crossley, R., & Cook, M. J. et al. (2014). Extending communication for patients with disorders of consciousness. *Journal of Neuroimaging*, *24*(1), 31–38. doi:10.1111/j.1552-6569.2012.00744.x PMID:22928842

Liberska, H. (2017). *Attachment and stress in adolescents during treatment in hospital* . Paper sent to the editor.

Liberska, H. (2004). *Perspektywy temporalne młodzieży. Wybrane uwarunkowania* [Temporar perspectives of adolescents. Selected determinants]. Poznań: Wydawnictwo Naukowe UAM.

Liberska, H., & Boniecka, K. (2016). Introduction: biopsychosocial approach to transplantation. In H. Liberska & K. Boniecka (Eds.), *Selected psychosocial and medical problems of transplantation* (pp. 9–18). Warszawa: Difin.

Lichtarski, H. Jagoda (red.), *Kierunki i dylematy rozwoju nauki i praktyki zarządzania przedsiębiorstwem*. Wrocław, CA: Uniwersytet Ekonomiczny.

Lisiecka, K. (2003). Zarządzanie jakością usług zdrowotnych. Warszawa, CA: Instytut Przedsiębiorczości i samorządności.

Lisowska, B. (n.d.). Zmiany w służbie zdrowia: Wizyta w kwadrans, kolejki przed gabinetami. *Gazeta prawna.pl*. Retrieved from http://serwisy.gazetaprawna.pl/zdrowie/artykuly/862915,zmiany-w-sluzbie-zdrowia-wizyta-w-kwadrans-kolejki-przed-gabinetami.html

Litwiejko, A. (2010). *The basics of public health in terms of legal and social Publishing House*. Wroclaw.

Longtin, Y., Sax, H., Leape, L. L., Sheridan, S. E., Donaldson, L., & Pittet, D. (2010). Patient Participation: Current Knowledge and Applicability to Patient Safety. *Mayo Clinic Proceedings*, *85*(1), 53–62. doi:10.4065/mcp.2009.0248 PMID:20042562

Luauté, J., Morlet, D., & Mattout, J. (2015). BCI in patients with disorders of consciousness: Clinical perspectives. *Annals of Physical and Rehabilitation Medicine*, *58*(1), 29–34. doi:10.1016/j.rehab.2014.09.015 PMID:25616606

Łuczak, A. (2011). *Standardization work on mental workload* (pp. 105–115). Kraków: PAN.

Luoma, M. (2006). Increasing the Motivation of Health-care Workers. Capacity Project Technical Brief 7.

Lush, M., Rosner, D., Zant, C., & Notte, S. (2016). Patient engagement strategies in a digital environment: Life sciences companies respond to changing patient expectations. *Delloite Review*, 18.

Luszczynska, A., Mazurkiewicz, M., Ziegelmann, J. P., & Schwarzer, R. (2007). Recovery self-efficacy and intention as predictors of running or jogging behavior: A cross-lagged panel analysis over a two-year period. *Psychology of Sport and Exercise*, *8*(2), 247–260. doi:10.1016/j.psychsport.2006.03.010

Macdonald, A. L., & Sevdalis, N. (2017, March). Patient safety improvement interventions in children's surgery: A systematic review. *Journal of Pediatric Surgery*, *52*(3), 504–511. doi:10.1016/j.jpedsurg.2016.09.058 PMID:27717565

Maciąg, A. 2004. Rola informacji w procesie tworzenia jakości usług medycznych. *Zdrowie i Zarządzanie*, *6*(6).

Mądrala, A. (Ed.). (2013). System ochrony zdrowia w Polsce - Diagnoza i kierunki reformy, AKADEMIA ZDROWIA 2030 [Health System in Poland - Diagnosis and directions of reform, HEALTH ACADEMY 2030].

Makoul, G., & Clayman, M. (2006). An integrative model of shared decision making in medical encounters. *Patient Education and Counseling*, *60*(3), 301–312. doi:10.1016/j.pec.2005.06.010 PMID:16051459

Makowska, H. (2001). Informing the patient by a doctor. Whether people ill want to know everything threatens? In The basics of Health Psychology. Publishing House of the University of Wrocław.

Mangia, A. L., Pirini, M., Simoncini, L., & Cappello, A. (2014). A feasibility study of an improved procedure for using EEG to detect brain responses to imagery instruction in patients with disorders of consciousness. *PLoS One*, *9*(6), e99289. doi:10.1371/journal.pone.0099289 PMID:24915148

Manias, E. (2012). Complexities of pain assessment and management in hospitalised older people: A qualitative observation and interview study. *International Journal of Nursing Studies*, *49*(10), 1243–1254. doi:10.1016/j.ijnurstu.2012.05.002 PMID:22640777

Manongi, R. N., Marchant, T. C., & Bygbjerg, I. C. (2006). Improving motivation among primary health care workers in Tanzania: A health worker perspective. *Human Resources for Health*, *4*(1), 6. doi:10.1186/1478-4491-4-6 PMID:16522213

Marciniak, J. (2011). *Mobbing, dyskryminacja, molestowanie – zasady przeciwdziałania* (p. 59). Warszawa: Wolters Kluwer Polska.

Mary, H. (2008). *Building a Culture of Patient Safety*. Department of Health & Children.

Masić, I., Ridanovic, Z., & Pandza H. (1995). Medical expert systems. *Med. Arh.*, *49*(3-4), 107-112.

Maslach, C. & Jackson, S. (1982). Burnout in health professions: A social psychological analysis. Social psychology of health and illness. New York: Erlbaum.

Maslach, C. A. (1998). Multidimensional theory of burnout. Theories of organizational stress. Oxford University Press 68-85, New York.

Maslach, C. (2001). What have we learned about burnout and health? *Psychology & Health.*

Maslach, C., & Jackson, S. (1981). The measurement of experienced burnout. *Journal of Occupational Behaviour, 2*(2), 99113. doi:10.1002/job.4030020205

Maslach, C., & Leiter, M. (1997). *The truth about burnout.* San Francisco, CA: Jossey-Bass.

Maslach, C., & Schaufeli, W. B. (1993). *Historical and conceptual development of burnout. Professional burnout: Recent developments in theory and research.* Washington, DC: Taylor and Francis.

Maslow, A. (1970). *Motivation and personality.* New York: Harper & Row.

Matthews, G., Deary, I., & Whiteman, M. (2003). *Personality traits.* Cambridge: Cambridge University Press. doi:10.1017/CBO9780511812736

Mayerscough, P. R., & Ford, M. (2003). *Jak rozmawiać z pacjentem. Podręcznik komunikacji interpersonalnej.* Warszawa: Wydawnictwo Naukowe PWN.

McEvans, B., & Kalia, M. (2010). The role of corticosteroids and stress in chronic pain conditions. *Metabolism: Clinical and Experimental, 59*(Suppl. 1), s9–s13. PMID:20837196

McEwan, B., & Kalia, M. (2010). The role of corticosteroids and stress in chronic pain conditions. *Metabolism: Clinical and Experimental, 59*(Suppl. 1), s9–s13. doi:10.1016/j.metabol.2010.07.012 PMID:20837196

McGuire [2000] – T. McGuire, Physician agency, w: Handbook of Health Economics, red. A. J. Culyer, J. P. Newhouse, vol. 1A. (2000). Amsterdam: Elsevier.

McKinstry, B. (1992). Paternalism and the doctor-patient relationship in general practice. *The British Journal of General Practice, 42*(361), 340–342. PMID:1457157

Mclean, J., & Page, M. (2005) Social Capital and Quality of Life. In *Proceedings of the 7th Australian Conference on Quality of Life.*

McLeod, S. A. (2010). *SRRS - Stress of Life Events.* Retrieved from www.simplypsychology.org/SRRS.html

Melamed, S., Ugarten, U., Shirom, A., Kahana, L., Lerman, Y., & Froom, P. (1999). Chronic burnout, somatic arousal and elevated salivatory cortisol levels. *Journal of Psychosomatic Research, 46*(6), 591–598. doi:10.1016/S0022-3999(99)00007-0 PMID:10454175

Meller, D., & Milik, A. (2014). Komunikacja interpersonalna w zakładach opieki zdrowotnej. *Zarządzanie i Finanse Journal of Management and Finance, 12*(2), 133–144.

Mellor, D., Cummins, R., & Loquet, T. (2012). Life quality and wealth: a qualitative and quantitative comparison of affluent and poor people. *Journal of Social Research and Policy, 3*(2), 7–18.

Messina, D. J., Scotti, D. J., Caney, R., & Zipp, G. P. (2009). The Relationship Between Patient Satisfaction and Inpatient Admissions Across Teaching and Nonteaching Hospitals. *Journal of Healthcare Management, 54*(3), 177–190. Retrieved from http://search.ebscohost.com/login.aspx?direct=true&db=buh&AN=41033454&lang=de&site=ehost-live PMID:19554798

Messner, S., Baumer, E., & Rosenfeld, R. (2004). Dimensions of Social Capital and Rates of Criminal Homicide. *American Sociological Review, 69*(6), 882–903. doi:10.1177/000312240406900607

Michalin, M. (2003). From ethics to business ethics. Foundation for Innovation, Higher Socio-Economic School.

Mikułowski Pomorski, J. (2003). *Komunikacja międzykulturowa. Wprowadzenie.* Kraków: Wyd. AE.

Miles, S., & Leinster, S. J. (2010). Identifying Professional characteristics of the ideal medical doctor: The laddering technique. *Medical Teacher*, *32*(2), 136–140. doi:10.3109/01421590903196987 PMID:20163229

Miller, D., & O'Callaghan, J. (2002). Neuroendocrine aspects of the response to stress. *Metabolism: Clinical and Experimental*, *51*(6 Suppl. 1), 5–10. doi:10.1053/meta.2002.33184 PMID:12040534

Miller, F. L., Bennett, S., & Kanfer, R. (2002). Health sector reform and public sector health worker motivation: A conceptual framework. *Social Science & Medicine*, *54*(8), 1255–1266. doi:10.1016/S0277-9536(01)00094-6 PMID:11989961

Miller, J. B., & Stiver, I. P. (1997). *The Healing Connection: How Women form Relationships in Therapy and in Life*. Boston: Beacon Press.

Miller, J. H., & Page, S. E. (Eds.). (2007). *Complex adaptive systems: An introduction to computational models of social life*. Princeton, NJ: Princeton University Press.

Miller, J. L., & Gros-Louis, J. (2013). Socially guided attention influences infants' communicative behavior. *Infant Behavior and Development*, *36*(4), 627–634. doi:10.1016/j.infbeh.2013.06.010 PMID:23906941

Ministry of Finance. (n.d.). Communication No. 23 of the Minister of Finance of 16 December 2009 on standards Management control for the public finance sector (Official Journal 2009.15.84).

Ministry of Finance. (n.d.). Communication No. 6 of the Minister of Finance dated 6 December, 2012 on detailed issues Guidelines for the public finance sector in planning and management of risk (Official Journal 2012.56).

Mintzberg H.; Managing on three planes. Journal: Leader To Leader, vol. 2010, no. 57, pp. 29-33.

Mishra, P. H., & Gupta, S. (2012). Study of patient satisfaction in a surgical unit of a tertiary care teaching hospital. *Journal of Clinical Orthopaedics and Trauma*, *3*(1), 43–47. doi:10.1016/j.jcot.2012.04.002 PMID:25983455

Mohrman, S. A., Cohen, S. G., & Mohrman, A. M. (1995). *Designing team based organizations: New forms for knowledge work*. San Francisco: Jossey-Bass.

Mommersteeg, P., Heijnen, C., Kavelaars, A., & van Doornen, L. J. P. (2006). Immune and endocrine function in burnout syndrome. *Psychosomatic Medicine*, *68*(6), 879–886. doi:10.1097/01.psy.0000239247.47581.0c PMID:17079708

Monaghan, J., Channell, K., McDowell, D., & Sharma, A. K. (2005). Improving patient and carer communication, multidisciplinary team working and goal-setting in stroke rehabilitation. *Clinical Rehabilitation*, *19*(2), 194–199. doi:10.1191/0269215505cr837oa PMID:15759535

Monkiewicz, J., & Gąsiorkiewicz, L. (2010). *Zarządzanie ryzykiem w działalności organizacji*. Warszawa, CA: C.H. Beck.

Montero-Marĭn, J., Garcĭa-Campayo, J., Fayó-Pascual, M., Carrasco, J., Gascón, S., Gili, M., & Mayoral-Cleries, F. (2011). Sociodemographic and occupational risk factors associated with the development of different burnout types: The cross-sectional University of Zaragoza study. *BMC Psychiatry*, *11*(1), 49–62. doi:10.1186/1471-244X-11-49 PMID:21447169

Montero-Marĭn, J., Garcĭa-Campayo, J., Mera, D., & del Hoyo, Y. (2009). A new definition of burnout syndrome based on Farber's proposal. *Journal of Occupational Medicine and Toxicology (London, England)*, *4*(1), 31–48. doi:10.1186/1745-6673-4-31 PMID:19948055

Moore, G. F., Audrey, S., & Barker, M. et al.. (2015). Process evaluation of complex interventions: Medical Research Council guidance. *BMJ (Clinical Research Ed.)*, *350*, h1258. PMID:25791983

Moore, S. E. (1992). Cultural sensitivity treatment and research issues with Black adolescent drug users. *Child & Adolescent Social Work Journal*, *9*(3), 249–260. doi:10.1007/BF00755864

Moos, R. H., & Schaefer, J. A. (1993). Coping Resources and Process: Current Concepts and Measures. In L. Goldberger & S. Breznits (Eds.), Handbook of Stress. Theoretical and Clinical Aspects (pp. 234–257). New York: The Free Press.

Moser, D., Kimble, L., Alberts, M., Alonzo, A., Croft, J., & Dracup, K. et al.. (2006). Reducing delay in seeking treatment by patients with acute coronary syndrome and stroke: A scientific statement from the American Heart Association Council on cardiovascular nursing and stroke council. *Circulation*, *114*(2), 168–182. doi:10.1161/CIRCULATIONAHA.106.176040 PMID:16801458

Mosley, I., Nicol, M., Donnan, G., Patrick, I., Kerr, F., & Dewey, H. (2007). The impact of ambulance practice on acute stroke care. *Stroke*, *38*(10), 2765–2770. doi:10.1161/STROKEAHA.107.483446 PMID:17717317

Motyka, H. (2010). Komunikacja interpersonalna w opiece medycznej. *Medycyna Rodzinna*, *4*, 124–128.

Murante, A. M. (2010). Patient satisfaction: a strategic tool for health services management. *Scuola Superiore Sant' Anna*.

Naci, L., Monti, M. M., Cruse, D., Kübler, A., Sorger, B., Goebel, R., & Owen, A. M. et al. (2012, September). Brain-computer interfaces for communication with nonresponsive patients. *Annals of Neurology*, *72*(3), 312–323. doi:10.1002/ana.23656 PMID:23034907

Naci, L., & Owen, A. M. (2013). Making every word count for nonresponsive patients. *JAMA Neurology*, *70*(10), 1235–1241. PMID:23939634

Naidu, A. (2009). Factors affecting patient satisfaction and healthcare quality. *International Journal of Health Care Quality Assurance*, *22*(4), 366–381. doi:10.1108/09526860910964834 PMID:19725209

Nakamura, H., Nagase, H., Yoshida, M., & Ogino, K. (1999). Natural killer (NK) cell activity and NK cell subsets in workers with a tendency to burnout. *Journal of Psychosomatic Research*, *46*(6), 569–578. doi:10.1016/S0022-3999(99)00009-4 PMID:10454173

Nakata, A., Takahashi, M., Irie, M., & Swanson, N. (2010). Job satisfaction is associated with elevated natural killer cell immunity among healthy white-collar employees. *Brain, Behavior, and Immunity*, *24*(8), 1268–1275. doi:10.1016/j.bbi.2010.05.004 PMID:20561922

Narodowa Agencja Programu „Uczenie się przez całe życie": Wprowadzenie do projektu Tuning Educational Structures in Europe – Harmonizacja struktur kształcenia w Europie. Wkład uczelni w Proces Boloński. (2008). Warszawa: Fundacja Rozwoju Systemu Edukacji.

National Audit Office. (2005). A safer place for patients: learning to improve patient safety. Retrieved from http://www.nao.org.uk/pn/05- 06/0506456.htm

Nęcki, Z. (1995). *Negocjacje w biznesie*. Kraków: Wydawnictwo Profesjonalnej Szkoły Biznesu.

Nelson, B. V., Patience, T. H., & MacDonald, D. C. (1999). Adolescent Risk Behavior and the Influence of Parents and Education. *Journal of the American Board of Family Medicine*, *12*(6), 436–443. doi:10.3122/jabfm.12.6.436 PMID:10612361

Nelson, J. E., Puntillo, K. A., Pronovost, P. J., Walker, A. S., McAdam, J. L., Ilaoa, D., & Penrod, J. (2010, March). In their own words: Patients and families define high-quality palliative care in the intensive care unit. *Critical Care Medicine*, *38*(3), 808–818. doi:10.1097/CCM.0b013e3181c5887c PMID:20198726

Neumar, R. W., Nolan, J. P., Adrie, C., Aibiki, M., Berg, R. A., Bottiger, B. W., & Vanden Hoek, T. et al. (2008). Post-cardiac arrest syndrome. *Circulation*, *118*(23), 2452–2483. doi:10.1161/CIRCULATIONAHA.108.190652 PMID:18948368

Nichols, A. L., & Cottrell, C. A. (2014, August). Cottrell Catherine A. What do people desire in their leaders? The role of leadership level on trait desirability. *The Leadership Quarterly*, *25*(4), 711–729. doi:10.1016/j.leaqua.2014.04.001

Nieszporska, S. (2008). Jakość usług szpitalnych w ocenie pacjenta. In K. Ryć, & Z. Skrzypczak (Ed.), Ochrona zdrowia i gospodarka. Mechanizmy rynkowe a regulacje publiczne (pp. 197-205). Warszawa, CA: Zarządzania Uniwersytetu Warszawskiego.

Nirel, N., Goldwag, R., Feigenberg, Z., Abadi, D., & Halpern, P. (2008). Stress, work overload, burnout, and satisfaction among paramedics in Israel. *Prehospital and Disaster Medicine*, *23*(06), 537–546. doi:10.1017/S1049023X00006385 PMID:19557971

Noble, R. (2002). Diagnosis of stress. *Metabolism: Clinical and Experimental*, *51*(6 Suppl. 1), 37–39. doi:10.1053/meta.2002.33190 PMID:12040539

Noghani, M., Asgharpour, A., Safa, S., & Kermani, M. (2009) *Quality of life and Social Capital in Mashhad City in Iran, Conference of health and society*. Retrieved 27 November 2012 from http://profdoc.um.ac.ir/paper-abstract-1021206.html

Nowaczyk, N., & Cierpiałkowska, L. (2016). Psychological profiles of patients with multiple sclerosis based on Hobfoll's conservation of resources theory. *Health Psychology Review*, *4*(4), 332–339. doi:10.5114/hpr.2016.59990

O'Brien, M., & Shea, J. (2011). Disparities in patient satisfaction among Hispanics: The role of language preference. *Journal of Immigrant and Minority Health*, *13*(2), 408–412. doi:10.1007/s10903-009-9275-2 PMID:19626440

O'Gara, P. T., Kushner, F. G., & Ascheim, D. D. et al.. (2012). ACCF/AHA Guidelines for the management of ST-Elevation of Mycocardial infraction: A report of American College of Cardiology Foundation/American Heart Association task force on practice guidelines. *Circulation*. doi:10.1161/CIR.0b013e3182742cf6

Obuchowski, K. (2000). *Galaktyka potrzeb. Psychologia dążeń ludzkich*. Poznań: Zysk i S-ka.

OECD. (2001). *The Well-Being of Nations: The Role of Human and Social Capital, Education and Skills*. Paris: OECD Centre for Educational Research and Innovation.

Official materials of the National health Fund in Poland. (2017). Koordynowana opieka zdrowotna w Polsce [Coordinated healthcare in Poland]. Retrieved from http://akademia.nfz.gov.pl/ook/

Ogińska-Bulik, N. (2013). The role of social support in people struggling with cancer. *Health Psychology Review*, *1*(1), 1–8. PMID:25793484

Ogińska-Bulik, N. (2016). The role of rumination in the occurrence of positive effects of experienced traumatic events. *Health Psychology Review*, *4*(4), 321–331.

Ogińska-Bulik, N., & Juczyński, Z. (2012). Resiliency as determinant of the positive and negative consequences of an experienced traumatic situation. *Polskie Forum Psychologiczne*, *2*(17), 395–410.

Őhlin, B., Berglund, G., Nilsson, P., & Melander, O. (2008). Job strain, job demands and adrenergic beta-1-receptor=polymorphism: A possible interaction affecting blood pressure in men. *Journal of Hypertension*, *26*(8), 1583–1589. doi:10.1097/HJH.0b013e328303df5f PMID:18622236

Okamoto, H., Tsunoda, T., Teruya, K., Takeda, N., Uemura, T., Matsiu, T., & Takashima, Y. et al. (2008). An occupational health study of emergency physicians in Japan: Health assessment by immune variables (CD4, CD8, CD56, and NK cell activity) at the beginning of work. *Journal of Occupational Health*, *50*(2), 136–146. doi:10.1539/joh.L6084 PMID:18403864

Olatunji, S.O. & Mokuolu, B.O. (2014). The Influence of Sex, Marital Status, and Tenure of Service on Job Stress, and Job Satisfaction of Health Workers in a Nigerian Federal Health Institution. An International Multidisciplinary Journal, 8(1), 126-133.

Oleksyn, T. (2006). *Zarządzanie kompetencjami. In Teoria i praktyka* (p. 30). Kraków: Oficyna Ekonomiczna.

Oleś, M. (2015). Resilience and quality of life in chronically ill youth. *Health Psychology Review*, *3*(3), 220–236. doi:10.5114/hpr.2015.53246

Oleś, P. (2000). *Psychologia przełomu połowy życia* [Psychology of the mid-life breakthrough]. Lublin: Towarzystwo Naukowe KUL.

Olson, J., & Masur, E. F. (2015). Mothers' labeling responses to infants' gestures predict vocabulary outcomes. *Journal of Child Language*, *3*, 1–23. PMID:25643656

Opolski, K., & Waśniewski, K. (2011). Zarządzanie jakością i ryzykiem w usługach zdrowotnych. Warszawa, CA: CeDeWu.

Opolski, K., Dykowska, G., & Możdżonek, M. (2005). Zarządzanie przez jakość w usługach zdrowotnych. Teoria i praktyka., Warszawa, CA: CeDeWu.

Osika G. (2000). Negocjacje-charakterystyka problemu *Organizacja i zarządzanie. Zeszyty naukowe politechniki śląskiej, 1467*(1), 55-65.

Ostasiewicz, W. (2004). *Ocena i analiza jakości życia*. Wroclaw: Wroclaw University of Economics Press.

Ostrowska, A. (2001). The relationship patient doctor-new quality. Health promotion. *Social Science & Medicine*, *21*, 109–121.

Otani, K., & Kurz, R. S. (2004, May). The impact of nursing care and other healthcare attributes on hospitalized patient satisfaction and behavioral intentions. *Journal of Healthcare Management*, *49*(3), 181–196. PMID:15190860

Ounagh, N., & Ounagh, M. (2011). A Comparative Study of Social Capital and Quality Of Life in Delhi and Tehran. *Journal of Exclusion Studies*, *1*(1), 19–35. doi:10.5958/j.2231-4547.1.1.002

Owen, A. M. (2013). Detecting consciousness: A unique role for neuroimaging. *Annual Review of Psychology*, *64*(1), 109–133. doi:10.1146/annurev-psych-113011-143729 PMID:23043305

P. Experience. (2010). Focus on the Patient Experience Save the Date.

Pagórski P., & Markiewicz D. (2015). Motivating employees of some hospital with a particular emphasis on nurses. *Pielęgniarstwo polskie, 2*(56),216-224.

Panesar Sukhmeet, S. (2009, July 1). Cleary Kevin, Sheikh Aziz. Reflections on the National Patient Safety Agency's database of medical errors. *Journal of the Royal Society of Medicine*, *102*(7), 256–258. doi:10.1258/jrsm.2009.090135 PMID:19605852

Parker, J. D. A., & Endler, N. S. (1994). Assessment of multidimensional coping: Task, emotion and avoidance strategies. *Psychological Assessment*, *6*(1), 50–60. doi:10.1037/1040-3590.6.1.50

Parkhurst, J. O., & Abeysinghe, S. (2016). What constitutes "good" evidence for public health and social policy-making? From hierarchies to appropriateness. *Social Epistemology*, *30*(5-6), 665–679. doi:10.1080/02691728.2016.1172365

Pascale, C., & Wood, K. E. (2010). Patient Safety: The Role of Human Factors and Systems Engineering. *Studies in Health Technology and Informatics*, *153*, 23–46. PMID:20543237

Pasowicz, M. (2012). Zarządzanie podmiotami leczniczymi – bezpieczeństwo pacjentów i sposoby ograniczania ryzyka szpitali. Kraków, CA: Krakowskie Towarzystwo Edukacyjne sp. z o.o. – Oficyna Wydawnicza AFM.

Patient Rights Patent and Patient Rights Act of 6 November 2008 (Journal of Laws, no. 2016.186t.j. With later meme).

Paul, J. (2002). PhD; Kravitz R.L., MD, MSPH, Physician Career Satisfaction Across Specialties. *Archives of Internal Medicine*, *162*(14), 1577–1584. doi:10.1001/archinte.162.14.1577 PMID:12123400

Pawlak, J. (2015). The Influence of Subjectivity and Employee Participation on Team Involvement and Responsibility during Times of Change. *Zeszyty Naukowe Uniwersytetu Ekonomicznego w Krakowie*, *944*(08), 57–67. doi:10.15678/ZNUEK.2015.0944.0805

Paxton, P. (1999). Is Social Capital Declining in the United States? A Multiple Indicator Assessment. *American Journal of Sociology*, *105*(1), 88–127. doi:10.1086/210268

Paxton, P. (2002). Social Capital and Democracy: An Interdependent Relationship. *American Sociological Review*, *67*(2), 254–277. doi:10.2307/3088895

Peabody, J. W., Taguiwalo, M. M., Robalino, D. A., & Frenk, J. (2006). Improving the Quality of Care in Developing Countries. In Disease Control Priorities in Developing Countries (2nd ed.). New York: Oxford University Press.

Peberdy, M. A., Callaway, C. W., Neumar, R. W., Geocadin, R. G., Zimmerman, J. L., Donnino, M., & Kronick, S. L. et al. (2010). Part 9: Post–Cardiac Arrest Care 2010 American Heart Association guidelines for cardiopulmonary resuscitation and emergency cardiovascular care. *Circulation*, *122*(18 Suppl. 3), S768–S786. doi:10.1161/CIRCULATIONAHA.110.971002 PMID:20956225

Peeva, K., & Kyosev, Y. (2004). *Fuzzy relational calculus, theory, application and software. In Advances in Fuzzy Systems – Applications and Theory* (Vol. 22). Singapore: World Scientific Publishing.

Penc, J. (2006). *Sztuka skutecznego zarządzania*. Kraków: Oficyna Ekonomiczna.

Per, B. (1998). Obesity: A chronic disease with alarming prevalence and consequences. *Journal of Internal Medicine*, *244*(4), 267–269. doi:10.1046/j.1365-2796.1998.00417.x PMID:9797490

Perechuda, K., & Kowalewski, M. (2008). *Zarządzanie komercyjną firmą medyczną*. Warszawa, CA: Wolters Kluwer.

Perry, J., Galloway, S., Bottorff, J. L., & Nixon, S. (2005). Nurse-patient communication in dementia: Improving the odds. *Journal of Gerontological Nursing*, *31*(4), 43–52. doi:10.3928/0098-9134-20050401-10 PMID:15839524

Peterson, C., Maier, S. F., & Seligman, M. E. P. (1996). *Learned Helplessness. A Theory for the Age of Personal Control*. Oxford: Oxford University Press.

Petticrew, M., Rehfuess, E., Noyes, J., Higgins, J. P. T., Mayhew, A., Pantoja, T., & Sowden, A. et al. (2013). Synthesizing evidence on complex interventions: How meta-analytical, qualitative, and mixed-method approaches can contribute. *Journal of Clinical Epidemiology*, *66*(11), 1230–1243. doi:10.1016/j.jclinepi.2013.06.005 PMID:23953082

Pezdek, K. (2010). Responsibility as a value in the work of physiotherapist. *Physiotherapy*, *18*(1), 72–77. doi:10.2478/v10109-010-0047-2

Piddington R.A. (2014). Health and diseases. In *The Limits of Mankind* (pp. 32-56).

Piegat, A. (1999). *Modelowanie i sterowanie rozmyte*. Warszawa: Akademicka Oficyna Wydawnicza EXIT.

Piercy, N., & Morgan, N. A. (1994). The marketing planning process: Behavioral problems compared to analytical techniques in explaining marketing plan credibility. *Journal of Business Research*, *29*(3), 167–168. doi:10.1016/0148-2963(94)90001-9

Piernas, C., & Popkin, B. M. (2011). Food portion patterns and trends among U.S. children and the relationship to total eating occasion size, 1977–2006. *The Journal of Nutrition*, *141*(6), 1159–1164. doi:10.3945/jn.111.138727 PMID:21525258

Pietrasiński, Z. (1990). *Rozwój człowieka dorosłego* [Development of an adult]. Warszawa: WP.

Pimental, P. A. (1986). Alterations in communication. Biopsychosocial aspects of aphasia, dysarthria, and right hemisphere syndromes in the stroke patient. *The Nursing Clinics of North America*, *21*(2), 321–337. PMID:3517820

Platonova, E. A., Kennedy, K. N., & Shewchuk, R. M. (2008). Understanding patient satisfaction, trust, and loyalty to primary care physicians. *Medical Care Research and Review*, *65*(6), 696–712. doi:10.1177/1077558708322863 PMID:18723450

Pledger, C. (2003). Discourse on disability and rehabilitation issues: Opportunities for psychology. *The American Psychologist*, *58*(4), 279–284. doi:10.1037/0003-066X.58.4.279 PMID:12866393

Plentara, R., Knyszyńska, A., Bażydło, M., Zabielska, P., Klim, A., Kotwas, A., . . . Karakiewicz, B. (2015). Satysfakcja pacjentów podstawowej opieki zdrowotnej z opieki medycznej i psychospołecznej [Patient satisfaction measure of the quality of primary health care]. *Pomeranian Journal of Life Sciences*, *61*(3), 335–340. Retrieved 08.05.2017 from https://www.pum.edu.pl/__data/assets/pdf_file/0014/111038/PomJLifeSci_61-03_335-340.pdf

Płużek, Z. (1997). Kryzysy psychologiczne i rodzaje kryzysów osobowościowych, [Psychological crises and types of personality crises]. In D. Kubacka-Jasiecka, & A. Lipowska–Teutsch (Eds.), Oblicza kryzysu psychologicznego i pracy interwencyjnej [Faces of the psychological crisis and intervention] (pp. 31-43). Kraków: Wyd. ALL.

Pommersbach, J. (1988). Wsparcie społeczne a choroba [Social support and illness]. *Przegląd Psychologiczny*, *31*(2), 503–525.

Popa, F., Arafat, R., Purcărea, V. L., Lală, A., Popa–Velea, O., & Bobirnac, G. (2010). Occupational burnout levels in emergency medicine – a stage 2 nationwide study and analysis. *Journal of Medicine and Life*, *3*(4), 449–453. PMID:21254747

Popa, F., & Arafat, R. (2010). Occupational Burnout levels in Emergency Medicine – a nationwide study and analysis. *Journal of Medicine and Life*, *3*(3), 207–215. PMID:20945809

Porter M.E. (2007). Competitive Strategy.

Potocki, A., Winkler, R., & Żbikowska, A. (2011). Komunikowanie w organizacjach gospodarczych. *Wydawnictwo Difin Warszawa,* 16-18.

Pound, P., & Ebrahim, S. (2000). Rhetoric and reality in stroke patient care. *Social Science & Medicine*, *51*(10), 1437–1446. doi:10.1016/S0277-9536(00)00040-X PMID:11077948

Powell, L. (2004). Patient satisfaction surveys for critical access hospitals. *National Rural Health Resource Center*, *1*, 26–45.

Prakash, B. (2010). Patient Satisfaction. *Journal of Cutaneous and Aesthetic Surgery*, *3*(3). Retrieved 02.05.2017 from ncbi.nlm.nih.gov/pcm/articles/PCM3047732

Prawelska-Skrzypek, G., & Lenartowicz, M. (2013). Badanie organizacji i zarządzania na gruncie humanistyki. *Problemy Zarządzania*, *11*(4), 45–57. doi:10.7172/1644-9584.44.4

Preuessner, J., Hellhammer, D., & Kirschbaum, C. (1999). Burnout, perceived stress, and cortisol responses to awakening. *Psychosomatic Medicine*, *61*(2), 197–204. doi:10.1097/00006842-199903000-00012 PMID:10204973

Preventing medication errors. Institute of Medicine, 2006

Pruessner, M., Boekestyn, L., Bèchard-Evans, L., Abadi, S., Vracotas, N., Joober, R., & Malla, A. et al. (2008). Sex differences in the cortisol response to awakening in recent onset psychosis. *Psychoneuroendocrinology*, *33*(8), 1151–1154. doi:10.1016/j.psyneuen.2008.04.006 PMID:18640785

Puchta, P. (2014). *Polish Healthcare System in Transition - Perceptions of the OLD and NEW Systems*. Dayton, Ohio: Wright State University.

Putnam, R. D. (1995). *Demokracja w działaniu*. Krakow, Warsaw: Znak Press, Batory Foundation.

Putnam, R. D. (2000). *Bowling Alone: The Collapse and Survival of American Community*. New York: Touchstone. doi:10.1145/358916.361990

Qu, H., Platonova, E., Kennedy, K. N., & Shewchuk, R. M. (2011). Primary care patient satisfaction segmentation. *International Journal of Health Care Quality Assurance*, *24*(7), 564–576. doi:10.1108/09526861111160599 PMID:22204089

Rabin, R. C. (2014). *15-Minute Visits Take A Toll On The Doctor-Patient Relationship*. Keiser Health News. Retrieved 07.05.2017 from http://khn.org/news/15-minute-doctor-visits/

Rahe, R. H., Mahan, J. L. Jr, & Arthur, R. J. (1970). Prediction of near-future health change from subjects' preceding life changes. *Journal of Psychosomatic Research*, *14*(4), 401–406. doi:10.1016/0022-3999(70)90008-5 PMID:5495261

Rahmqvist, M. (2001). Patient satisfaction in the relation to age, health status and background factors. A model for comparisons of care unit. *International Journal for Quality in Health Care*, *13*(5), 385–390. doi:10.1093/intqhc/13.5.385 PMID:11669566

Ramuszewicz, M., Krajewska-Kułak, E., Rolka, H., Łukaszuk, C., & Kułak, K. (2005). Problem of professional burnout among operative nurses. *Surgery Poland*, *VII*, 244–251.

Redo, K., & Bielawska-Batorowicz, E. (2014). Expectations towards medical personnel – a study with infertility clinic patients. *Health Psychology Review*, *2*(3), 218–226. doi:10.5114/hpr.2014.45197

Reetz-Wasielewska, A. E., Kretowicz, K., & Zarzeczna-Baran, M. (2016). Konflikt w zespole pielęgniarskim. *Problemy Pielęgniarstwa*, *24*(2), 125–130.

Regel, S. (2007). Post-trauma support in the workplace: The current status and practice of critical incident stress management (CISM) and psychological debriefing (PD) within organizations in the UK. *Occupational Medicine (Philadelphia, Pa.)*, *57*(6), 411–416. PMID:17728314

Reid, J., & Bromiley, M. (2012). Clinical human factors: The need to speak up to improve patient safety. *Nursing Standard*, *26*(35), 35–40. doi:10.7748/ns2012.05.26.35.35.c9084 PMID:22708165

Riddle, M. C., & Karl, D. M. (2012). Individualizing targets and tactics for high-risk patients with type 2 diabetes. Practical lessons from ACCORD and other cardiovascular trials. *Diabetes Care*, *35*(10), 2100–2107. doi:10.2337/dc12-0650 PMID:22996182

Rider, E. A., & Keefer, C. H. (2006). Communication skills competencies: Definitions and a teaching toolbox. *Medical Education*, *40*(7), 624–629. doi:10.1111/j.1365-2929.2006.02500.x PMID:16836534

Rittel, H. W. J., & Webber, M. M. (1973). Dilemmas in a general theory of planning. *Policy Sciences*, *4*(2), 155–169. doi:10.1007/BF01405730

Robbins, S. (2001). *Zasady zachowania w organizacji*. Poznań: Zysk i S-ka.

Roberts, A. R. (2005). Bridging the past and present to the future of crisis intervention and crisis management. In A. R. Roberts (Ed.), *Crisis intervention handbook: Assessment, treatment, and research* (3rd ed., pp. 3–34). New York: Oxford University Press.

Robin, H. (2008). Making sense of medical paternalism. *Medical Hypotheses, 70*(5), 910–913. doi:10.1016/j.mehy.2007.09.002 PMID:17959323

Rogoda, B. (2013). Zarządzanie konfliktem i przeciwdziałanie mobbingowi a intensyfikacja procesów innowacyjnych. *Nierówności Społeczne a Wzrost Gospodarczy, 46*(2), 289–301. doi:10.15584/nsawg.2016.2.16

Rogoziński, K. (2000). *Nowy marketing usług*. Poznań: Wydawnictwo Akademii Ekonomicznej.

Rohleder, N., Wolf, J., & Wolf, O. (2010). Glucocorticoid sensitivity of cognitive and inflammatory processes in depression and posttraumatic stress disorders. *Neuroscience and Biobehavioral Reviews, 35*(1), 104–114. doi:10.1016/j.neubiorev.2009.12.003 PMID:20005894

Rosenberg, C., E. (1998). Patologies of Progress: The Idea of Civilization as Risk. *Medicine & Health, 72*(4).

Rosiek A et al. (2015). A Comparison of Direct and Two-Stage Transportation of Patients to Hospital in Poland. IJERPH.

Roughead, E.E., & Semple, S. (2002). Second national report on patient safety: improving medication safety.

Rowe, A. K., de Savigny, D., Lanata, C. F., & Victora, C. G. (2005). How can we achieve and maintain high-quality performance of health workers in low-resource settings? *Lancet, 366*(9490), 1026–1035. doi:10.1016/S0140-6736(05)67028-6 PMID:16168785

Rozkwitalska, M. (2011). *Bariery w zarządzaniu międzykulturowym*. Warszawa: Wolters Kluwer Polska.

Rozwój zarządzania ryzykiem w medycynie (2017). Retrieved 01.03.2017 from http://www.madanes.pl

Ruhstaller, T., Roe, H., Thürlimann, B., & Nicoll, J. J. (2006). The multidisciplinary meeting: An indispensable aid to communication between different specialities. *European Journal of Cancer (Oxford, England), 42*(15), 2459–2462. doi:10.1016/j.ejca.2006.03.034 PMID:16934974

Rusin, M. (2012). Model bed modern physiotherapist. *Medical Rehabilitation, 16*(2), 34-46.

Rusin, M. (2013). *Attitude and ethical principles of physiotherapist*. Bielsko-Biała: WSA.

Rutter, H. R., Savona, N., Glonti, K., Cummins, S., Finegood, D., & Greaves, F. (2017). The need for a complex systems model of evidence for public health. *Lancet*. doi:10.1016/S0140-6736(17)31267-9 PMID:28622953

Ryff, C. D. (2014). Psychological well-being revisited: Advances in the science and practice of eudaimonia. *Psychotherapy and Psychosomatics, 83*(1), 10–28. doi:10.1159/000353263 PMID:24281296

Ryff, C. D., & Spencer, B. (2002). Ironies of the human condition: well-being and health on the way to mortlity. In L. G. Aspinwal & U. M. Staudinger (Eds.), *A psychology of human strengths: Fundamental questions and future directions for a positive psychology* (pp. 271–287). Washington, D.C.: American Psychological Association.

Rymaszewska, J., Kiejna, A., & Hadryś, A. (2003). Depression and anxiety in coronary artery by pass grafting patients. *European Psychologist, 18*(4), 155–160. doi:10.1016/S0924-9338(03)00052-X PMID:12814847

Rynekzdrowia.pl. (2009). Ile-minut-lekarz-powinien-rozmawiac-z-pacjentem. Retrieved 07.05.2017 from http://www.rynekzdrowia.pl/Uslugi-medyczne/Ile-minut-lekarz-powinien-rozmawiac-z-pacjentem,11641,8.html

Rzeźnik, M. (2011). *Zarządzanie komunikacją w zespole projektowym. Warszawa: Wydawnictwo PJWSTK.*

Safar, P. (1988). Resuscitation from clinical death: Pathophysiologic limits and therapeutic potentials. *Critical Care Medicine*, *16*(10), 923–941. doi:10.1097/00003246-198810000-00003 PMID:3048894

Sajid, A., & Ali, H. (n.d.). Impact of Process Improvement on Patient Satisfaction in Public Health Care Facility in Pakistan.

Salch, P., & Shapiro, C. (2008). Disturbed sleep and burnout: Implications for long-term health [editorial]. *Journal of Psychosomatic Research*, *65*(1), 1–3. doi:10.1016/j.jpsychores.2008.05.028 PMID:18582605

Sallis, J. F., & Glanz, K. (2009). Physical activity and food environments: Solutions to the obesity epidemic. *The Milbank Quarterly*, *87*(1), 123–154. doi:10.1111/j.1468-0009.2009.00550.x PMID:19298418

Salovey, P., & Birnbaum, D. (1989). Influence of mood on health-relevant cognitions. *Journal of Personality and Social Psychology*, *57*(3), 539–551. doi:10.1037/0022-3514.57.3.539 PMID:2778638

Salovey, P., Detweiler, J. B., Steward, W. T., & Bedell, B. T. (2001). Affect and health-relevant cognition. In J. Forgas (Ed.), *Handbook of Affect and Social Cognition* (pp. 344–370). Mahwah, NJ: Lawrence Erlbaum and Associates.

Sandoval, G. A., Brown, A. D., Sullivan, T., & Green, E. (2006). Factor that influence cancer patients; overall perception of the quality of care. *International Journal for Quality in Health Care*, *18*(4), 266–274. doi:10.1093/intqhc/mzl014 PMID:16809400

Sarason, I. G., & Sarason, B. R. (1982). Concomitants of social support: Attitudes, personality characteristics, and life experiences. *Journal of Personality*, *50*(3), 331–344. doi:10.1111/j.1467-6494.1982.tb00754.x PMID:7143186

Schaufeli, W., & Enzmann, D. (1998). *The burnout companion to study and practice: A Critical Analysis*. London: Taylor & Francis.

Scheffert, D. R., Hornvedt, J., & Chazdon, S. (2008). *Social Capital and Our Community*. Minnesota: University of Minnesota Press.

Scholl, J. C., Wilson, J. B., & Hughs, P. C. (2011). Expression of patients' and providers' identities during the medical interview. *Qualitative Health Research*, *21*(8), 1022–1032. doi:10.1177/1049732310393748 PMID:21263064

Schwarzer, R., & Luszczynska, A. (2015). Health Action Process Approach. In M. Conner & P. Norman (Eds.), *Predicting health behaviours* (3rd ed., pp. 252–278). Maidenhead, UK: McGraw Hill Open University Press.

Seccareccia, D., Wentlandt, K., Kevork, N., Workentin, K., Blacker, S., Gagliese, L., & Zimmermann, C. et al. (2015). Communication and Quality of Care on Palliative Care Units: A Qualitative Study. *Journal of Palliative Medicine*, *18*(9), 758–764. doi:10.1089/jpm.2014.0408 PMID:26069934

Sędek, G. (1991). Jak ludzie radzą sobie z sytuacjami, na które nie ma rady? [How do people deal with situations that are not solved?]. In M. Kofta & T. Szustrowa (Eds.), Złudzenia, które pozwalają żyć [Illusions that allow you to live] (pp. 226-248). Warszawa: Wydawnictwo Naukowe PWN.

Segal, S. (2012). Saving patients from Internet health information. Retrieved from: http://www.kevinmd.com/blog/2012/02/saving-patients-internet-health-information.html

Sęk, H., & Cieślak, R. (2004). Wsparcie społeczne - sposoby definiowania, rodzaje i źródła wsparcia, wybrane koncepcje teoretyczne [Social Support - Ways to Defining, Types and Sources of Support, Selected Theoretical Concepts]. In H. Sęk & R. Cieślak (Eds.), Wsparcie społeczne, stres i zdrowie [Social Support, Stress, Health] (pp. 11-28).Warszawa: Wydawnictwo Naukowe PWN.

Sęk, H. (2012). *Professional burnout. Reasons and prevention*. Warsaw: PWN.

Sęk, H., & Cieślak, R. (2005). *Wsparcie społeczne, stres i zdrowie (Social Support, Stress and Health)*. Warsaw: PWN.

Sekhri, N. K. (2000). Managed care: The US experience. *Bulletin of the World Health Organization*, 830–844. PMID:10916920

Seligman, M. (1995). *Optymizmu można się nauczyć (Optimism Can Be Learned)*. Poznan: Media Rodzina.

Seligman, M. E. P. (1975). *Helplessness: on depression, development, and death*. San Franciso: Freeman.

Seligman, M. E. P., & Maier, S. (1967). Failure to escape traumatic shock. *Journal of Experimental Psychology*, *74*(1), 1–9. doi:10.1037/h0024514 PMID:6032570

Seligman, M. E. P., Steen, T. A., Park, N., & Peterson, C. (2005). Positive Psychology Progress: Empirical Validation of Interventions. *The American Psychologist*, *60*(5), 410–421. doi:10.1037/0003-066X.60.5.410 PMID:16045394

Semuel, H., Siagian, H., & Octavia, S. (2017, February). The Effect of Leadership and Innovation on Differentiation Strategy and Company Performance. *Procedia: Social and Behavioral Sciences*, *237*(21), 1152–1159. doi:10.1016/j.sbspro.2017.02.171

Sertoz, O., Binbay, I., Koylu, E., & Noyan, A. (2008). The role of BDNF and HPA axis in the neurobiology of burnout syndrome. *Progress in Neuro-Psychopharmacology & Biological Psychiatry*, *32*(6), 1459–1465. doi:10.1016/j.pnpbp.2008.05.001 PMID:18541357

Service quality and customer satisfaction. (1994). Customer based definitions for Quality: Value based definitions for Quality (Ch. 4, 109–133).

Shannon, C. (1948). A Mathematical Theory of Communication. *The Bell System Technical Journal*, *27*(3), 379–423, 623–656. doi:10.1002/j.1538-7305.1948.tb01338.x

Shortliffe, E. H. (1986). *Medical Expert Systems—Knowledge Tools for Physicians,* Western Journal of Medicine, *145*(6). Retrieved 06.05.2017 from https://www.ncbi.nlm.nih.gov/pmc/articles/PMC1307157/

Shu-Hsien, L. (2004). Expert system methodologies and applications—a decade review from 1995 to 2004. In *Expert Systems with Applications*. Retrieved 19.09.2012 from http://www.dca.fee.unicamp.br/~gomide/courses/EA072/artigos/ExpertSystemMethodologiesApplicationsReview1995to2004Liao2004.pdf

Shusaku, T., & Hiroshi, T. (1996). Automated Discovery of Medical Expert System Rules from Clinical Databases based on Rough Sets. In *Proceedings of KDD '96*. Retrieved 06.05.2017 from http://www.aaai.org/Papers/KDD/1996/KDD96-011.pdf

Siemiński, M., Nitka-Siemińska, A., & Nyka, W. (2007). Zespół wypalenia. *Centrum Medycyny Rodzinnej*, *1*(1), 45–49.

Silberfein, E. J., Zhou, W., Kougias, P., El Sayed, H. F., Huynh, T. T., Albo, D., & Lin, P. H. et al. (2007). Percutaneous cholecystostomy for acute cholecystitis in high-risk patients: Experience of a surgeon-initiated interventional program. *American Journal of Surgery*, *194*(5), 672–677. doi:10.1016/j.amjsurg.2007.07.019 PMID:17936433

Simon, H., & Dietl, M. (2007). *Tajemniczy mistrzowie XXI wieku. Strategie sukcesu nieznanych liderów na światowych rynkach*. Warszawa, CA: Difin.

Sirota, R. L. (2000, November). The Institute of Medicine's report on medical error. Implications for pathology. *Archives of Pathology & Laboratory Medicine*, *124*(11), 1674–1678. PMID:11079023

Slort, W., Blankenstein, A. H., Deliens, L., & van der Horst, H. E. (2011). Facilitators and barriers for GP-patient communication in palliative care: A qualitative study among GPs, patients, and end-of-life consultants. *The British Journal of General Practice*, *61*(585), 167–172. doi:10.3399/bjgp11X567081 PMID:21439174

Śmiatacz, K., Michalska, A., & Samek, K. (2014). Rola komunikacji w unikaniu błędów menedżerskich. *Marketing i Rynek, 10*, 484–489.

Smith, R. (2001). Why are doctors so unhappy? *British Medical Journal, 322*(7294), 1073–1074. doi:10.1136/bmj.322.7294.1073 PMID:11337419

Sniehotta, F. F., Schwarzer, R., Scholz, U., & Schüz, B. (2005). Action planning and coping planning for long-term lifestyle change: Theory and assessment. *European Journal of Social Psychology, 35*(4), 565–576. doi:10.1002/ejsp.258

Snyder, C. R. (1994). *The Psychology of Hope: You Can Get There from Here*. New York: The Free Press.

Snyder, M., Stephan, W., & Rosenfield, D. (1976). Egotism and attribution. *Journal of Personality and Social Psychology, 33*(4), 435–441. doi:10.1037/0022-3514.33.4.435 PMID:1271219

Sobkowiak, B. (1998). Procesy komunikowania się w organizacji. In B. Dobek-Ostrowska (Ed.), *Współczesne systemy komunikowania* (pp. 22–40). Wrocław: Wyd. UW.

Spetz, J., & Keane, D. (2009). Information technology implementation in a rural hospital: A cautionary tale. *Health Management, 54*, 337–347, discussion 348. PMID:19831118

Stanford Encyclopedia of Philosophy. (n.d.). Logic classical. Retrieved 25.04.2017 from https://plato.stanford.edu/entries/logic-classical/

Staniec, K. Klimczak, M. (2008). Panorama ryzyka. W: I.Staniec& J. Zawiła-Niedźwiecki (red.), *Zarządzanie ryzykiem operacyjnym.* Warszawa, CA: C.H. Beck.

Stanisz-Busch, E. (2010). *Podstawy zarządzania marketingowego w placówce Medycznej*. Poznań: Wolters Kluwer.

Stankiewicz, J. (1999). *Komunikowanie się w organizacji*. Wrocław: Wyd. Astrum.

Starosta, P., & Frykowski, M. (2008). Typy kapitału społecznego i wzory partycypacji obywatelskiej w wiejskich gminach centralnej Polski (Types of social capital and models of the civic participation in the rural communities of central Polish). In M. S. Szczepański, K. Bierwiaczonek, & T. Nawrocki (Eds.), *Kapitały ludzkie i społeczne a konkurencyjność regionów [Human and social capitals vs. region's competitiveness]*. Katowice: Silesian University Press.

Steg, P. G., James, S. K., Atar, D., Badano, L. P., Blomstrom-Lundqvist, C., & Borger, M. A. et al.. (2012). ESC Guidelines for the management of acute mycocardial infraction in patients presenting with ST-segment elevation. *European Heart Journal, 33*(20), 2569–2619. doi:10.1093/eurheartj/ehs215 PMID:22922416

Stein, K. V. (2016). *Integrated Care around the world. Examples to help improve (primary) health care in Poland.* Warszawa: Narodowy Fundusz Zdrowia – Centrala Departament Analiz i Strategii.

Stewart, J. (2010). *Mosty zamiast murów. Podręcznik komunikacji interpersonalnej*. Warszawa: Wydawnictwo Naukowe PWN.

Stille, C. J., Mazor, K. M., Meterko, V., & Wasserman, R. C. (2011). Development and validation of a tool to improve paediatric referral/consultation communication. *BMJ Quality & Safety, 20*(8), 692–697. doi:10.1136/bmjqs.2010.045781 PMID:21339312

Stille, C. J., McLaughlin, T. J., Primack, W. A., Mazor, K. M., & Wasserman, R. C. (2006). Determinants and impact of generalist specialist communication about pediatric outpatient referrals. *Pediatrics, 118*(4), 1341–1349. doi:10.1542/peds.2005-3010 PMID:17015522

Stone, W., & Hughes, J. (2002) Social Capital: Empirical Meaning and Measurement Validity (Research Paper 27). Australian Institute of Family Studies, Melbourne.

Stone, J. (2009). Cultural considerations in disability and rehabilitation. *Disability and Rehabilitation*, *31*(14), 1109–1110. doi:10.1080/09638280902773679 PMID:19479534

Straburzyńska-Lupa,A.Straburzyński,G. (2007). *Physiotherapy*. PZWL.

Strawbridge, W. J., Cohen, R. D., Shema, S. J., & Kaplan, G. A. (1997). Frequent attendance at religious services and mortality: A 28-year follow-up. *American Journal of Public Health*, *87*(6), 957–961. doi:10.2105/AJPH.87.6.957 PMID:9224176

Street, R. L. Jr, Makoul, G., Arora, N. K., & Epstein, R. M. (2009). How does communication heal? Pathways linking clinician–patient communication to health outcomes. *Patient Education and Counseling*, *74*(3), 295–301. doi:10.1016/j.pec.2008.11.015 PMID:19150199

Strelau, J. (2000). Temperament. [Temperament] In J. Strelau (Ed.), *Psychologia. Podręcznik akademicki* [Psychology. Academic manual] (Vol. 1, pp. 683–719). Gdańsk: Gdańskie Wydawnictwo Psycholgiczne.

Stychlerz, A. (2008). Dyplom to nie wszystko. *Magazyn Pielęgniarki i Położnej*, *1-2*, 15.

Suddick, K. M., & De Souza, L. (2006). Therapists' experiences and perceptions of teamwork in neurological rehabilitation: Reasoning behind the team approach, structure and composition of the team and teamworking processes. *Physiotherapy Research International*, *11*(2), 72–83. doi:10.1002/pri.325 PMID:16808088

Sulch, D., Melbourn, A., Perez, I., & Kalra, L. (2002). Integrated care pathways and quality of life on a stroke rehabilitation unit. *Stroke*, *33*(6), 1600–1604. doi:10.1161/01.STR.0000017144.04043.87 PMID:12052998

Sundquist, J., & Johannsson, S. E. (2000). High demand, low control, and impaired general health: Working conditions in a sample of Swedish general practitioners. *Scandinavian Journal of Public Health*, *28*(2), 123–131. doi:10.1177/140349480002800208 PMID:10954139

Suresh, S., Kodikal, R., & Kar, S. (2015). Measuring job satisfaction and impact of demographic characteristics among Doctors of Teaching Hospitals. *International Multispecialty Journal of Health*, *1*(9). Retrieved from http://www.imjhealth.org/admin/issues_detail/gallery/IMJH-NOV-2015-5.pdf

Surman, G., Lambert, T. W., & Goldacre, M. (2016). Doctors' enjoyment of their work and satisfaction with time available for leisure: UK time trend questionnaire-based study. *Postgraduate Medical Journal*. doi:10.1136/postgradmedj-2015-133743

Sutton, S. (2005). Stage models of health behaviour. In M. Conner & P. Norman (Eds.), *Predicting health behaviour: Research and practice with social cognition models* (2nd ed., pp. 223–275). Maidenhead, England: Open University Press.

Świątek, W. (2016). Rola lidera w innowacyjnej organizacji. *Zarządzanie Zasobami Ludzkimi*, *1*, 9–23.

Syrkiewicz, O., Ewitała, M., Holecki, T., & Kotowski, P. (2012). Koncepcja marketingowego zarządzania organizacją świadczącą usługi medyczne. *Zarządzanie i Edukacja*, *82*.

Szary, S., & Knotowicz, J. (2014). Different aspects of holism in medicine and physiotherapy. In Fizjoterapia wobec nowych wyzwań (pp. 7-17). Poznań: Wydawnictwo WSEiT.

Szary, S. (2013). Nowoczesna medycyna w służbie człowiekowi. *Hygeia Public Health*, *48*(1), 17–20.

Szelènyi, J., & Vizi, S. (2007). The catecholamine-cytokine balance interaction between brain and the immune system. *Annals of the New York Academy of Sciences*, *1113*(1), 311–324. doi:10.1196/annals.1391.026 PMID:17584982

Szmaus-Jackowska, A. (2011). *Troska o siebie osób w starszym wieku* [Caring for oneself in old age]. Bydgoszcz: Wydawnictwo Uniwersytetu Kazimierza Wielkiego.

Szreter, S., & Woolcock, M. (2004). Health by association? Social capital, social theory, and the political economy of public health. *International Journal of Epidemiology*, *33*(4), 650–667. doi:10.1093/ije/dyh013 PMID:15282219

Sztompka, P. (2002) Integracja europejska jako szansa kulturowa. O moralności, tożsamości, zaufaniu [European Integration as a Cultural Opportunity. On Morality, Identity and Trust]. Nauka, 2, 59–66.

Sztompka, P. (2007). *Zaufanie. Fundament społeczeństwa [Trust. The Cornerstone of Society]*. Krakow: Znak Press.

Targosz-Krysik, B. (1997). *Urzeczywistnienie zasad demokratycznych w uczącej się organizacji*. Edukacja Dorosłych.

Tempest, S., & McIntyre, A. (2006). Using the ICF to clarify team roles and demonstrate clinical reasoning in stroke rehabilitation. *Disability and Rehabilitation*, *28*(10), 663–667. doi:10.1080/09638280500276992 PMID:16690581

Terkelsen, C. J., Lassen, J. F., Norgaard, B. L., Gerdes, J. C., Poulsen, S. H., Bendix, K., & Andersen, H. R. et al. (2005). Reduction of treatment delay in patients with ST-elevation myocardial infarction: Impact of pre-hospital diagnosis and direct referral to primary percutaneous coronary intervention. *European Heart Journal*, *26*(8), 770–777. doi:10.1093/eurheartj/ehi100 PMID:15684279

Teutsch, C. (2003, September). Patient-doctor communication. *The Medical Clinics of North America*, *87*(5), 1115–1145. doi:10.1016/S0025-7125(03)00066-X PMID:14621334

The Act of 6 November 2008 on Accreditation in Health Care (Journal of Laws No. 2016.2135).

The National Program. (n.d.). Educational Program—Treatment to Reduce Frequencies. The Prevalence of Overweight and Obesity in Children and Adolescents. Retrieved 6 August 2015 from http://wsd.org.pl/Ogloszenia/

The Scottish Doctor. (2011). *Outcomes for Communication*. Retrieved 20.04.2017 from http://www.scottishdoctor.org/node.asp?id=0501010000

Theiss, M. (2007). *Krewni – Znajomi – Obywatele. Kapitał społeczny a lokalna polityka społeczna [Relatives – Friends – Citizens. Social Capital and the Local Policy]*. Torun: Adam Marszałek Press.

Tobiasz-Adamczyk, B. (2002). Relacje lekarz-pacjent w perspektywie socjologii medycyny, Wyd. *UJ Kraków*, *19*, 81–85.

Tobin, C. (1997) What is managed health care? Retrieved from https://nfb.org/images/nfb/publications/vodold/mngdcare.htm

Tomaszewska M. (2008). Możliwości doskonalenia zawodowego pielęgniarek – potrzeby a rzeczywistość. *Problemy pielęgniarstwa*, *16*(1-2).

Tops, M., Boksem, M., Wijers, A., van Duinen, H., Den Boer, J., Meijman, T., & Korf, J. (2007). The psychobiology of burnout: Are the two different syndromes? *Neuropsychobiology*, *55*(3-4), 143–150. doi:10.1159/000106056 PMID:17641533

Trela, A. (2016). Zarządzanie jakością w działalności leczniczej. Warszawa, CA: Wiedza i Praktyka.

Trempała, J. (Ed.) (2011). Psychologia rozwoju człowieka [Psychology of human development]. Warszawa: Wydawnictwo Naukowe PWN.

Trenner M., Haller B., Storck M., Reutersberg B., Kallmayer M.A., Eckstein H.-H. Trends in Patient Safety of Intact Abdominal Aortic Aneurysm Repair: German Registry Data on 36,594 Procedures. *European Journal of Vascular and Endovascular Surgery, Available online 19 January 2017*

Trippner-Hrabi, J. (2014). Etapy rozwoju zespołów zadaniowych w organizacjach. *Przedsiębiorczość i Zarządzanie, 15*(6), 189–2001.

Truog, R. D., Meyer, E. C., & Burns, J. P. (2006). Toward interventions to improve end-of-life care in the pediatric intensive care unit. *Critical Care Medicine, 34*(11 Suppl.), S373–S379. doi:10.1097/01.CCM.0000237043.70264.87 PMID:17057601

Tsao, K. J., & Browne, M.Tsao KuoJen. (2015, December). Browne Marybeth. Culture of safety: A Foundation for patient care. *Seminars in Pediatric Surgery, 24*(6), 283–287. doi:10.1053/j.sempedsurg.2015.08.005 PMID:26653161

Tsou, A. Y., Creutzfeldt, C. J., & Gordon, J. M. (2013). Chapter 9- The good doctor: Professionalism In the 21 st century. *Handbook of Clinical Neurology, 118*, 119–132. doi:10.1016/B978-0-444-53501-6.00009-3 PMID:24182371

Tvp.info. (2015). 90 pacjentów w siedem godzin. „Średni czas wizyty to 4,5 minuty. Retrieved 08.05.2017 from https://www.tvp.info/18329897/90-pacjentow-w-siedem-godzin-sredni-czas-wizyty-to-45-minuty

Ulrey, K. L., & Amason, P. (2001). Intercultural communication between patients and health care providers: An exploration of intercultural communication effectiveness, cultural sensitivity, stress, and anxiety. *Health Communication, 13*(4), 449–463. doi:10.1207/S15327027HC1304_06 PMID:11771806

US Joint Commission. (1998). Patient safety incident Events: Approaches to error reduction and prevention. *Journal Quality Improvement, 11*(6), 290–294.

Vadhana, M. (2012). assessment of patient satisfaction in an outpatient department of an autonomous hospital in Phnom Penh, Cambodia [Thesis]. *Public Health Management*, (September).

Vahdat, S., Hamzehgardeshi, L., Hessam, S., & Hamzehgardeshi, Z. (2014). Patient Involvement in Health Care Decision Making: A Review. *Iranian Red Crescent Medical Journal, 16*(1), e12454. doi:10.5812/ircmj.12454 PMID:24719703

van den Brink-Muinen A, van Dulmen SM, de Haes HC, Visser AP, Schellevis FG, Bensing

van den Brink-Muinen, A., van Dulmen, S. M., de Haes, H. C. J. M., Visser, A. P., Schellevis, F. G., & Bensing, J. M. (2006). Has patients' involvement in the decision-making process changed over time? *Health Expectations, 9*(4), 333–342. doi:10.1111/j.1369-7625.2006.00413.x PMID:17083560

Van Gerven, E., Deweer, D., Scott, S. D., Panella, M., Euwema, M., Sermeus, W., & Vanhaecht, K. (2016, July). Personal, situational and organizational aspects that influence the impact of patient safety incidents: A qualitative study. *Revista de Calidad Asistencial, 31*(Suppl. 2), 34–46. doi:10.1016/j.cali.2016.02.003 PMID:27106771

van Woerkum, C. M. (2003). The Internet and primary care physicians: Coping with different expectations. *The American Journal of Clinical Nutrition, 77*(4 Suppl.), 1016S–1018S. PMID:12663310

Van, K. A., Nogueira, L., Gustafson, D., Tieu, W., Averch, T. D., & Kim, F. J. (2016, October). The Culture of Patient Safety Practice: Systematic Review. *Urology Practice*, 22.

Vanltallie, T. (2002). Stress: A risk factor for serious illness. *Metabolism: Clinical and Experimental, 51*(6 Suppl. 1), 40–45. doi:10.1053/meta.2002.33191 PMID:12040540

Voelker, R. (1995). Speaking the languages of medicine and culture. *Journal of the American Medical Association, 273*(21), 1639–1641. doi:10.1001/jama.1995.03520450007003 PMID:7752395

Vogelzangs, N., Beekman, A., Milaneschi, Y., Bandinelli, S., Ferrucci, L., & Penninx, B. W. J. H. (2010). Urinary cortisol and six-year risk of all-cause and cardiovascular mortality. *The Journal of Clinical Endocrinology and Metabolism, 95*(11), 4959–4964. doi:10.1210/jc.2010-0192 PMID:20739384

Vogus, T., & McClelland, L. (2016). When the customer is the patient: Lessons from healthcare research on patient satisfaction and service quality ratings. *Human Resource Management Review, 26*(1), 37–49. doi:10.1016/j.hrmr.2015.09.005

von Bertalanffy, K.L. (1952). Problems of Life: An Evaluation of Modern Biological and Scientific Thought. New York: Harper.

von Känel, R., Bellingrath, S., & Kudielka, B. (2008). Association between burnout and circulating levels of pro- and anti-inflammatory cytokines in schoolteachers. *Journal of Psychosomatic Research, 65*(1), 51–59. doi:10.1016/j.jpsychores.2008.02.007 PMID:18582612

Vujicic, M., & Zurn, P. (2006). The dynamics of the health labour market. *The International Journal of Health Planning and Management, 21*(2), 101–115. doi:10.1002/hpm.834 PMID:16846103

Wagner Edward H. The role of patient care teams in chronic disease management. British Medical Journal 320.7234:569.

Wahlberg, K., Ghatan, P., Modell, S., Nygren, A., Ingvar, M., Åsberg, M., & Heiling, M. (2009). Suppressed neuroendocrine stress response in depressed women on job-stress related long-term sick-leave: A stable marker potentially suggestive of pre-existing vulnerability. *Biological Psychiatry, 65*(9), 742–747. doi:10.1016/j.biopsych.2008.10.035 PMID:19058782

Wald, H. S., Dube, C. E., & Anthony, D. C. (2007). Untangling the Web – The Impact of Internet Use on Health Care and the Physician-Patient Relationship. *Patient Education and Counseling, 68*(3), 218–224. doi:10.1016/j.pec.2007.05.016 PMID:17920226

Wallace, P. (2001). Improving palliative care through effective communication. *International Journal of Palliative Nursing, 7*(2), 86–90. doi:10.12968/ijpn.2001.7.2.8919 PMID:12271254

Walton, R. E., & Dutton, J. M. (1969). The management of interdepartmental conflict: A model and review. *Administrative Science Quarterly, 14*(1), 73–84. doi:10.2307/2391364

Wang, H.-J., Demerouti, E., & Le Blanc, P. (2017). Transformational leadership, adaptability and job crafting: The moderating role of organizational identification. *Journal of Vocational Behavior, 100*(June), 185–195. doi:10.1016/j.jvb.2017.03.009

Waszkiewicz, P. (2009). Zasady mediacji. In E. Gmurzyńska & R. Morka (Ed.), *Mediacje. Teorie i praktyka* (pp. 91-105). Warszawa: Oficyna a Wolters Kluwer business.

Wciórka, J. (2010). Psychopatologia: objawy i zespoły zaburzeń psychicznych. In J. Rybakowski, S. Pużyński, & J. Wciórka (Eds.), *Psychiatria. T.1.Podstawy psychiatrii* (pp. 305–398). Wrocław: Elsevier Urban & Partner.

Wciórka, J., Pużyński, S., & Rybakowski, J. (Eds.). (2012). *Psychiatria. T.3. In Metody leczenia. Zagadnienia etyczne, prawne, publiczne, społeczne* (pp. 385–405). Wrocław: Elsevier Urban & Partner.

Weiner, J. S., & Cole, S. A. (2004). Three principles to improve clinician communication for advance care planning: Overcoming emotional, cognitive, and skill barriers. *Journal of Palliative Medicine, 7*(6), 817–829. doi:10.1089/jpm.2004.7.817 PMID:15684849

Weiss Gary, B. (1985). Paternalism modernized. *Journal of Medical Ethics, 11*(4), 184–187. doi:10.1136/jme.11.4.184 PMID:4078856

Werachowska, L., Damps-Konstańska, I., Janowicz, A., & Krakowiak, P. (2013). Medical caregiver as a new member of the therapeutic team for chronic ill and elderly patients. *Problemy Pielęgniarstwa*, *21*(2), 235–241.

White, B. (1999). Measuring Patient Satisfaction: How to Do It and Why to Bother. *Family Practice Management.* Retrieved 08.05.2017 from http://www.aafp.org/fpm/1999/0100/p40.html

WHO. (1994, March 28–30). A Declaration on the Promotion Rights of Patients in Europe, European Consultation on the Rights of Patients. Retrieved from http://www.who.int/genomics/public/eu_declaration1994.pdf?ua=1

WHO. (n.d.). World Alliance for patient safety. Retrieved from http://www.who.int/patientsafety/worldalliance/alliance/en/

Wiedemann, A. U., Lippke, S., Reuter, T., Ziegelmann, J. P., & Schwarzer, R. (2011). How planning facilitates behaviour change: Additive and interactive effects of a randomized controlled trial. *European Journal of Social Psychology*, *41*(1), 42–51. doi:10.1002/ejsp.724

Wijndaele, K., Brage, S., Besson, H., Khaw, K. T., Sharp, S. J., Luben, R., & Ekelund, U. et al. (2010). Increased cardiometabolic risk is associated with increased TV viewing time. *Medicine and Science in Sports and Exercise*, *42*(8), 1511–1518. doi:10.1249/MSS.0b013e3181d322ac PMID:20139784

Williams, S. L., Haskard, K. B., & DiMatteo, M. R. (2007). The therapeutic effects of the physician-older patient relationship: Effective communication with vulnerable older patients. *Clinical Interventions in Aging*, *2*(3), 453. PMID:18044195

Wilski, M., & Sienkiewicz-Wilowska, J. A. (2014). Social support as regulator of self-care attitude in persons with myocardial infraction. *Polish Psychological Bulletin*, *45*(4), 521–532. doi:10.2478/ppb-2014-0062

Wirtz, P., Ehlert, U., Emini, L., & Suter, T. (2008). Higher body mass index (BMI) is associated with reduced glucocorticoid inhibition of inflammatory cytokine production following acute psychosocial stress in men. *Psychoneuroendocrinology*, *33*(8), 1102–1110. doi:10.1016/j.psyneuen.2008.05.002 PMID:18644679

Włodarczak, W. (2009). Pielęgniarstwo w Polsce i na świecie. Kompendium wiedzy dla studentów pielęgniarstwa. In *Państwowa Wyższa Szkoła Zawodowa im. Stanisława Staszica w Pile.* Wyd. Tekst Bydgoszcz.

Wojciech, K., Sławomir, C., & Stefan, H. (n.d.). Oczekiwania pacjentów hospitalizowanych na oddziałach zabiegowych wobec personelu pielęgniarskiego. *Pielęgniarstwo Chirurgiczne i Angiologiczne*, *208*(1), 12-18.

Wolf, Z. R., & Hughes, R. G. (2008). Error Reporting and Disclosure. In R.G. Hughes (Eds.), *Patient Safety and Quality: An Evidence-Based Handbook for Nurses* (Ch. 35). Retrieved from: https://www.ncbi.nlm.nih.gov/books/NBK2652/

Wolniak, R. (2012). *Wymiary kulturowe polskich organizacji a doskonalenie zarządzanie jakością.* Warszawa: Ce-DeWu.

Woolcock, M. (2001). The Place of Social Capital in Understanding Social and Economic Outcomes. *Canadian Journal of Policy Research*, *2*(1), 11–17.

Woolock, M. (1998). Social Capital and Economic Development: Toward and Theoretical Syntesis and Policy Framework. *Theory and Society*, *27*(2), 151–208. doi:10.1023/A:1006884930135

World Alliance for Patient Safety. (2004, October 27). The Launch of the World Alliance for Patient Safety.

World Alliance for Patient Safety. (2008). WHO surgical safety checklist and implementation manual.

World Health Organisation. (2006). London Declaration: Patients for Patient Safety. Retrieved from http://www.who.int/patientsafety/patients_for_patient/London_ Declaration_EN.pdf

World Health Organization. (2006). The world health report: 2006: working together for health. *World Health Organization.* Retrieved from http://www.who.int/whr/2006/en/

World Health Organization. (2007). Strengthening health systems to improve health outcomes.

Wrońska, I., & Krajewska-Kułak, E. (2007). Selected issues in European nursing. Czelej, Lublin.

Wrześniewski, K., & Włodarczyk, D. (2004). Rola wsparcia społecznego w leczeniu i rehabilitacji osób po zawale serca. [Role of Social Support in Treatment and Rehabilitation of Persons After Heart Failure] In H. Sęk & R. Cieślak (Eds.), *Wsparcie społeczne, stres i zdrowie* [Social Support, Stress, Health]. (pp. 170–189). Warszawa: Wydawnictwo Naukowe PWN.

Wu, H., Zhao, X., Fritzsche, K., Leonhart, R., Schaefert, R., Sun, X., & Larisch, A. (2015). Quality of doctor-patient relationship in patient with high somatic symptom severity in China. *Complementary Therapies in Medicine, 23*(1), 23–31. doi:10.1016/j.ctim.2014.12.006 PMID:25637149

Wutzke, S., Morrice, E., Benton, M., & Wilson, A. (2016). Systems approaches for chronic disease prevention: Sound logic and empirical evidence, but is this view shared outside of academia? *Public Health Research & Practice, 26*(3), e2631632. doi:10.17061/phrp2631632 PMID:27421344

Xu, W., Zhao, Y., Guo, L., Guo, Y., & Gao, W. (2009). Job stress and coronary heart disease: A case-control study using a Chinese population. *Journal of Occupational Health, 51*(2), 107–113. doi:10.1539/joh.L8060 PMID:19179802

Yagil, D., Biron, M., Pat, D., Mirzahi-Reuveni, M., & Zoller, L. (2015). Accurate diagnosis of patient's distress levels: The effect of family physicians' ability to take the patient's perspective. *Patient Education and Counseling, 98*(12), 1631–1635. doi:10.1016/j.pec.2015.07.008 PMID:26215572

Yami, A., Hamza, L., Hassen, A., Jira, C., & Sudhakar, M. (2011). Job satisfaction and its determinants among health workers in Jimma University specialized hospital, southwest Ethiopia. Ethiopian journal of health sciences, 21(3). PMID:22435005

Yellowlees, P. M., Chorba, K., Burke Parish, M., Wynn-Jones, H., & Nafiz, N. (2010). Telemedicine can make healthcare greener. *Telemedicine Journal and e-Health, 16*(2), 229–232. doi:10.1089/tmj.2009.0105 PMID:20156125

Yoshiaki, N. S. K., Onoda, K., Hamano, T., & Kimura, K. (2015). Job and life satisfaction and preference of future practice locations of physicians on remote islands in Japan. *Human Resources for Health, 13*(1), 39. doi:10.1186/s12960-015-0029-z PMID:26008624

Yoshikawa, R. (1997). Hyperactivity at 18 months of age and attention-deficit hyperactivity disorder before entry to school - follow up study from 18 months to 6 years. *Seishin Shinkeigaku Zasshi. Psychiatria et Neurologia Japonica, 99*(2), 47–67. PMID:9086845

Young, L. R., & Nestle, M. (2002). The contribution of expanding portion sizes to the U.S. obesity epidemic. *American Journal of Public Health, 92*(2), 246–249. doi:10.2105/AJPH.92.2.246 PMID:11818300

Young, L. R., & Nestle, M. (2003). Expanding portion sizes in the U.S. marketplace: Implications for nutrition counseling. *Journal of the American Dietetic Association, 103*(2), 231–234. doi:10.1053/jada.2003.50027 PMID:12589331

Zadeh, L. A. (1965). Fuzzy sets. *Information and Control, 8*(3), 338–353. doi:10.1016/S0019-9958(65)90241-X

Zakariasen Kenneth, L. (2006, Summer). The importance of process in building an executive leadership team: A case study. *Healthcare Management Forum, 19*(2), 6–10. doi:10.1016/S0840-4704(10)60816-2 PMID:17017759

Założenia do projektu ustawy o jakości w ochronie zdrowia i bezpieczeństwie pacjentów. (n.d.). Project of 20 January 2017. Retrieved 21.01.2017 from http://www.legislacja.rcl.gov.pl

Zandbelt, L. C., Smets, E., Oort, F. J., Godfried, M. H., & Haes, H. C. J. M. (2004). Satisfaction with the outpatient encounter. *Journal of General Internal Medicine, 19*(11), 1088–1095. doi:10.1111/j.1525-1497.2004.30420.x PMID:15566437

Zayas, V., & Hazan, C. (Eds.). (2015). *Bases of Adult Attachment: Linking Brain, Mind and Behavior.* New York: Springer. doi:10.1007/978-1-4614-9622-9

Zizza, C., Siega-Riz, A. M., & Popkin, B. M. (2001). Significant increase in young adults' snacking between 1977–1978 and 1994–1996 represents a cause for concern! *Preventive Medicine, 32*(4), 303–310. doi:10.1006/pmed.2000.0817 PMID:11304090

Żuchowski, I. (2009). Wybrane aspekty procesu szkoleniowego w praktyce działalności małych i średnich przedsiębiorstw. *Przegląd organizacji*, 7-8.

About the Contributors

Aleksandra Rosiek-Kryszewska has, since 2007, worked at the Nicolaus Copernicus University in Toruń, Faculty of Pharmacy. Scientific work is closely related to the author's interest in health issues and a broad range of issues aimed at improving the functioning of medical institutions. A degree of doctor of health of health science received in 2016 at the Nicolas Copernicus University in Toruń, Collegium Medicum in Bydgoszcz. Author of several manuscripts and chapters concerning public health. She is also the initiator, co-creator and coordinator of research project and monographs. She is taking part in an international project as an expert in Public Health and coordinator of this project at the international area.

Krzysztof Leksowski, Full Professor, DSc, PhD, MD, graduated from Military Medical Academy of Łódź, Faculty of Medicine. At present the Head of the Department of General, Thoracis and Vascular Surgery Military Hospital in Bydgoszcz, and Chair of Public Health Collegium Medicum in Bydgoszcz, Nicolaus Copernicus in Toruń. Experience in practical application of non-invasive surgery gained during courses, seminaries and workshops in Poland and abroad. Member of national and international science associations and editorial boards of medical journals. Author of many scientific works on the subject of the use of non-invasive techniques in various branches of surgery. Well known academic teacher and mentor of young scientists. He is the initiator, co-creator and coordinator of research projects, monographs and conferences. Author of more than one hundred articles and chapters.

* * *

Karolina Czarnecka, PhD, Assistant Professor at Medical University of Lodz (Poland). Graduated from Biotechnology (Faculty of Biology, Warsaw University, Poland); postgraduate studies in Science Commercialization (Stanford University, USA) and Health Service Management (Technical University of Lodz, Poland). Karolina H. Czarnecka has conducted for the last 12 years research focused on molecular mechanisms underlying cancers (lung, breast, thyroid, prostate, renal carcinoma), autoimmune diseases (sarcoidosis, asthma, allergy, psoriasis, MS), chronobiology and osteoporosis. In years 2013-2015 she was also Vice-President of Young Scientists' Council (advisory body at the Ministry of Science and Higher Education). For the last 5 years she has been working in the field of commercialization as Innovation Broker. She has focused on creating cooperation between Academia and business, and boosting the technology transfer. Karolina H. Czarnecka is involved in mentoring startups realizing projects, related to the implementation of coordinated care solutions and telemedicine.

Tomasz Komendziński, PhD, is senior lecturer at Department of Cognitive Science and Epistemology, Nicolaus Copernicus University in Toruń, and researcher at Neurocognitive Laboratory, Center for Modern Interdisciplinary Technologies, Nicolaus Copernicus University in Toruń. He is the initiator, co-creator and coordinator of InterRDoCTor research team, well known from many previous research projects and conferences. She has a Master's degree and a doctorate in philosophy, human perception, sensory and cognitive processes.

Hanna Liberska, psychologist and biologist, professor at the Institute of Psychology at Kazimierz Wielki University in Bydgoszcz (Poland), chair of the Department of Social psychology and Youth Research. Her research includes many aspects of social development of adolescents, young adults and people in old age. She is also interested in very specific problem of health and illnesses as biopsychosocial functioning of human before and after transplantation. Hanna Liberska - psychologist and biologist, professor at the Institute of Psychology at ul. Kazimierz Wielki in Bydgoszcz, Faculty of Social Psychology and Youth Research. Her studies cover many aspects of the social development of adolescents, young adults and the elderly. He is interested in specific health and disease problems, namely biopsychosocial human functioning before and after transplantation. Author and co-author of more than 160 scientific publications in polish, English, Russian, Ukrainian: monographs, articles, chapters; Editor or co-editor of eighteen monographs. She publishes in Poland, German, Great Britain, Russia, Ukrainian, Hungary and Australia.

Emilia Mikołajewska, PhD, is physiotherapist, assistant professor in Department of Physiotherapy, Ludwig Rydygier Collegium Medicum of the Nicolaus Copernicus University in Bydgoszcz, senior assistant in Rehabilitation Clinic, Military Clinical Hospital No. 10 with Policlynic in Bydgoszcz, and researcher in Neurocognitive Laboratory, Centre for Modern Interdisciplinary Technologies, Nicolaus Copernicus University in Toruń. She is also member of the Inter RDoCT or research team. Author of ten books, 40 book chapter, 210 articles in the area rehabilitation and physiotherapy. Reviewer in 40 scientific journals (also member of five Editorial Boards), several book chapter, and many grant applications. She also teaches courses on neurorehabilitation and assistive technology and acts as supervisor of specialization candidates. Her research interests cover areas: rehabilitation of adult patients and children, increasing of patients' quality of life using novel technologies (assistive devices, telemedicine, telerehabilitation, cybertherapy, rehabilitative robotics, applications of IT, AI and integrated systems in medicine), co-operation within therapeutic multidisciplinary team, evidence based medicine in clinical practice, biomedical engineering in rehabilitation.

Dariusz Mikołajewski, MSc Eng., PhD candidate, is engineer and scientist, specialist in IT, applications of IT in medical sciences, biocybernetics, and medical robotics. He works for three research centers: 1) Institute of Mechanics and Applied Computer Science, Kazimierz Wielki University in Bydgoszcz, 2) Department of Informatics, Nicolaus Copernicus University in Toruń, 3) Neurocognitive Laboratory, Centre for Modern Interdisciplinary Technologies, Nicolaus Copernicus University in Toruń. He is also member of the InterRDoCTor research team. Author of more than one hundred articles and chapter in the area of medical IT, biocybernetics, and biomedical engineering.

Aleksandra Mreła, PhD, was born in Żnin, Poland. She took her degree in Mathematics (1988) at the Higher Pedagogical School in Bydgoszcz (Poland), and earned her Ph.D. in Mathematics at the University of Łódź, Poland, in 1994. Currently she is an adjunct in Kujawy and Pomorze University in Bydgoszcz in the Technical Department. Her research interests are: Fuzzy Logic, Decision Support Systems, Test Theory, Mathematics.

Monika Mularska-Kucharek is a PhD graduate in Sociology. She graduated in sociology from the Faculty of Economics and Sociology, University of Lodz. She is a student of postgraduate studies in career counseling and the Psychological Training School. She participates in Professional Psychotherapy Studies at the Brief Therapy Center. Her research interests include social capital, quality of life and entrepreneurship. She is the author of "Kapitał społeczny a postawy i działania przedsiębiorcze mieszkańców Łodzi" ("Social capital versus entrepreneurial attitudes and actions of Lodz residents"), "Kapitał społeczny a jakość życia. Na przykładzie zbiorowości wielkomiejskiej"("Social capital and quality of life. A study of a metropolitan population"); "Social capital and quality of life" The Role of Social Capital in the Development of Entrepreneurship" and over fifty scholarly articles.

Agata Pasternak, Master of nursing, health management specialist. Lecturer at the medical school in Inowrocław.

Filip Pawliczka, Faculty of medicine graduate & PhD student in II Department of Cardiology at Medical University of Łódź. Student at XXI edition of Postgraduate Studies of Healthcare Management at Warsaw School of Economics. Alumnus of III edition of "Leaders of healthcare" project at Lesław A. Paga Foundation. Member of "Young Managers of Medicine" team cooperating with The Polish Hospital Federation. Member of "Young Doctors and Dentists Club" at Regional Medical Chamber in Łódź.

Bożena Pieczka has many years of professional experience in working in medical institutions. Holder of a university degree in law; Postgraduate studies in Unit Management in Health Care - Health Manager; Numerous competence certificates, including: Certificate of improvement of internal auditors in health care institutions, ISO / IEC internal auditor certificate, Certificate: Internal Auditor of Information Security Management System according to PN-ISO / IEC 27001: 2014.

Anna Rosiek has completed research work closely connected with her interests in health care and in solving problems in public health care. Scientific work is closely related to the author's interest in health issues and a broad range of issues aimed at improving the functioning of medical institutions. Science 2002 author worked for both the medical community and the business community. Opportunity to exchange experience in the medical and business field with countries such as Switzerland, the United States and United Kingdom has contributed to the start of author's research in the field of Public Health. A degree of doctor of health of health science received in 2012 at the Nicolas Copernicus University in Toruń, Collegium Medicum in Bydgoszcz. Since 2012 she is a member of Society for the Promotion of Quality of Health Care in Poland. Author of several manuscripts and chapters concerning public health.

Dorota Rutkowska graduated from Wroclaw Medical University, the Faculty of Medicine in 2011. After graduation, she began her emergency medicine residency training. Currently she is a fourth-year resident at A. Jurasz University Hospital No. 1 in Bydgoszcz. She also maintains a teaching schedule at the Collegium Medicum in Bydgoszcz as part of the University of Torun. Drawing upon her international experience, gained at multiple EM conferences, coupled with her volunteer work in the USA, she continues to focus her efforts on encouraging young doctors in Poland to actively participate in the growth and further development of the specialty. In the future she would like to concentrate on the advancement of emergency medicine in Poland, as well as strengthening her homeland's overall system of medical education.

Łukasz Sielski left Medical Academy in Bydgoszcz in 2001 in the Department of Theories about the Health - obtaining the title of the physiotherapist. The title got the doctor of medicine in Collegium Medicum in Bydgoszcz in 2007. About 2006 he/she is working as the university teacher in Collegium Medicum in Bydgoszcz. He is an active member of the Polish Company of the Rehabilitation, the Polish Company of Physiotherapy and the Polish Company of Sports Traumatology. From 2014 a Centre Rehabilitation of the Hospital is a Manager for them.

Julita Soczywko graduated from the Medical Academy of Bydgoszcz, the Faculty of Pharmacy in 2001, earning a master's degree in the science of laboratory medicine. In 2015, she earned her PhD in medical science at the Collegium Medicum of Bydgoszcz. Beginning in 2001, she has been practicing as a laboratory diagnostician while teaching at the Department of Emergency Medicine and Disasters at the Collegium Medicum in Bydgoszcz. Her scientific interests include: laboratory medicine in relation to clinical science, emergency medicine, toxicology and quality control management.

Oleksandr Sokołov, Professor, Dr of Science, PhD, was born in Kharkiv, Ukraine. He took his degree in Applied Mathematics at Kharkiv Aviation Institute, and earned his PhD in Control Theory at the Institute of Machinery Building of Academy of Science of Ukraine, and earned his Dr of Science in Control Theory at National Aerospace University, Kharkiv. Currently, he is a professor in the Nicolaus Copernicus University in Toruń in the Department of Informatics, Faculty of Physics, Astronomy and Informatics. His research interests are: Fuzzy Logic, Decision Support Systems, Intelligent Control Systems, Test Theory, Multiagent systems, Simulation of biological systems.

Anita Wójcik, Master of Public Health, a graduate of the Nicolaus Copernicus University in Toruń (Poland), operating nursing, nurse specialist. She works in the Military Clinical Hospital in Bydgoszcz in the Integrated Operational Unit. Conducts research among patients suffering from Parkinson's disease treated with deep brain stimulation. The results will from the material of her doctoral dissertation. She is also teaching as a teacher and lecturer in the field of nursing and health.

Nafazi Vaz has worked for seven years in the healthcare industry at a managerial position. She is currently working as a faculty at Goa Institute of Management.

Index

www.ingramcontent.com/pod-product-compliance
Lightning Source LLC
LaVergne TN
LVHW062136300926
849161LV00010B/2548
* 9 7 8 1 5 2 2 5 3 9 4 6 9 *